AF597485

Cardiac Reconstructions with Allograft Valves

R.A. Hopkins

Cardiac Reconstructions with Allograft Valves

With Contributions by
V.J. Ferrans S.L. Hilbert M. Jones
P.L. Lange L. Wolfinbarger, Jr.

Illustrations by Thomas Xenakis

With 169 Figures

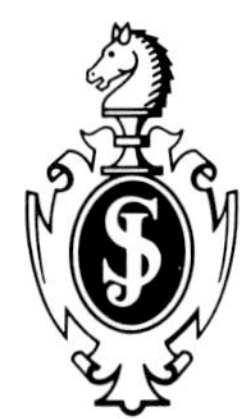

Springer-Verlag
New York Berlin Heidelberg
London Paris Tokyo

RICHARD A. HOPKINS, M.D.
Department of Surgery
Georgetown University Medical Center
Washington, DC 20007, USA

Library of Congress Cataloging-in-Publication Data
Cardiac reconstructions with allograft valves.
Includes bibliographies and index.
1. Heart—Valves—Surgery. 2. Homografts.
I. Hopkins, Richard A. [DNLM: 1. Heart Valves—transplantation. 2. Transplantation, Homologous.
WG 169 C2667]
RD598.C3435 1989 617'.4120592 88-29466

Printed on acid-free paper

Typeset by Arcata Graphics/Kingsport, Kingsport, Tennessee.
Printed and bound by Arcata Graphics/Halliday, West Hanover, Massachusetts.
Printed in the United States of America.

9 8 7 6 5 4 3 2 1

ISBN 0-387-96855-5 Springer-Verlag New York Berlin Heidelberg
ISBN 3-540-96855-5 Springer-Verlag Berlin Heidelberg New York

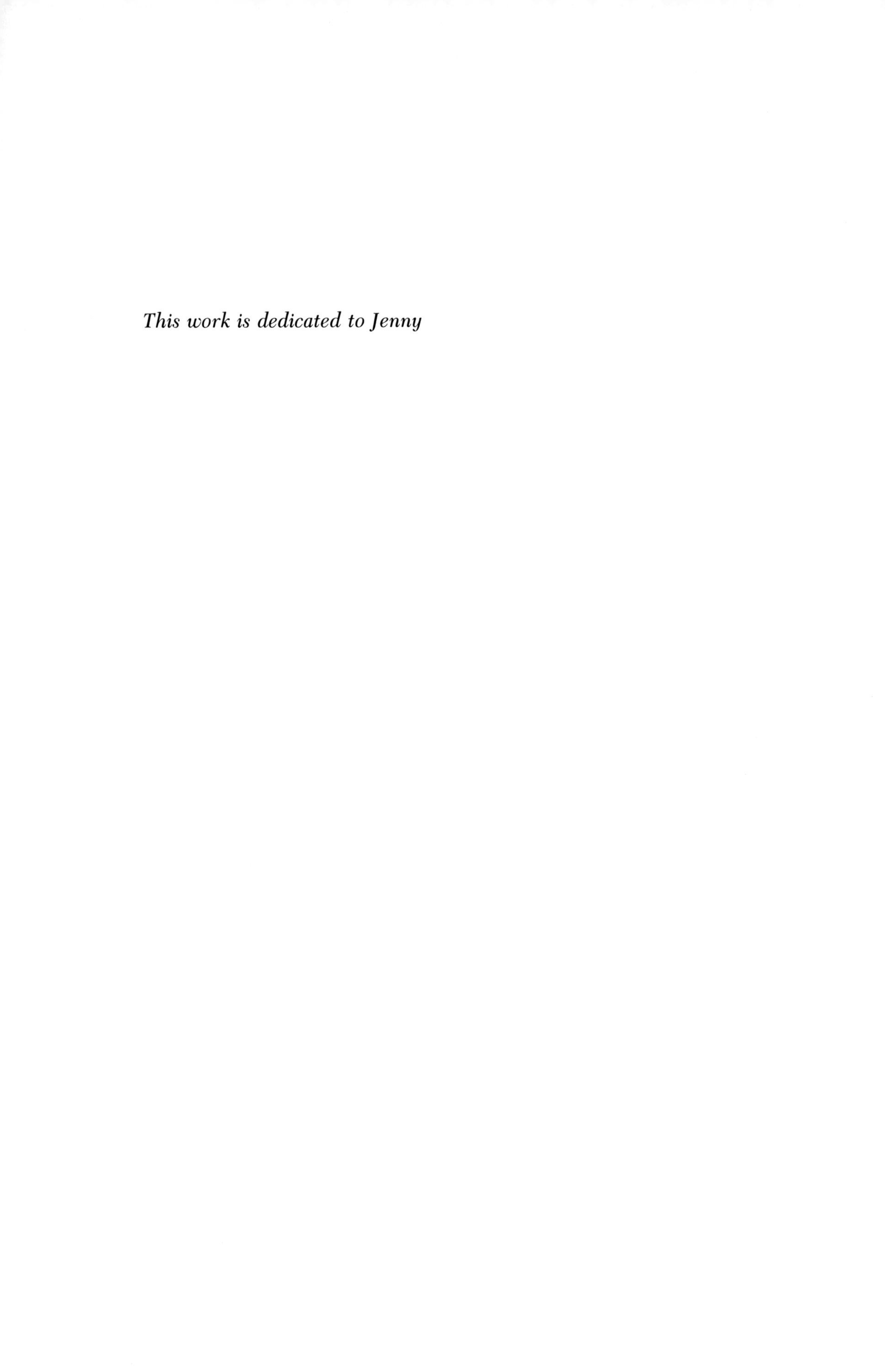

This work is dedicated to Jenny

Preface

Human cadaver tissues (homografts) were used clinically for vascular reconstructions as initially reported by Gross in 1948 and based on the experimental work of Carrel and others earlier in the century. An aortic homograft allowed the first abdominal aneurysm operation by DuBost in 1951, and valved tissues were utilized during the 1950s and early 1960s prior to the general availability of mechanical or xenograft valve prostheses. However, the continued use of homograft valves (allografts) in cardiac reconstructions has subsequently been limited to a few centers. This limitation has been partly because processing homograft valves for sterility and preservation (e.g., irradiation, glutaraldehyde) resulted in poor durability, and "fresh" valves stored in nutrient media with antibiotics were logistically difficult to bank and probably not truly viable.

Now, however, use is increasing and interest greatly heightened for a number of reasons. First, human allograft valves do indeed have hydraulic performance superior to that of synthetic prostheses when harvested, sized, and implanted properly. Second, availability is increasing owing to the expanded use of multiple organ harvests. Third, cardiologists and cardiac surgeons are increasingly dissatisfied with "prosthetic valvular disease" in regard to thromboembolic and anticoagulation complications associated with mechanical prostheses and the poor durability of xenografts, especially in young patients. Lastly, improved performance and durability of allograft valves are being demonstrated with new cryopreservation techniques that result in cellular viability of valves "banked" in vapor-phase liquid nitrogen. It is clear that these allograft cardiovascular tissues have special advantages in certain anatomic situations, for many patients requiring aortic or pulmonary valve replacements, and for pediatric cardiac reconstructions requiring conduit procedures. Thus we are entering a new era of cardiac reconstructions that utilize transplanted viable human tissues—distinct from the era of nonviable homografts and mechanical/xenograft prosthetics.

Although allograft cardiovascular tissues are being used in a number of applications, the focus of this volume is on valved ventricular outflow tract reconstructions. As with all materials used in surgery, surgeons must learn the technical features specific to the new materials in order to fully exploit their potential benefits and unique characteristics. For allograft valves and conduits, this knowledge involves an amalgamation of old and new methods. Viable allograft tissue is a more forgiving and easier material with which to reconstruct outflow tracts than rigid prostheses. Allografts lend themselves to somewhat different reconstructive techniques that solve tricky anatomic problems while preserving physiological principles.

This book is primarily designed as a guide to the practicing cardiac surgeon for the use of allograft valves and conduits in cardiac reconstructions. Full descriptions are given for their use in various lesions, including indications, sizing, and specific surgical techniques for both simple implants and complex reconstructions. The cryobiology of viable human cardiovascular tissue cryopreservation is reviewed in Chapters 3, 4 and 5. An understanding of the principles and techniques is necessary for the safe participation in harvesting, thawing, preparation, and handling of these allografts.

Certain conventions are used in the book. Half-tone or carbon dust figures are used to depict surgical techniques as viewed from the surgeon's perspective. When figures are drawn from a nonsurgical view to make anatomic or other points, pen-and-ink line drawings are used. There is some repetition of steps in the depiction of various surgical techniques so readers can be spared page flipping to follow a procedure from beginning to end. The older term "homograft" is used generically, particularly when referring to information gained from the precryopreservation era (when the term was universally used), and the term "allograft" is adopted for more recent series, particularly when there is an expectation, or intention, of some element of donor cellular viability in the transplanted tissues. While not inherent in the vocabulary, this convention nicely separates the older from the current literature.

All surgeons performing valve replacements and congenital cardiac surgery should be interested in these methods. Cardiothoracic residents will hopefully benefit from the illustrations and descriptions as well. Cardiologists who time the referral of patients for valve surgery based on expected performance of various types of valve replacements will also be interested in human valve transplants.

All of the techniques depicted have been used by the author; they are based on original classic descriptions but as modified by a modest experience of 85 personally performed surgeries in neonates, children, and adults. The surgical techniques are, of course, derived from those of the pioneers in the field—Sir Brian Barratt-Boyes, Mr. Donald Ross, Dr. William W. Angell, Dr. Mark O'Brien, Mr. Magdi Yacoub, Professor Francis Fontan, Mr. Jaroslav Stark, and Dr. John Kirklin—as well as others cited in the text. One of the goals of this volume was to collate techniques into one resource. Our own variations are noted. When these techniques vary significantly from those previously promulgated, the rationale is given as well as indications for alternative methods. Allograft valve transplants involve the use of biologic tissues, which lend themselves to many creative reconstructions. Learning and mastering a flexible range of techniques is important and allows improved solutions to complex problems in ventricular outflow reconstructions. Expanding the ranks of surgeons facile with the use of cardiovascular allografts is the fundamental purpose of this book.

RICHARD A. HOPKINS

Acknowledgments

This work could not have been finished without the help of numerous people. The collaboration with Tom Xenakis, the illustrator, has been a superb intellectual exercise, and his contributions cannot be overemphasized. I am especially grateful to the London teachers who first introduced me to the use of homografts, Jaroslav Stark and Marc de Leval. It is with great appreciation that I acknowledge Professor David C. Sabiston, Jr., for whose support, teaching and training I am grateful. My Norfolk colleagues contributed with thoughts and suggestions. Contributors to Chapters 3, 4, and 5, Perry Lange, Lloyd Wolfinbarger, Stephen Hilbert, Victor Ferrans, and Michael Jones, are all experts in their fields, and their contributions are superb. The dedicated professionals at the Virginia Tissue Bank have invested tremendously in the development of improved cryopreservation techniques and have given freely of their time and expertise. In addition to Perry Lange and Lloyd Wolfinbarger, special thanks go to Scott Bottenfield, Helen Leslie, Bill Anderson, and Dr. Richard Hurwitz. The assistance of Debbie Davenport with the typing is gratefully acknowledged.

Contents

Contributors

VICTOR J. FERRANS, Ph.D., M.D.
Chief, Ultrastructural Section, Pathology Branch, National Heart, Lung, and Blood Institute, National Institutes of Health, Bethesda, MD 20892, USA

STEPHEN L. HILBERT, Ph.D.
Experimental Pathologist, Office of Science and Technology, Center for Devices and Radiological Health, Food and Drug Administration, Rockville, MD 20852, USA

RICHARD A. HOPKINS, M.D.
Director, Pediatric Cardiac Surgery, Department of Surgery, Georgetown University Hospital and Medical School, Washington, DC 20007, USA; Medical Director, Cardiovascular Tissues Program, Virginia Tissue Bank, Virginia Beach, VA 23455, USA

MICHAEL JONES, M.D.
Senior Surgeon, Surgery Branch, National Heart, Lung, and Blood Institute, National Institutes of Health, Bethesda, MD 20892, USA

PERRY L. LANGE, B.S., C.S.A.
Technical Coordinator, Cardiovascular Services, Virginia Tissue Bank, Virginia Beach, VA 23455, USA

LLOYD WOLFINBARGER, JR., Ph.D.
Director, Center for Biotechnology, Research and Development, Virginia Tissue Bank, Virginia Beach, VA 23455, USA

Section I—Principles

1—Historical Development of the Use of Homograft Valves

RICHARD A. HOPKINS

In 1956 Gordon Murray reported the use of fresh aortic valve homografts transplanted into the descending thoracic aorta for amelioration of the consequences of native aortic valve insufficiency. His initial operations preceded by 5 years the availability of the Starr-Edwards mechanical aortic valve prosthesis.[1–7] Although this operation was only partially successful hemodynamically, the homograft valves had remarkable durability and performance. Four patients cited by Heimbecker had no calcification or gradient, with normal leaflet function for up to 13 years, and two patients continued to demonstrate excellent valve function for up to 20 years. Kerwin's subsequent reports support the contention that aortic leaflet homograft pliability and performance were well preserved in these early patients.[3] These clinical trials were preceded by laboratory investigations, especially that of Lam and coworkers.[8] Hemodynamic improvements were demonstrated in both stenotic and regurgitant aortic valve disease by the various early methods of reconstructing diseased aortic valves, and the results ultimately obtained with replacement utilizing the Starr-Edwards and other prostheses supported replacement treatment for ventricular outflow valvular disease, with excellent results continuing to be reported today with both mechanical and bioprosthetic valves.[9]

In 1962 the initial clinical use of aortic valve homografts was reported independently by Donald Ross in England and Sir Brian Barratt-Boyes in New Zealand.[10,11] Duran and Gunning developed a technique in the laboratory for implanting the aortic valve homograft utilizing a single running suture line technique.[12] A two suture line running freehand suturing technique was devised by Barratt-Boyes and is still used in various modifications today.[13] Interestingly, the initial homograft valve transplants were performed utilizing freshly harvested valves that are minimally treated and inserted into the orthotopic position relatively quickly after harvest with no attempt at ABO blood group matching, and so on. These intitial valves had remarkable performance and durability and gave great impetus to the early workers for pursuing this method of aortic valve replacement.

Limitation of donor availability led to preservation attempts to increase storage time and to establish homograft valve "banks." Storage techniques included freeze-drying and antibiotic sterilization with prolonged refrigeration at 4°C. Concerns about transmission of infection led to aggressive sterilization techniques, including multiple antibiotic incubation, irradiation, and glutaraldehyde pretreatment. Unfortunately, although they increased the availability, these techniques resulted in shortened functional survival of homograft valves and caused significant disenchantment with the technique during the 1960s and early 1970s.[14]

It is the purpose of this chapter to examine in detail the earlier experiences with valve homografts and to elucidate valuable lessons pertinent to valve transplantation today.

Early Homograft Work

In 1952 Lam and his associates demonstrated that it was technically possible to tranpslant canine aortic valve homografts into the descending aorta of a recipient animal; however, if the cusps were not "used" and were constantly in the open position, they deteriorated. If aortic insufficiency was induced in the recipient dog, thereby "forcing" the transplanted valve to function, valve integrity was greatly enhanced.[8] This fascinating study has great clinical relevance today and was the basis on which Murray and others developed the technique for clinical use. The studies of Heimbecker and colleagues demonstrated that treatment with gamma radiation or β-propiolactone markedly diminished the durabilty of transplanted homograft valves.[5] The use of radiation was confirmed by others as having deleterious effects and has been completely abandoned.[15]

Flash freezing was one of the harsher preservation methods tested, but it resulted in poor clinical results and laboratory evidence of damage to the elastic properties of the native valves.[16] Other groups found great difficulties in the durability of frozen irradiated aortic valve homografts and advised against their use because of the increased failure rates beginning around the fifth to sixth postoperative year.[17] With some of these less harsh methods, patient valve survival was in the 50% range at 7 years, which was equivalent to contemporaneous series of xenograft and mechanical prosthetic replacements performed during the mid-1970s.[18,19] Valves prepared with the harsher methods were markedly inferior to mechanical valve replacements in terms of durability.

Fresh Wet-Stored Homograft Valves

During the late 1970s attention turned to the use of fresh aortic allografts in which the valves were harvested (usually from cadavers) with variable ischemic times and then antibiotic-sterilized and stored at 4°C in nutrient media. Although donor cellular viability was probably not preserved, these gentler techniques improved valve and patient survival. The contrast between the use of exceedingly fresh valve tissue for transplant and the use of harsh chemical sterilization or storage techniques was stark, and thus the greatest experience has been gained with the relatively gentler methods of storage: antibiotic-sterilized, "fresh wet-stored" valves.

A number of series have been reported that demonstrated good medium-term (7–10 years) results with the wet-storage technique.[20–24] Ross' group from the National Heart Hospital (London) in 1980 reported on 615 valves followed for up to 15 years, including 145 freeze-dried homografts, 89 frozen homografts, 202 fresh homografts, and 179 pulmonary autografts. The study clearly demonstrated the superiority of the autografts and fresh homografts; there were excellent clinical results with up to 90% of patients free of valve-related death at 10 years.[25] Others have also reported good results with the pulmonary autograft transplant to the aortic position.[26]

The Stanford series of 114 patients receiving fresh aortic homografts between March 1967 and March 1971 revealed ten operative deaths (8.8%): six deaths during the first year (5.8%) and then a mortality rate of 1.5% per year. Of the late deaths, only six were due to valve dysfunction, whereas 12 were due to other cardiac causes. A total of 3.2% of patients per year required re-replacement for regurgitation (n = 20), and only one valve developed calcific stenosis. Of 53 patients followed for 5 years or more, 47 had minimal or no disability.[21] In 1986 The Stanford group reexamined 83 patients of this original series such that 773 patient-years of follow-up were available with a maximum to 19 years.[22] For this subgroup the calculated actuarial estimate of freedom from all modes of valve failure was 83 ± 4% at 5 years, 62 ± 6% at 10 years, and 43 ± 7% at 15 years; 92 ± 3% of patients were free from endocarditis at 8 years after operation. Freedom from reoperation was 88 ± 4% at 5 years, 67 ± 6% at 10 years, and 45 ± 7% at 15 years. Interestingly, 94 ± 3% of patients were free of valve-related deaths 5 years following surgery.[23] Thus satisfactory results were achieved with the wet-storage freehand technique and were comparable to results with xenografts.[24]

Another pioneer in the use of allografts has been Yacoub and his group in Harefield, England, who summarized their experience in 1979–1980.[24,27,28] The homografts were procured and prepared similarly to the fresh wet-stored and antibiotic-sterilized protocol of Ross at the National Heart Hospital, with a storage time of 1–42 days, with most being used within 1 week of procurement. This remarkable series of 679 patients demonstrated a 3.9% perioperative mortality rate and actuarial patient survival rates of 87% (5 years) and 81% (8 years). Importantly, these authors noted the superb hydraulic performance of these valves, even in the smaller sizes, and suggested that they "provide almost ideal hemodynamic characteristics."[28,29]

In 1984 the Harefield group published a 10- to 13-year follow-up (mean 11 years) of 140 of their aortic valve replacements with fresh wet-stored homografts.[25] This series demonstrated 71.6% freedom from valve failure at 10 years. Valve degeneration occurred in 19.3% and endocarditis in 6.4%. In this series older age of recipient and prolonged warm ischemia time at procurement (interval between death and dissection of the homograft) were correlated with increased risk for valve degeneration ($p > 0.01$). Although this series had a slightly higher incidence of subacute bacterial endocarditis (SBE) than other homograft experiences and a significant valve degeneration rate that gradually increased from 0.8% at 3 years to 5.2% at 10 years, patient survival (65% at 10 years) compared favorably with the 10-year survival of a classic mechanical series with Starr-Edwards valves (56%).[25,30]

A comparable series from Southampton, England, utilizing antibiotic-sterilized homografts (but not cryopreservation), demonstrated that for the adult aortic valve replacements there was 95% patient survival at 7 years and a regurgitation-free-valve rate of 74% at 7 years. A 0.6% reoperation rate was also reported.[31]

Prosthetic Valve Disease

With the development of the Starr and subsequent models and types of valves, prosthetic valvular disease has been substituted for native valve dysfunction despite the demonstration that patient survival is far superior with treated valve disease when indicators for surgical correction are observed.[32] The controversy of mechanical versus xenograft valves has generated a vast literature, but for adults it can be summarized as follows: Lumping morbidity/mortality and prosthetic durability together, there is an advantage for xenografts over mechanical valves for the first 5 years following replacement, but thereafter the mechanical valves' greater durability confers an advantage.[33] Specifics such as the age of the patient and valve location, e.g., left versus right ventricular outflows versus atrioventricular (AV) valve location, can favor various types or models, and the "trade-offs" of durability versus morbidity must be carefully evaluated clinically.[34]

Hydraulic dysfunction, to a critical degree, can occur when only a small mechanical prosthesis can be inserted into a small aortic annulus. It results in high gradients that worsen with exercise and result in elevated perioperative mortality rates.[35,36] Schaff and colleagues have suggested that a 19-mm Bjork-Shiley valve has satisfactory hemodynamics,[37] but otherwise most authorities recommend against placing a mechanical valve smaller than 21-mm. Valvuloplasty has not been a frequently applicable alternate solution.[38] Porcine-pericardial prostheses have the advantage of reducing the need for anticoagulation, but hydraulic performance is still limited in the smaller sizes.[39]

The related problems of thromboembolism and anticoagulation complications are a tremendous factor in late complications following treatment of aortic valve disease in both children and adults. After cardiac failure, thromboembolism is the leading cause of death following aortic valve replacement.[35] Potential fatal anticoagulation and complications occur at a rate of approximately 5% per year.[40]

The rapidity of calcific degeneration of xenografts in young adults has been emphasized by a number of investigators. Currently, most cardiac surgeons try to implant mechanical prostheses in patients younger than 60 years.[41–45] Valve replacement in children presents even greater difficulties.[46] Mechanical valves in children are associated with anticoagulation complications and hemodynamic dysfunction.[47–51] The introduction of xenograft tissue valves resulted in their enthusiatic use in young patients in the hope of avoiding anticoagulation. Their use was soon followed by widely reported high early failure rates as a consequence of calcification.[52–60] Annulus size constraints and the unsuitability of bioprostheses resulted in techniques to enlarge the aortic root, thereby allowing placement of a large mechanical prosthesis in children with aortic stenosis.[55,61] However, this solution accepts the complications associated with mechanical valves.[62] Homografts offer some solutions and improvements for the problem of prosthetic valvular disease: (1) better hydraulic performance; (2) reduced thromboembolic complications; (3) resistance to endocarditis; and (4) acceptable to superior valve durability.

The two clinical originators of the orthotopic homograft aortic valve replacement, Ross and Barratt-Boyes, have maintained a strong commitment to its use. In multiple publications their two centers have shared much of the developing knowledge. Their series' warrant special attention for the many lessons on the use of "fresh wet/cold-stored" homografts.

London Homografts

Ross and colleagues have produced a number of reports over the past 20 years on the evolution of their results and techniques with aortic valve homografts.[63–71] In 1979 their group reported an 89% graft survival in the aortic position at 6 years for fresh antibiotic-sterilized allografts.[72] In this same series the frozen allograft survival rate at 6 years was reported at 79%. Although they did not claim persistent cellular viability in any of these valves, they were able to show valve functional survival far exceeding the actual native cell survival.

Although the London preservation techniques have been various over the years, the predominant one has been fresh antibiotic-sterilized valves stored at 4°C. On the basis of tritiated thymidine studies of fibroblast viability, Ross's group has shown that no donor fibroblasts are viable after 600 days in the patient when wet-stored homografts are used. Although "fresh" wet-stored homografts can appear histologically and by some metabolic tests to possess cellular viability, those that are stored for more than a few days are most likely not viable months after implantation.[73,74] Ross and coworkers have shown that valve survival following implantation is better in right-sided reconstructions than left-sided ones but that the survival has not been particularly affected by storage times or warm ischemia times.[75] This finding is not surprising, as a wet-stored valve for 6 days is probably ultimately just as nonviable as one stored for 26 days.[76] Utilizing their methods of storage and harvesting, which often included a relatively long warm ischemia time, with cadaveric recovery being delayed for up to 24–48 hours, there was only a 23 ± 6% rate of valve survival at 15 years and a rate of 50% at 12 years.[75] In their hands, this method has produced better results than those seen with prosthetic valves. Patient survival, however, has been markedly superior to valve survival, with the former averaging 75% at 15 years.

The hypothesis that cellular viability at the time of implantation is related to prolonged optimal function is suggested by the unique series of autologous transplants by Ross and colleagues.[69,77] This series demonstrated an 82% actuarial survival of the allograft valve at 14 years and an 81 ± 5% event-free survival of the concomitantly implanted aortic homograft in the right ventricular outflow tract.[69,70]

During the early years of homograft valve use, technical factors were noted to play a significant role in early valve failure, e.g., dehiscence, prolapse, tears, and perforations.[78] The importance of such surgical techniques as the careful two-suture freehand technique and attention to ensuring commissural post suspension for semilunar cusp function were determined.[79]

New Zealand Homografts

The New Zealand group headed by Barratt-Boyes summarized their experience in a selected series of 252 isolated aortic homograft valve replacements with a 9- to 16.5-year follow-up (mean 10.8 years), which represents perhaps the classic summary of the fresh wet-storage era.[80] These valves were all inserted with the original freehand "subcoronary" technique. All of the valves were sterilized in antibiotic solution, stored in nutrient media at 4°C, and considered nonviable.

The results of this New Zealand series are exemplary.[80] Their careful analysis of one of the most important series in the world has many nuggets of information. First, the results are superb, with only 20 valve-related deaths (8.4%) of which eight were due to endocarditis, seven to cusp rupture, and five to incompetence resulting in reoperation and death. Actuarial analysis demonstrated freedom from significant incompetence to be 95% at 5 years, 78% at 10 years, and 42% at 14 years. Factors increasing the risk of significant incompetence due to valve deterioration were donor valve age greater than 55 years, a young recipient age, and aortic root diameters over 30 mm. Poor results with chemical sterilization were noted by the group. Overall actuarial survival was 77% at 5 years, 57% at 10 years, and 38% at 14 years, which is comparable to results from xenograft or mechanical prostheses series.

It is of note that when aortic insufficiency developed it usually progressed slowly, allowing elective reoperation for replacement at low risk of mortality. No specific embolism was proved to have originated from the valve. No stenosis occurred in any of the valves, and the authors had no difficulties with hemodynamic performance in the small valve sizes (17–19 mm). The development of aortic insufficiency was rarely due to rupture, more often being caused by either technical problems at the time of insertion, progressive dilation of an aortic root, central incompetence due to improper commissural suspension, allograft degeneration, or bacterial endocarditis.[80]

Interestingly, Barratt-Boyes and his group did not find increased valve failure related to older recipient age, longer valve salvage times (warm ischemia time), or insertion into an aortic root afflicted with stenotic disease. The New Zealand group thus recommeded this valve as the valve of choice for virtually all patients and suggested the following donor characteristics: age less than 50 years, aortic valve internal diameter (ID) of 28 mm or less, a valve free of imperfections, and a valve stored no longer than 50 days when wet-stored at 4°C.[80] They believed that allografts are particularly valuable in women of childbearing age, patients unsuitable for anticoagulation, and those with small aortic roots. The resistance to endocarditis by the homograft valve, whatever its method of preservation, has been consistent in all series; although not absolute, it is most marked during the postoperative period when compared to mechanical prostheses. Risk-hazard analysis demonstrated much lower risk of prosthetic endocarditis in these valves, especially during the early postoperative phase.[81] Their listed contraindications to its use were the presence of an aortic root aneurysm, aortic root dilatation due to diffuse medial disease, cystic medial necrosis, and aortic root dilatation not amenable to aortic root tailoring (see Chapter 6).[80]

Right Ventricular Outflow Tract Reconstructions

In contrast to the merely "quite good" results in the more stressful aortic position, the nonviable aortic homograft has been used with "superb" results for reconstruction of the right ventricular outflow tract, particularly in children, beginning in 1966.[82]

Conduit surgery revolutionized the repairs of complex congenital cardiac defects; the ability to anatomically rebuild ventricular outflow tracts has allowed repair of lesions previously not amenable to surgery.[83–89] Unfortunately, conduit malfunction has been a frustratingly frequent occurrence following initial operative successes with synthetic prostheses and is associated with significant morbidity and mortality.[90] Conduit malfunction has been due to calcification and degeneration of the xenograft valve, peel formation within the Dacron tube, and thromboembolic occurrences.[91] Hancock valve replacement in children has an optimal calculated replacement of 7% per year, which suggests the projected probability of a Hancock valve remaining replacement-free to be only 50% at 5 years.[56] The Stanford group reported similar pessimistic durability in studies of porcine xenografts when used as intracardiac xenografts or conduits; their linearized reoperation rates were 10% and 4% per patient-year, respectively; the rate of valve failure due to leaflet fibrocalcification was 8% per patient-year.[57] The Mayo Clinic, Toronto group, and investigators at other major centers have found that the porcine valve containing conduits fail relatively rapidly owing to both conduit peel and cumulative valve degeneration.[62] In a study from The Hospital for Sick Children (London), in which the mean age of the patients was 6.5 years, only 27% of the xenograft bioprostheses did *not* require replacement by the fifth year.[92]

One of the synthetic conduit series with representative results comes from Boston, where 201 children underwent reconstructions of the right ventricular outflow tract with porcine valve–tightly woven Dacron conduits.[93] Actuarial patient survival of perioperative survivors was 83% at 8 years. Valve durabilty was actuarially reported, 50% of patients being valve-replacement-free at 8 years; however, most of the late complications in these patients were due to *valve conduit* problems. Analysis suggested zero durability after 10 years.[93]

In contrast, Fontan and associates, on the basis of 103 aortic valve homograft implantations in children with complex congenital heart disease since 1968, postulated an expected graft valve survival rate of 10–15 years. Their data demonstrated an actuarial survival of 80% at 9 years.[94] The Great Ormond Street group has also demonstrated that the antibiotic-sterilized, wet-stored homografts have good durabilty; in 65 patients with a mean age of 6.5 years, there was 85% homograft valve survival at 5 years and 75% valve survival at 9 years.[95] Although the aortic wall calcifies with time, the valve leaflet tissue of the homografts appear to remain pliable without stenosis.[20,95–98] Kay and Ross have reported a 13% replacement (for obstruction) rate at 10 years.[99] These results with fresh antibiotic-sterilized aortic homografts contrast markedly with results with irradiated or otherwise harshly preserved homograft conduits.[14,100,101] The homograft is now the prosthesis of choice for right ventricular outflow tract reconstructions, especially for children.[75] In the latest report from Great Ormond Street on 249 right ventricular outflow tract reconstructions (72 with aortic homografts from Ross's bank at the National Heart Hospital), homograft obstructions have occurred but seemed to have often been related to the concomitant use of Dacron tubes and extensions: Only one of 29 homografts implanted without Dacron became stenotic.[102] The more common mode of failure appears to be the gradual development of insufficiency, which allows leisurely elective replacement. The role of the immune response relative to failure is not yet clear and may play no role in the deterioration of valve leaflets, although it does participate in calcification of the aortic wall.[73,74,103]

Summary

Beginning in 1962 there have been four eras related to method of procurement, sterilization, and storage of aortic valve homografts. During the first era, fresh aseptic harvesting with immediate transplantation (within hours or a few days—"fresh fresh") was the rule. This method appears to have given excellent results, both initially and in terms of long-term durability. The second era saw a clean harvest with harsh sterilization and storage techniques, clearly resulting in poor durabilty. The third and predominant era saw the clean harvest with gentle antibiotic sterilization and wet 4°C storage for up to 6 weeks ("fresh wet-stored"). This method of preparing "nonviable" aortic homografts has had the most extensive experience and the best results. The fourth technique, which is discussed in Chapter 2, involves aseptic harvest with a short warm ischemia time, gentle antibiotic sterilization, and cryopreservation with liquid nitrogen storage utilizing cyroprotectants ("cryopreserved").[104] As was pointed out by O'Brien and associates, when evaluating results of "homograft" series one must clearly identify whether viable or nonviable valves are being implanted, and when "fresh" valves are used how fresh they are.[105] All homografts have not been alike at the time of implantation.

The results chronicled in this chapter relate to homografts implanted without cryopreservation. Many relevant lessons have been learned and a number of advantages of fresh wet-stored homograft valves determined despite their likely lack of viability.

1. These valves provide optimal hydraulic function with central nonobstructive flow resulting in excellent hemodynamic performance even in small sizes; thus a large, effective valve for a small recipient annulus can be achieved as a consequence of optimal hemodynamics.[24,27,28]
2. Thromboembolism and hemolysis rates are reduced despite no anticoagulation.
3. It is a relatively simple surgical implant.
4. Calcification rarely affects the leaflets.
5. Resistance to endocarditis is enhanced.[81]

As Kirklin and Barratt-Boyes have discussed, although there are multiple causes for prosthesis-related late deaths following aortic valve replacements, only two are relevant to homograft aortic valve replacement: incompetence and endocarditis. Endocarditis rates are lower with allografts than with any other prosthesis.[81] When early technical failures are avoided and appropriate donor and recipient criteria are followed, incompetence is not an early problem. Valve failure does not equate with patient mortality, the latter being far superior to that reported for most other prostheses series at medium term.

The surgical lessons from the fresh wet-storage era fall into three categories.

1. "Freehand" surgical technique must account for semilunar valve functional anatomy, thereby avoiding early technical failures. It requires attention to the following.
   a. Accurate sizing.
   b. Effective commissural post suspension—important for retaining semilunar function.
   c. "Normalized" aortic root geometry.
   d. Careful trimming of the allograft.
   e. Seating of the annulus without deformation.
2. It is necessary to understand the factors that have been found to lead to *decreased* durability of homografts.[82]
   a. Older donor age.
   b. Dilated aortic root (unless corrected by aortoplasty).
   c. Aortic root disease, e.g., Marfan's syndrome and cystic medial necrosis.
   d. Technically imperfect implant.
   e. Prolonged storage of wet-stored allografts prior to use.
   f. Harsh sterilization, harvesting, or preservation techniques.
3. Conduct of aortic valve surgery has improved results of all types of aortic valve replacements and includes attention to the following.[106]
   a. Cardioplegia-myocardial protection.
   b. Coronary artery disease.
   c. Shorter cross-clamp times.

These lessons continue to be relevant, and their applications are discussed in detail in the appropriate chapters of this book. Results of the antibiotic-sterilization/wet-storage era of homograft valve transplants proved that homografts were an important alternative with distinct advantages for certain subgroups of patients needing valve replacement.

References

1. Murray G: Homologous aortic valve segment transplants as surgical treatment for aortic and mitral insufficiency. *Angiology* 7:466–471, 1956.
2. Murray G: Aortic valve transplants. *Angiology* 11:99–102, 1960.
3. Kerwin AG, Lenkei SC, Wilson DR: Aortic valve homograft in the treatment of aortic insufficiency: report of nine cases with one follow-up for 6 years. *N Engl J Med* 266:852–857, 1962.
4. Heimbecker RO: The homograft cardiac valve. In Marendino KA (ed): *Prosthetic Valves for Cardiac Surgery*. Springfields, Ill: Charles C Thomas, 1961, pp. 157–159.
5. Heimbecker RO, Aldridge HE, Lemire G: The durability and fate of aortic valve grafts. *J Cardiovasc Surg* 9:511–517, 1968.
6. Heimbecker RO: Whither the homograft valve? *Ann Thorac Surg* 9:487–488, 1970.
7. Heimbecker RO: Durability of fresh homograft. *Ann Thorac Surg* 42:602–603, 1986.
8. Lam CR, Aram HH, Mennell ER: An experimental study of aortic valve homografts. *Surg Gynecol Obstet* 94:129–135, 1952.
9. Borkon AM, Soule LM, Baughman KL, et al: Comparative analysis of mechanical and bio-

prosthetic valves after aortic valve replacement. *J Thorac Cardiovasc Surg* 94:20–33, 1987.
10. Ross DN: Homograft replacement of the aortic valve. *Lancet* 2:487, 1962.
11. Barratt-Boyes BG: Homograft aortic valve replacement and aortic incompetence and stenosis. *Thorax* 19:131–150, 1964.
12. Duran CG, Gunning AJ: A method for placing a total homologous aortic valve in the subcoronary position. *Lancet* 2:488–489, 1962.
13. Barratt-Boyes BG: A method for preparing and inserting a homograft aortic valve. *Br J Surg* 52:847–856, 1965.
14. Merin G, McGoon DC: Reoperation after insertion of aortic homograft-right ventricular outflow tract. *Ann Thorac Surg* 16:122–126, 1973.
15. Malm JR, Bowman FO Jr, Harris PD, Kovalick ATW: An evaluation of aortic valve homografts sterilized by electron beam energy. *J Thorac Cardiovasc Surg* 54:471–477, 1967.
16. Parker R, Nandakumaran K, Al-Janabi N, Ross DN: Elasticity of frozen aortic valve homografts. *Cardiovasc Res* 11:156–159, 1977.
17. Beech PM, Bowman FO Jr, Kaiser GA, Malm JR: Frozen irradiated aortic valve homografts. *NY State J Med* 19:651–654, 1973.
18. Wain WH, Greco R, Ignegeri A, et al: Fifteen years experience with 615 homograft and autograft aortic valve replacements. *Int J Artif Organs* 3:169–172, 1980.
19. Barratt-Boyes BF, Roch ABG, Whitlock RML: Six year review of results of freehand aortic valve replacement using an antibiotic sterilized homograft valve. *Circulation* 55:353–361, 1977.
20. Saravalli OA, Somerville J, Jefferseon KE: Calcification of aortic homografts used for reconstruction of the right ventricular outflow tract. *J Thorac Cardiovasc Surg* 80:909–920, 1980.
21. Anderson ET, Hancock EW: Long-term follow up of aortic valve replacement with fresh aortic homograft. *J Thorac Cardiovasc Surg* 72:150–156, 1976.
22. Miller DC: Fresh aortic homografts: long-term results with freehand aortic valve replacement. *J Cardiac Surg* 2:185–191, 1987.
23. Barratt-Boyes BG: Cardiothoracic surgery in the antipodes. *J Thor Cardiovasc Surg* 78:804–822, 1979.
24. Thompson R, Yacoub M, Ahmed M, et al: The use of "fresh" unstented homograft valves for replacement of the aortic valve. *J Thorac Cardiovasc Surg* 79:896–903, 1980.
25. Penta A, Qureshi S, Radley-Smith R, Yacoub MH: Patient status 10 or more years after "fresh" homograft replacement of the aortic valve. *Circulation* 70(suppl I): I182–I186, 1984.
26. Stelzer P, Elkins RC: Pulmonary autograft: an American experience. *J Cardiac Surg* 2:429–433, 1987.
27. Thompson R, Yacoub M, Seabra-Gomes R, et al: Influence of preoperative left ventricular function on results of homograft replacement of aortic valve for aortic regurgitation. *J Thorac Cardiovasc Surg* 77:411–421, 1979.
28. Thompson R, Yacoub MH, Ahmed M, et al: Influence of preoperative left ventricular function on results of homograft replacement of the aortic valve for aortic stenosis. *Am J Cardiol* 43:929–938, 1979.
29. Ross D, Yacoub MH: Homograft replacement of the aortic valve: a critical review. *Prog Cardiovasc Dis* 11:275–293, 1969.
30. Teply JF, Grunkemeier GL, D'Arcy SH, et al: The ultimate prognosis after valve replacement: an assessment of twenty years. *Ann Thorac Surg* 32:111–119, 1981.
31. Khanna SK, Ross JK, Monro JL: Homograft aortic valve replacement: seven years' experience with antibiotic-treated valves. *Thorax* 36:330–337, 1981.
32. Selzer A: Changing aspects of the natural history of valvular aortic stenosis. *N Engl J Med* 317:91–98, 1987.
33. Hammond GL, Geha AS, Kopf GS, Hashim SW: Biological versus mechanical valves: analysis of 1,116 valves inserted in 1,012 adult patients with a 4,818 patient-year and 5,327 valve-year follow-up. *J Thorac Cardiovasc Surg* 93:182–198, 1987.
34. Schoen FJ: Cardiac valve prostheses: pathological and bioengineering considerations. *J Cardiac Surg* 2:65–108, 1987.
35. Dale J, Levang O, Eng I: Long-term results after aortic valve replacement with four different prostheses. *Am Heart J* 99:155–162, 1980.
36. Bjork VO, Henze A, Holmgren A: Five years' experience with the Bjork-Shiley tilting-disc valve in isolated aortic valvular disease. *J Thorac Cariovasc Surg* 68:393–404, 1974.
37. Schaff HV, Borkon AM, Hughes C, et al: Clinical and hemodynamic evaluation of the 19 mm Bjork-Shiley aortic valve prosthesis. *Ann Thorac Surg* 32:50–57, 1981.
38. Mindich BP, Guarino T, Goldman ME: Aortic valvuloplasty for acquired aortic stenosis. *Circulation* 74(suppl I):I130–I135, 1986.
39. Yoganathan AP, Woo YR, Sung HW, et al: In vitro hemodynamic characteristics of tissue bio-

prostheses in the aortic position. *J Thorac Cardiovasc Surg* 92:198–209, 1986.

40. Horst-Kotte D, Korfer R, Seipel L, et al: Late complications in patients with Bjork-Shiley and St. Jude Medical Heart Valve replacements. *Circulation* 68(suppl II):II175–II184, 1983.
41. Gabbay S, Frater RWM: In vitro comparison of the newer heart valve bioprostheses in the mitral and aortic positions. In Cohn LH, Gallucci V (eds): *Cardiac Bioprostheses.* New York: Yorke, 1982, pp. 457–468.
42. Villani M, Bianchi T, Vanini V, et al: Bioprosthetic valve replacement in children. In Cohn LH, Gallucci V (eds): *Cardiac Prostheses.* New York: Yorke, 1982, pp. 248–255.
43. Carpentier A, Dubost C, Lane E, et al: Continuing improvements in valvular bioprostheses. *J Thorac Cardiovasc Surg* 83:27–42, 1982.
44. Magilligan DJ, Lewis JW, Tilley B, Peterson E: The porcine bioprosthetic valve. *J Thorac Cardiovasc Surg* 89:499–507, 1985.
45. Schaff HV, Danielson GK, DiDonato RM, et al: Late results after Starr-Edwards valve replacement in children. *J Thorac Cardiovasc Surg* 88:583–589, 1984.
46. Milano A, Vouhe PR, Baillot-Vernant F, et al: Late results after left-sided cardiac valve replacement in children. *J Thorac Cardiovasc Surg* 92:218–225, 1986.
47. Sade, RM, Ballenger JF, Hohn HR, et al: Cardiac valve replacement in children. *J Thorac Cardiovasc Surg* 78:123–127, 1979.
48. Williams WG, Pollock JC, Geiss DM, et al: Experience with aortic and mitral valve replacement in children. *J Thorac Cardiovasc Surg* 81:326–333, 1981.
49. Wada J, Yokoyama M, Hashimoto A, et al: Long-term follow-up of artificial valves in patients under 15 years old. *Ann Thorac Surg* 29:519–521, 1980.
50. Mathews RA, Park SC, Neches WH, et al: Valve replacement in children and adolescents. *J Thorac Cardiovasc Surg* 73:872–876, 1977.
51. Klint R, Hernandez A, Weldon C, et al: Replacement of cardiac valves in children. *J Pediatr* 80:980, 1972.
52. Berry BE, Ritter DB, Wallace RB, et al: Cardiac valve replacement in children. *J Thorac Cardiovasc Surg* 68:705–710, 1974.
53. Geha AS, Laks H, Stansel HC, et al: Late failure of porcine valve heterografts in children. *J Thorac Cardiovasc Surg* 78:351–364, 1979.
54. Gardner TJ, Roland JMA, Neill CA, Donahoo JS: Valve replacement in children. *J Thorac Cardiovasc Surg* 83:178–185, 1982.
55. Manouguian S, Seybold-Epting W: Patch enlargement of the aortic valve ring by extending the aortic incision into the anterior mitral leaflet. *J Thorac Cardiovasc Surg* 78:402–412, 1979.
56. Williams DB, Danielson GK, McGoon DC, et al: Porcine heterograft valve replacement in children. *J Thorac Cardiovasc Surg* 84:446–450, 1982.
57. Miller DC, Stinson EB, Oyer PE, et al: The durability of porcine xenograft valves and conduits in children. *Circulation* 66(suppl I):172–185, 1982.
58. Dunn JM: Porcine valve durability in children. *Ann Thorac Surg* 32:357–368, 1981.
59. Silver MM, Pollock J, Silver MD, et al: Calcification in porcine xenograft valves in children. *Am J Cardiol* 45:685–688, 1980.
60. Odell JA: Calcification of porcine bioprostheses in children. In Cohn LH, Gallucci V (eds): *Cardiac Bioprostheses.* New York: Yorke, 1982, pp. 231–237.
61. Konno S, Imai I, Iida Y, et al: A new method for prosthetic valve replacement in congenital aortic stenosis associated with hypoplasia of the aortic valve ring. *J Thorac Cardiovasc Surg* 70:909–917, 1976.
62. Williams WG, Pollock LC, Geiss DM, et al: Experience with aortic and mitral valve replacement in children. *J Thorac Cardiovasc Surg* 81:326–333, 1981.
63. Ross DN: Homograft replacement of the aortic valve. *Lancet* 2:487, 1962.
64. Ross DN, Martelli V, Wain WH: Allograft and autograft valves used for aortic valve replacement. In Ionescu MI (ed): *Tissue Heart Valves.* Boston: Butterworth, 1979, pp. 127–172.
65. Al-Janabi N, Ross DN: Long-term preservation of fresh viable aortic valve homografts by freezing. *Br J Surg* 61:229–232, 1974.
66. Wain WH, Greco R, Ignegeri A, et al: Fifteen years experience with 615 homograft and autograft aortic valve replacements. *Int J Artif Organs* 3:169–172, 1980.
67. Khanna SK, Ross JK, Monro JL: Homograft aortic valve replacement: seven years' experience with antibiotic-treated valves. *Thorax* 36:330–337, 1981.
68. Wain WH, Pearce HM, Riddell RW, Ross DN: A re-evaluation of the antibiotic sterilization of heart valve allografts. *Thorax* 32:740, 1977.
69. Ross DN: Replacement of the aortic and mitral

valve with a pulmonary autograft. *Lancet* 2:956, 1967.
70. Bodnar E, Wain WH, Martelli V, Ross DN: Long-term performance of homograft and autograft valves. *Artif Organs* 4:20, 1980.
71. Ashwood-Smith, Farrant J: *Low Temperature Preservation in Medicine and Biology.* London: Pitman, 1980.
72. Ross DN, Martelli V, Wain WH: Allograft and autograft valves used for aortic valve replacement. In Ionescu MI (ed): *Tissue Heart Valves.* Boston: Butterworth, 1979, pp. 127–172.
73. Livi V, Abdulla AK, Parker R, et al: Viability and morphology of aortic and pulmonary homografts. *J Thorac Cardiovasc Surg* 93:755–760, 1987.
74. Yankeh AC, Wotlage HU, Muller-Hermelink HIC, et al: Transplantation of aortic and pulmonary allografts, enhanced viability of endothelial cells by cryopreservation, importance of histocompatability. *J Cardiac Surg* 2(suppl):209–220, 1987.
75. Ross DN: Applications of homografts in clinical surgery. *J Cardiac Surg* 2 (suppl):175–183, 1987.
76. Bodnar A, Ross DN: Mode of failure in 226 explanted biologic and bioprosthetic valves. In Cohn LH, Gallucci V (eds): *Cardiac Bioprostheses.* New York, Yorke, 1982, pp. 401–407.
77. Robles A, Vaughan M, Lau JK, et al: Long-term assessment of aortic valve replacement with autologous pulmonary valve. *Ann Thorac Surg* 39:238–142, 1985.
78. Lefrak EA, Starr A: Aortic valve homograft. In: *Cardiac Valve Prostheses.* New York: Appleton-Century-Crofts, 1979, pp. 273–300.
79. Moore ECH, Martelli V, Al-Janabi N, Ross DN: Analysis of homograft valve failure in 311 patients followed up to 10 years. *Ann Thorac Surg* 20:274–281, 1975.
80. Barratt-Boyes BG, Roche AHG, Subramanyan R, et al: Long-term follow-up on patients with the antibiotic-sterilized aortic homograft valve inserted freehand in the aortic position. *Circulation* 75:768–777, 1987.
81. Kirklin JW, Barratt-Boyes BG: Aortic valve disease. In: *Cardiac Surgery.* New York: Wiley, 1986, pp. 398–416.
82. Ross DN, Somerville J: Correction of pulmonary atresia with homograft aortic valve. *Lancet* 2:1446–1447, 1966.
83. Revuelta JM, Val F, Duran CMG: Reconstruction of right ventricular outflow and pulmonary artery with a composite pericardial monocusp patch: an experimental study. *Ann Thorac Surg* 37:150–153, 1984.
84. Goor DA, Hoa TQ, Mohr R, et al: Pericardial-mechanical valved conduits in the management of right ventricular outflow tracts. *J Thorac Cardiovasc Surg* 87:236–243, 1984.
85. Danielson GK: Introduction—conduit operations in surgery. In Anderson RH, Shinebourne EA (eds): *Paediatric Cardiology.* New York: Churchill Livingstone, 1978, pp. 537–539.
86. McGoon DC: Left ventricular and biventricular extracardiac conduits. *J Thorac Cardiovasc Surg* 72:7–14, 1976.
87. Ciaravella JM, McGoon DC, Danielson GF, et al: Experience with extracardiac conduit. *J Thorac Cardiovasc Surg* 78:920–930, 1979.
88. McGoon DC, Danielson GK, Schaff HV, et al: Factors influencing late results of extracardiac conduit repair for congenital cardiac defects. In Cohn LH, Gallucci V (eds): *Cardiac Bioprostheses.* New York: Yorke, 1982, pp. 217–230.
89. McGoon PC, Danielson GK, Puga FJ, et al: Late results after extracardiac conduit repair for congenital cardiac defects. *Am J Cardiol* 49:1741–1749, 1982.
90. Castaneda AR, Norwood WI: Valved conduits: a panacea for complex congenital heart defects? In Cohn LH, Gallucci V (eds): *Cardiac Bioprostheses.* New York: Yorke, 1982, pp. 205–216.
91. Agarwal KC, Edwards WD, Feldt RH, et al: Clinicopathological correlates of obstructed right-sided porcine-valved extracardiac conduits. *J Thorac Cardiovasc Surg* 81:591–601, 1981.
92. Shore DF, de Leval MR, Stark J: Valve replacement in children: biologic versus mechanical valves. In Cohn LH, Gallucci V (eds): *Cardiac Bioprostheses.* New York: Yorke, 1982, pp. 239–247.
93. Jonas RA, Freed MD, Mayer JE, Castaneda AR: Long-term follow-up of patients with synthetic right heart conduits. *Circulation* 72(suppl II):II77–II83, 1985.
94. Fontan F, Choussat A, Deville C, et al: Aortic valve homografts in surgical treatment of complex cardiac malformations. *J Thorac Cardiovasc Surg* 87:649–657, 1984.
95. Di Carlo D, Stark J, Revignas A, de Leval MR: Conduits containing antibiotic preserved homografts in the treatment of complex congenital

heart defects. In Cohn LH, Gallucci V (eds): *Cardiac Bioprostheses*. New York: Yorke, 1982, pp. 259–265.

96. Di Carlo D, de Leval MR, Stark J: "Fresh," antibiotic sterilized aortic homografts in extracardiac valved conduits: long-term results. *Thorac Cardiovasc Surg* 32:10–14, 1984.
97. Moore CH, Martelli V, Ross DN: Reconstruction of right ventricular outflow tract with a valved conduit in 75 cases of congenital heart disease. *J Thorac Cardiovasc Surg* 71:11–19, 1976.
98. Saravalli OA, Somerville J, Jefferson KE: Calcification of aortic homografts used for reconstruction of the right ventricular outflow tract. *J Thorac Cardiovasc Surg* 80:909–920, 1980.
99. Kay PH, Ross DN: Fifteen years' experience with the aortic homograft: the conduit of choice for right ventricular outflow tract reconstruction. *Ann Thorac Surg* 40:360–364, 1985.
100. Castaneda AR, Norwood WI: Valve conduits: a panacea for complex congenital heart defects. In Cohn LH, Gallucci V (eds): *Cardiac Bioprostheses: Proceedings of the Second International Symposium*. New York: Yorke, 1982, pp. 205–216.
101. Schaff HV, DiDonato RM, Danielson GK, et al: Reoperation for obstructed pulmonary ventricle-pulmonary artery conduits: early and late results. *J Cardiovasc Surg* 88:334–343, 1984.
102. Bull C, MaCartney FJ, Horvath P, et al: Evaluation of long-term results of homograft and heterograft valves in extracardiac conduits. *J Thorac Cardiovasc Surg* 94:12–19, 1987.
103. Bodnar E, Olsen WGJ, Florio R, et al: Heterologous antigenicity induced to human aortic homografts during preservation. *Eur J Cardiothorac Surg* 2:43–47, 1988.
104. Angell WW, Angell JD, Oury JH, et al: Long-term follow-up of viable frozen aortic homografts: a viable homograft valve bank. *J Thorac Cardiovasc Surg* 83:815–822, 1987.
105. O'Brien MF, Stafford G, Gardner M, et al: The viable cryopreserved allograft aortic valve. *J Cardiac Surg* 2(suppl):153–167, 1987.
106. Selzer A: Changing aspects of the natural history of valvular aortic stenosis. *N Engl J Med* 317:91–98, 1987.

2—Rationale for Use of Cryopreserved Allograft Tissues for Cardiac Reconstructions

Richard A. Hopkins

As outlined in Chapter 1 definite advantages were realized with the use of "fresh" wet-stored antibiotic-sterilized human homograft valves for the reconstruction of left and right ventricular outflow tracts. However, problems with availability and lack of certainty concerning preservation and storage techniques limited their widespread use. The combination of their resistance to infection, excellent hydraulic function, absence of need for anticoagulation, and versatility in difficult outflow reconstructions made them optimal choices for many categories of patients—beyond the single issue of durability. The durability of the nonviable but gently preserved homografts was certainly as good as xenografts in adults and even better than xenografts in children. If durability could be improved, a homograft would combine the superior attributes of xenografts with the superior attributes of mechanical prostheses and thus be the valve of choice.

Evaluation of data from the fresh, wet-stored series suggested that tissue viability at the time of transplantation was associated with increased durability.[1–3] This impression that short, warm ischemia times and shorter, cold storage periods contributed to prolonged graft durability has been difficult to prove with retrospective analyses. Attention to such issues was not what it is today in the era of multiple-organ donor retrievals.[4] Nevertheless, there does appear to be some suggestion that it has indeed been the case when looking at the larger series from the 1960s and 1970s. For example, many of the original recipients of homografts had prolonged durability of their prostheses, and these patients were the very ones in whom prolonged cold storage did not precede the implant. Also, comparing the Harefield series with the National Heart Hospital series of Ross suggested better durability in the former series.[38] The techniques of preservation and harvesting were essentially the same, with the primary difference being that the Harefield group tended to use homografts sooner following procurement; they reported their 8-year actuarial patient survival at 72%, with homograft valve failure occurring in only 19.3% of their patients by 13 years.[5–9] The Harefield group suggested by logistic analysis a significant negative contribution ($p < 0.01$) of warm ischemia time (defined by them as the death-to-dissection interval) to valve durability.[9] Thus these intriguing tidbits plus the teleological thinking that transplanting a viable fibroblast that can remodel and repair by synthesizing structural proteins would confer greater durability have led to cryopreservation techniques and alterations in retrieval protocols designed to enhance cellular viability.[10]

Brisbane Experience

Beginning in June 1975, O'Brien from Brisbane, Australia began a series of valve replacements utilizing allograft valves that had undergone gentle antibiotic sterilization after retrieval, with attention to short, warm ischemia times; they were then cryopreserved with a dimethylsulfoxide (DMSO) controlled-rate freezing technique with storage in liquid nitrogen at −190°C. His group has published histologic as well as biochemical data confirming viability.[4,11] In addition, the Brisbane center recovered cryopreserved valves from patients dying of unrelated causes 2 months to 9.5 years following implant; the tissue culture results from these valves suggested fibroblast viability, and chromosomal analysis confirmed donor origin of the fibroblasts. Thus O'Brien has undertaken the logical extension of the previous methods—capitalizing on the known advantages of the homograft valve and intensifying attention to techniques designed to increase durability by promoting donor fibroblast viability. This work is so important that we focus on his data.

Because the maturation of transplantation biology and surgery has occurred concomitantly with the evolution of valve transplantation, the newer terminology "allograft" is appropriately applied and provides a shorthand distinction between previous valve preparation protocols and present cryopreservation (viable) techniques. Henceforth in this book the term "allograft" is used in reference to valves prepared and transplanted with the principles of cellular preservation; such usage conveniently distinguishes current work from the previous "homograft" literature.

Angell and associates have reported on their early use of DMSO cryopreserved aortic allografts inserted between 1973 and 1975. Thirty-two such valves were placed, some of which were mounted on stents and 23 sewn freehand. At 10 years' follow-up, 80% of the freehand valves were functional in alive patients.[10] This early clinical application of the cryopreservation process was followed by an intensive and consistent effort by the Brisbane group under the direction of O'Brien. His group has reported on 192 valves placed between June 1975 and December 1986. A number of important points are made in review of their data.[4,11]

Their series had remarkable results. For the cryopreserved aortic valves, there was 100% freedom from reoperation because of valve degeneration at 10 years. There was minimal thromboembolism and a 4% prosthetic endocarditis rate. Ninety-two percent of patients were free of reoperation (actuarial) at 10 years for viable cryopreserved valves. The reason for reoperation was usually technical malalignment leading to insufficiency, never a consequence of allograft valve degeneration.

A most fascinating aspect of the reports by O'Brien's group is the demonstration by chromosomal analysis of the donor origin of the allograft fibroblasts demonstrated in a valve that had been in situ for more than 9 years. Incremental risk factor analysis demonstrated that the combination of young recipient age and old donor age were associated with a greater risk of degeneration of fresh, wet-stored allograft valves, but it was not applicable to the cryopreserved valves.

The resistance to prosthetic endocarditis and the pattern of its occurrence, being primarily late rather than early, was demonstrated not only in the O'Brien series but also in the experience of the Alabama and New Zealand groups.[12a]

Because the fresh wet-stored homograft valve was overall generally comparable to other prosthesis choices, the improvements achieved with cryopreservation are remarkable indeed. If other series support the O'Brien data, increased utilization is warranted.[12b] The role of the pulmonary valve implanted in the aortic position is still to be defined. Although technically it can be implanted easily, as proved by the autotransplant series of Ross, the pulmonary valve is structurally different and has yet to be proved a suitable allograft replacement in the aortic position.[12c,13]

Studies comparing xenografts and mechanical prostheses (Bjork-Shiley) in the aortic position have revealed a lower incidence of valve-related morbidity for the bioprosthesis, but no difference in valve-related mortality or valve failure at 5 years could be demonstrated between the two valves.[14] However, after 7 years the deterioration of porcine valves has been shown to increase, and the durability curves diverge.[15,16] This "knee" in the curve, indicating a later tendency for deterioration, has not yet been shown with the cryopreserved allografts but is present in the nonviable homograft aortic replacement series.

Putative Advantages of Cryopreserved Allografts

Combining what was learned from the use of fresh wet-stored valves with the lessons emerging from the early stages of the "viable" era of left ventricular outflow tract reconstructions with allograft valve transplants, the following statements can be made.[39]

1. Allograft durability may be superior to any other valve except a native undiseased valve.
2. Strict attention to harvesting, preservation, thawing, and storage methods enhance cellular viability—and *probably* graft durability.
3. Optimal hydraulic function due to central nonobstructed flow minimizes the problem of small aortic roots.
4. Allografts have low thromboembolism rates without anticoagulation. This fact is a clear advantage of the cryopreserved allograft in the aortic position for patients in whom anticoagulation is contraindicated, e.g., children, young women, and workers with traumatic occupations.
5. Allografts have resistance to prosthetic bacterial endocarditis.
6. From a material standpoint, an allograft is a flexible prosthesis for complex left ventricular outflow tract reconstructions, e.g., aortic root replacements and small aortic roots in children or adults. It also solves many problems for the surgeon when dealing with markedly deformed aortic roots.
7. Immunosuppression has not been necessary, but its future role is presently unclear.

Right Ventricular Outflow Reconstructions with Allografts

As has been clearly demonstrated in a number of centers, human tissue is superior material for reconstructions of the right ventricular outflow tract.[17–21] Fontan and associates[17] have reported 103 homograft reconstructions between 1968 and 1983 with no episodes of valvular dysfunction, thromboembolism, or hemolysis, although one-third of the patients died either early or late. None of these deaths was due to the aortic valve allograft itself, and only one replacement was required for the development of obstruction. The Alabama group has reported a significant series of 128 patients with cryopreserved aortic allograft reconstructions of the pulmonary outflow tract.[22] This important series demonstrated excellent short-term results, with a 94% actuarial freedom from reoperation at 3.5 years.

Most authorities agree that right-sided valve–Dacron conduits have limited durability, with obstruction inevitably developing and progression resulting in ultimate failure. Such failure can occur as quickly as 18–24 months, although, to be fair, excellent palliation may be achieved. The Mayo Clinic series of approximately 1,100 patients led Danielson to cite a failure-free rate of 94% at 5 years and to estimate a 10-year rate of approximately 75%.[22] Kirklin and colleagues cited a 15-year replacement-free rate of only 11%.[23]

The San Francisco group has reported good short-term palliation with the small Hancock prosthesis (12mm) in infant reconstructions for up to 44 months.[24] Valve survival is not equivalent to patient survival (which is better), or to a complication-free life (which is often worse). Allografts are easier to place in small infants and do not become obstructive as rapidly.

When utilizing a valve for reconstruction of the right ventricular outflow tract in young children, evidence to date suggests that a porcine valve conduit might have a projected useful life to the patient for as little as 4 years as a consequence of poor hemodynamic function and limited durabilty, whereas homograft reconstruction could last 10–20 years.[9,22]

Ross and others have noted that the right-sided position is less stressful than the left-sided position for transplanted valve tissues. If the encouraging results with aortic valve replacements utilizing cryopreserved allografts have a similar contribution to right-sided reconstructions, valve durability approaching 20 years might very well be achievable. Initially, most groups have used aortic allografts for right-sided reconstructions, but pulmonary allografts can also be used.[25]

Although it has long been known that a normal right ventricle can dispense with a pulmonary valve and pulmonary regurgitation is a lesion that is well tolerated for many years, there is increasing evidence that valved reconstructions are superior. Thus an argument can be made for using valves in reconstructions of the right ventricular tract because: (1) the long-term effects of pulmonary insufficiency lead to right ventricular dysfunction and right ventricular dilatation; (2) right ventricular outflow tract reconstructions must not be obstructive, and allografts have superior hemodynamic performance; (3) protection of the compromised right ventricle from pulmonary insufficiency helps prevent tricuspid regurgitation, and tricuspid incompetence clearly adds to the hemodynamic compromise of pulmonary regurgitation, leading to rapid and persistent right ventricular failure, which is often difficult to manage medically; and (4) many patients presenting for right ventricular outflow tract reconstructions already have less than normal right ventricular function (e.g., pulmonary atresia).[26]

All 13 patients in the San Francisco series of right ventricular outflow tract patches with preoperative tricuspid regurgitation required attention to the tricuspid valve.[27] In addition, right-sided prosthetic valves of either mechanical or xenograft materials are notoriously prone to calcification and failure. These factors, coupled with the increased durability of the cryopreserved allograft valves, presently mandates their use in such reconstructions in both adults and children.

Valve replacements in children tend to magnify problems with prostheses, and xenograft durability is poor.[28,29] Size constraints are exaggerated.[30] Thromboembolic/anticoagulation problems may be more difficult to manage, although the risk of emboli from the aortic position appears to be significantly less than the mitral position.[31–33]

Ilbawi and associates have reported that porcine prostheses have fared better in right-sided applications in young patients than on the systemic side, but with reduced durability compared to that in older adults.[34] Thus the xenograft is preferable to a mechanical graft for the right-sided atrioventricular (AV) valve position, but we prefer the allograft for the pulmonary outflow tract position. It is technically easier to insert, is probably more resistant to subacute bacterial endocarditis (SBE), has superior hemodynamic performance, has longer durability when Dacron extensions are avoided, and does not require anticoagulation.[35] Ilbawi's group, as others, have demonstrated excellent performance by the St. Jude prosthesis in the aortic position, with 88.7% actuarial freedom from prosthesis-related complications at 5 years in that position in the pediatric age group.[36] In comparison, the allograft appears to be as good or better and avoids the problem of anticoagulation in children.[36]

Allograft tissues are the optimal choice for all right ventricular outflow reconstructions in children for the reasons defined in this chapter and in Chapter 1, and probably for most left ventricular outflow tract repairs as well. Presently, the only apparent reasons not to use allografts are lack of availability and the rare instance in which a rigid conduit offers an advantage against compression or distortion.

Clinical Use of Allograft Valve Transplants: Unresolved Issues

Despite tantalizing data that suggest markedly improved results with the use of cyropreserved allograft valves, there are numerous areas of controversy and mystery. Are they really "viable," and if so, for how long? The reason for the partially immunologically privileged position of the valve fibroblast is not clearly understood, although the hypothesis that lack of vascular ingrowth and the ability for these hypoxia-resistant cells to live from passive diffusion suggests that their failure to be rejected is due to lack of exposure to the host's immune system. The role of the endothelium is clearly not understood. It can be argued that it protects the physicochemical balance of the matrix, but it can be counterargued that the endothelium is antigenic and incites host rejection, and that processing and storage techniques that result in gentle disposal of the graft endothelium are optimal. O'Brien has proved the donor origin of fibroblasts; recipient origin of endothelium may be key to avoiding antigen exposure.[4] It appears that many cryopreserved valves contain viable cells at implantation. How long the fibroblasts remain viable and the reasons for their later loss are not yet understood.

What percentage are viable appears to be variable. The hypothesis is that viable fibroblasts contain the ability to synthesize structural proteins, hence participate in the maintenance and repair of the valve leaflets over time. This is actually not been convincingly proven to occur consistently. While the clinical data suggest that these valves have superior durability while retaining the other advantages of the nonviable homografts, this could be possibly due to improved matrix preservation by the cryopreservation process, rather than fibroblast cellular function. While the latter seems more likely, the actual reasons still need to be proven.

The role of ABO and HLA tissue matching has clearly not been defined, as most series have ignored standard tissue typing criteria. It can be reasonably hypothesized that tissue matching may extend durability from "very good" (12–18 years) to "outstanding" (more than 20 years) if it leads to greater long-term fibroblast viability.

As with all transplantation fields, interesting legal issues arise, such as whether an allograft is a prosthetic device by U.S. Federal Drug Administration regulations or is in a category different from that of other valve replacements.[37]

Finally, the optimal cryopreservation techniques have not been ultimately defined and are actively being refined by all centers active in the process. Efforts to increase viability appear to be warranted, but if there is increasing benefit to viability above a certain arbitrary percentage has yet to be demonstrated. At present, attention is focused on the length of the warm ischemia times at procurement and the antibiotic sterilization phase during processing, as it is believed that these factors are the most cytotoxic elements of most preparation protocols (see Chapters 3 and 4).

Summary

The cyropreserved, *presumably viable* allograft is the replacement of choice for right ventricular outflow tract reconstructions in children and adults. It is also probably the first choice for complex left ventricular outflow reconstructions: (1) aortoventriculoplasty; (2) small aortic roots; (3) aortic root replacements; and (4) valve or root replacements for bacterial endocarditis. For aortic valve replacements in other situations it is considered competitive or superior to the porcine graft in young patients and those with contraindications to anticoagulation, with life expectancy exceeding the expected durability of the xenograft. Its role in routine aortic valve replacement has yet to be defined and may be inappropriate owing to limited availability, which may limit its use to the specific patient and indication categories in which clear advantages have been demonstrated.

References

1. O'Brien MF, Stafford EG, Gardner MAH, et al: The viable cryopreserved allograft aortic valve. *J Cardiac Surg* 2(suppl):153–167, 1987.
2. Barratt-Boyes BG: Long-term follow-up of aortic valvar grafts. *B Heart J* 33(suppl):60–65, 1971.
3. Kosek JC, Iben AB, Shumway NE, et al: Morphology of fresh heart valve homografts. *Surgery* 66:269–277, 1969.
4. O'Brien MF, Stafford EG, Gardner MAH, et al: A comparison of aortic valve replacement with viable cryopreserved and fresh allograft valves with a note on chromosomal studies. *J Thorac Cardiovasc Surg* 94:812–823, 1987.
5. Thompson R, Yacoub M, Ahmed M, et al: The use of "fresh" unstented homograft valves for replacement of the aortic valve. *J Thorac Cardiovasc Surg* 79:896–903, 1980.
6. Thompson R, Yacoub M, Seabra-Gomes R, et al: Influence of preoperative left ventricular function on results of homograft replacement of aortic valve for aortic regurgitation. *J Thorac Cardiovasc Surg* 77:411–421, 1979.
7. Thompson R, Yacoub MH, Ahmed M, et al: Influence of preoperative left ventricular function on results of homograft replacement of the aortic valve for aortic stenosis. *Am J Cardiol* 43:929, 1979.
8. Ross D, Yacoub MH: Homograft replacement of the aortic valve: a critical review. *Prog Cardiovasc Dis* 11:275–293, 1969.
9. Jonas RA, Freed MD, Mayer JE Jr, Castaneda AR: Long-term follow-up of patients with synthetic right heart conduits. *Circulation* 72(suppl II):II77–II83, 1985.
10. Angell WW, Angell JD, Oury JH, et al: Long-term follow-up of viable frozen aortic homografts: a viable homograft valve bank. *J Thorac Cardiovasc Surg* 93:815–822, 1987.
11. O'Brien MF, Stafford G, Gardner M, et al: The viable cryopreserved allograft aortic valve. *J Cardiac Surg* 2(suppl 1):153–167, 1987.

12a. Kirklin JW, Barratt-Boyes BG: *Cardiac Surgery*, New York: Wiley, 1986, pp. 409–412.

12b. Matsuki O, Okita Y, Almeida RS, McGoldrick JP, Hooper TL, Robles A, Ross DN. Two decades' experience with aortic valve replacement with pulmonary autograft.

12c. J. Thorac Cardiovasc Surg 95:705–711, 1988. O'Brien MF, Stafford EG, Gardner AH, Pohlner

P, McGiffin DC, Johnston N, Tesar P, Brosnan A, Duffy P. Cryopreserved viable allograft valves in Yonkah AC, Hetzer R, Miller DC, et al (eds) Cardiac Valve Allografts 1962–1987. New York: Springer Verlag 1988, pp 311–321.

13. Livi U, Abdulla AK, Parker R, et al: Viability and morphology of aortic and pulmonary homografts. *J Thorac Cardiovasc Surg* 93:755–760, 1987.
14. Borkon AM, Soule LM, Baughman KL, et al: Comparative analysis of mechanical and bioprosthetic valves after aortic valve replacement. *J Thorac Cardiovasc Surg* 94:20–33, 1987.
15. Hammond GL, Geha AS, Kopf GS, Hashim SW: Biological versus mechanical valves: analysis of 1,116 valves inserted in 1,012 adult patients with a 4,818 patient-year and a 5.327 valve-year follow-up. *J Thorac Cardiovasc Surg* 93:182–198, 1987.
16. Oyer PE, Stinson EB, Griepp RB, Shumway NE: Valve replacement with Starr-Edwards and Hancock prosthesis: comparative analysis of late morbidity and mortality. *Ann Surg* 186:301–309, 1977.
17. Fontan F, Choussat A, Deville C, et al: Aortic valve homografts in surgical treatment of complex cardiac malformations. *J Thorac Cardiovasc Surg* 87:649–657, 1984.
18. Shabbo FB, Wain WH, Ross DN: Right ventricular outflow reconstructions with aortic homograft: analysis of long-term results. *Thorac Cardiovasc Surg* 29:21–27, 1981.
19. Saravalli O, Somerville J, Jefferson KE: Calcification of aortic homografts used for reconstruction of the right ventricular outflow tract. *J Thorac Cardiovasc Surg* 80:909–920, 1980.
20. DiCarlo D, Stark J, Revignas A, DeLeval MR: Conduits containing antibiotic preserved homografts in the treatment of complex congenital heart defects. In Cohn LH, Gallucci V (eds): *Cardiac Bioprostheses.* New York: Yorke, 1982, pp. 259–265.
21. Kay PH, Ross DN: Fifteen years' experience with the aortic homograft; the conduit of choice for right ventricular outflow tract reconstructions. *Ann Thorac Surg* 40:360–364, 1985.
22. Danielson DK Jr: Discussion of Kay PH, Ross DN: Fifteen years experience with aortic homograft: the conduit of choice for right ventricular outflow tract reconstructions. *Ann Thorac Surg* 40:360–364, 1985.
23. Kirklin JW, Blackstone EH, Maehara T, et al: Intermediate-term fate of cryopreserved allograft and xenograft valved conduits. *Ann Thorac Surg* 44:598–606, 1987.
24. Boyce SW, Turley K, Yee ES, et al: The fate of the 12 mm porcine valved conduit from the right ventricle to the pulmonary artery. *J Thorac Cardiovasc Surg* 95:201–207, 1988.
25. McGrath LB, Gonzalez-Lavin L, Graf D: Pulmonary homograft implantation for ventricular outflow tract reconstruction: early phase results. *Ann Thorac Surg* 45:273–277, 1988.
26. Ebert PA: Second operations for pulmonary stenosis or insufficiency after repair of tetralogy of Fallot. *Am J Cardio* 50:637–640, 1982.
27. Ebert PA: Second operations for pulmonary stenosis or insufficiency after repair of tetralogy of Fallot. In Engle MA, Perloff JK (eds): *Congenital Heart Disease After Surgery: Benefits, Residua, Sequela.* New York: Yorke, 1983, pp. 202–209.
28. Iyer KS, Reddy KS, Rao IM, et al: Valve replacement in children under twenty years of age. *J Thorac Cardiovasc Surg* 88:217–224, 1984.
29. Williams DB, Danielson GK, McGoon DC, et al: Porcine heterograft valve replacement in children. *J Thorac Cardiovasc Surg* 84:446–450, 1982.
30. Williams WG, Pollock JC, Geiss DM, et al: Experience with aortic and mitral valve replacement in children. *J Thorac Cardiovasc Surg* 81:326–333, 1981.
31. Makhlouf AE, Friedli B, Oberhansli I, et al: Prosthetic heart valve replacement in children. *J Thorac Cardiovasc Surg* 93:80–85, 1987.
32. Edmonds LH: Thrombotic and bleeding complications of prosthetic heart valves. *Ann Thorac Surg* 44:430–445, 1987.
33. Robbins RC, Bowman FO Jr, Malm JR: Cardiac valve replacement in children: a twenty year series. *Ann Thorac Surg* 45:56–61, 1988.
34. Ilbawi MN, Idriss FS, DeLeon SY, et al: Valve replacement in children: guidlelines for selection of prosthesis and timing of surgical intervention. *Ann Thorac Surg* 44:398–403, 1987.
35. Hopkins, RA: Right ventricular outflow tract reconstructions—the role of valves in the viable allograft era. *Ann Thorac Surg* (in press).
36. Pass HI, Sade RM, Crawford FA, Hohn AR: Cardiac valve prostheses in children without anticoagulation. *J Thorac Cardiovasc Surg* 87:832–835, 1984.
37. Kessler DA, Pape SM, Sundwall DN: The federal regulation of medical devices. *N Engl J Med* 317:357–366, 1987.
38. Penta A, Qureshi S, Radley Smith R, Yacoub MH: Patient status 10 or more years after "fresh" homograft replacement of the aortic valve.
39. Barratt-Boyes BG, Roche AHG, Subramanyan R, et al: Long-term follow-up of patients with the antibiotic-sterilized aortic homograft valve inserted freehand in the aortic position. *Circulation* 75:768–777, 1987.

3—Biology of Heart Valve Cryopreservation

Lloyd Wolfinbarger Jr. and Richard A. Hopkins

Great advances have been made in the cryopreservation of living cells since the early works of Smith and Parkes during the 1950s. These advances have included development of sophisticated computer-controlled freezing equipment, characterization of a variety of cryprotective agents, and establishment of major research and development programs in cryobiology within academia and industry. Most of this research and technologic development has focused on the preservation of dispersed cell suspensions, and it has successfully enlarged our understanding of the basic principles of cryopreservation of biologic systems.

Complex tissues, however, are different from cell suspensions and require more sophisticated procedures for freezing. Consequently, research in this area has lagged behind. In heart valves the cellular component is surrounded by and attached to a mixture of proteins and proteoglycans that may be considered essentially insoluble and that serve to inhibit the free movement of solutes in the hydrating solvent. Cryopreservation protocols must ensure retention of this noncellular component in addition to maintaining cellular viability. Furthermore, it is relatively easy to quantitate cellular viability following cryopreservation of cell suspensions but more difficult to determine what constitutes viability in the more complex tissue. A "viable" tissue is regarded as one that retains function equal to that of tissues in their normal state, a characteristic that may or may not be dependent on cellular viability. Indeed, a fundamental question regarding the cryopreservation of heart valves concerns the need to retain cellular viability in order to retain valve durability: Is it necessary?

A typical mammalian cell contains low-molecular-weight solutes at concentrations equivalent to approximately 0.15 *M* NaCl. Consequently, their freezing point is about $-0.6°C$. Most cells, however, do not freeze internally unless cooled to $-10°C$ or lower. This supercooling effect means that the cells are not in thermodynamic equilibrium with the external solution, and eventually this equilibrium must be restored. The preponderance of research to date suggests that this disequilibrium can be restored by one of several mechanisms, including the formation of intracellular ice crystals either independently within the cell or by intrusion from the extracellular environment. Considering that ice crystals grow by accretion at their surfaces, it is improbable that ice crystals "grow" through a hydrophobic domain such as the plasma membrane. Rather, for transmembrane growth of an extracellular ice crystal, the crystal would need to pass through a hydrophilic domain such as an aggregation of phase-separated cell surface glycoproteins (or similar structues) expected to occur at reduced temperatures.

Alternatively, the disequilibrium may be restored by movement of intracellular water across the plasma membrane to add to the growing ice crystals forming outside the cell. Because the movement of water molecules across the plasma membrane occurs more rapidly than solute movement (e.g., Na^+, K^+, Cl^-) the cell(s) become progressively more dehydrated as a function of extracellular ice crystal formation until the eutectic point is reached. The eutectic point is defined as the temperature at which both solvent and solute solidify (crystallize).

For single cells, it is possible to calculate the movement of solvent and solutes across the plasma membrane as a function of temperature and thus to predict "accurately" the time required to effectively dehydrate the cell without the formation of intracellular ice.[1] However, with more complex tissues, these calculations are not as easily performed. The definition of "extracellular environment" becomes more difficult, and the movement of solvent and solutes must involve additional layers of cells and boundaries before their appearance in the "extracellular environment."

The intention of this chapter is to deal with the issues associated with the cryopreservation of heart valves and to review some of the approaches taken to resolve these issues. Cryopreservation protocols have been arrived at empirically, derived from knowledge gained from the cryobiology of single-cell suspensions; and they have consistently provided valves that perform adequately for extended periods of time.[2] It now becomes important to find out why they perform so well.

Factors Affecting Cellular Viability

It is well established that cooling in the absence of solvent freezing is normally not harmful to the typical cell. Exceptions to this general rule are found in specific cell systems, e.g., pig spermatozoa and embryos,[3] and is described as thermal or cold shock. Cold shock is normally classified as due to either direct or indirect chilling injury.[4] Direct chilling injury depends on the rate of cooling, and a rapid cooling rate appears to induce more cellular damage than a slow cooling rate. Damage is generally associated with loss of selective membrane permeability and cytoplasmic streaming, cell volume changes, alterations in the cytoskeleton components (actin), and differential loss of membrane components (phospholipids are preferentially lost compared to cholesterol[5]). Indirect chilling injury occurs after a long period (days) at the reduced temperature. This injury is independent of the rate of cooling, and injury may be more closely associated with ionic imbalance and osmotic changes. Of importance to cryopreservation of heart valves is the suggestion that dimethylsulfoxide (DMSO) may actually increase sensitivity to cold shock.[6] Hence DMSO should be added to cells after the initial cooling and prior to freezing. (See ref. 4 for a review of this subject.)

Freezing of cells can be accomplished rapidly or slowly, in a continuous or a discontinuous manner, and in the absence or presence of cryoprotective agents (e.g., glycerol and DMSO). The actual freezing of dilute aqueous solutions is governed by chemical and physical parameters rather than any biologic consideration. At the point at which nucleation of ice occurs, only a portion of the water in the solution actually undergoes the transition to type Ih ice. The molarity of the unfrozen solution is governed by the relation:

$$\mathrm{T\ C}/1.86\ (\text{osmols liter}^{-1})$$

Where T C is the depression of the freezing point. In the case of 0.15 *M* sodium chloride (initial molarity), the molarity of NaCl in the unfrozen fraction is a linear function of temperature (to its eutectic point), whereas the percent (volume) of unfrozen water is curvilinear, decreasing rapidly initially and then less rapidly at lower temperatures (see ref. 5). The proportion of unfrozen solution is directly related to the initial osmolality of that solution.

The presence of dissolved gases in the freezing solution may also complicate subsequent cellular viability. The solubility of gases actually increases over the temperature range 0°C to −20°C; and as water is converted to ice, these gases become concentrated in the unfrozen solution. Hobbs[7] has shown that ice bubbles are formed ahead of the ice–water interface and are excluded from the ice crystal lattice. Although these dissolved gases may be harmful during the freezing process, it is suggested that the appearance of ice bubbles during the thawing process may do considerable damage, particularly as the gases become concentrated in the unfrozen fraction. Research into the effects of solvent degassing prior to cryopreservation might be informative.

The effects of different freezing conditions are

considered separately. To optimize viability, an appropriate combination of parameters must be chosen, and the technology must address thawing as well as freezing conditions.

Rapid Cooling

Rapid cooling during cell freezing is generally regarded as harmful to the viability of cells. We may conveniently define "rapid cooling" as a freezing rate consistent with an absence of cell shrinkage due to osmotic imbalances. Consequently, the random formation of ice crystals during rapid freezing may occur either within the cellular cytoplasm or in the extracellular space, as a function of their respective volumes. Because the volume of the extracellular solvent is greater, nucleation preferentially occurs there, and ice crystal growth spreads rapidly. The membrane barrier surrounding each cell restricts the spread of ice into the cell; and as ice formation continues, the concentration of solute outside the cells increases and the cells begin to lose water by osmotically induced shrinkage. At a rapid rate of cooling, however, the random formation of intracellular ice would be expected to also occur in a large number of cells prior to a significant degree of cell shrinkage. Cells that are therefore rapidly cooled during freezing generally appear unshrunken and contain intracellular ice. As is discussed later, the damage to the cells caused by the intracellular ice probably occurs during thawing rather than during the actual freezing process.

Vitrification is an example of extremely rapid cooling during freezing. In this instance, cells are cooled so rapidly as to preclude ice crystal formation, and the solvent–solute mixture solidifies as an amorphous solid. The subject of vitrification has been extensively reviewed[8,9] and is not discussed in this chapter as it is not at present a viable technique for cryopreservation of heart valves.

Slow Cooling

Slow cooling during freezing is also harmful to cells, albeit via mechanisms different from rapid cooling. Slow cooling may be defined as the rate of cooling during freezing that permits significant cell shrinkage (dehydration) without the formation of intracellular ice. As with rapid cooling, the preferential formation of extracellular ice during slow cooling increases the extracellular solute concentration. As water is osmotically drawn from the cells, they shrink until their osmolality reaches that of the external solution at each successively lower temperature. For example, the NaCl concentration in nonfrozen iso-osmotic saline is 0.15 *M*, but the eutectic concentration (at −21.6°C) is 5.2 *M*. The importance of this observation lies in the solute-induced reduction of the temperature at which the cellular components actually solidify. As mentioned earlier, the eutectic point is that temperature at which the solvent and solute mixture freezes; the formation of natural eutectic mixtures probably aids in cell survival following slow cooling by avoiding the formation of intracellular ice. However, with slow cooling during freezing, high intracellular and extracellular solute concentrations occur, and these conditions are the most probable cause of cell damage. High salt concentrations are generally regarded as being disruptive to cell membrane and protein structure, and certain ionic components are more harmful than others.

The work of van den Berg and associates[10,11] has provided phase diagrams of eutectic temperatures and associated pH changes in a variety of salt combinations. They reported that pH changes occur with eutectic changes and are relatively independent of temperature.

It is well known that calcium and potassium precipitate during the initial stages of freezing, and sodium ions cause considerable fluctuations in pH during freezing. Potassium ions, to the contrary, cause little change in pH during freezing. The temperature and concentration dependence of phosphate buffers, associated with the appropriate activity coefficient (0.98 at 0.001 *M* H_2PO_4 versus 0.74 at 0.1 *M* H_2PO_4) readily explains the dramatic pH changes observed.

That cell damage occurring during freezing correlates with solute concentration changes is supported by the work of Lovelock[12] in which hemolysis produced by freezing red blood cells could also be produced by exposing these same cells to salt concentrations equivalent to those experienced at successively lower temperatures.

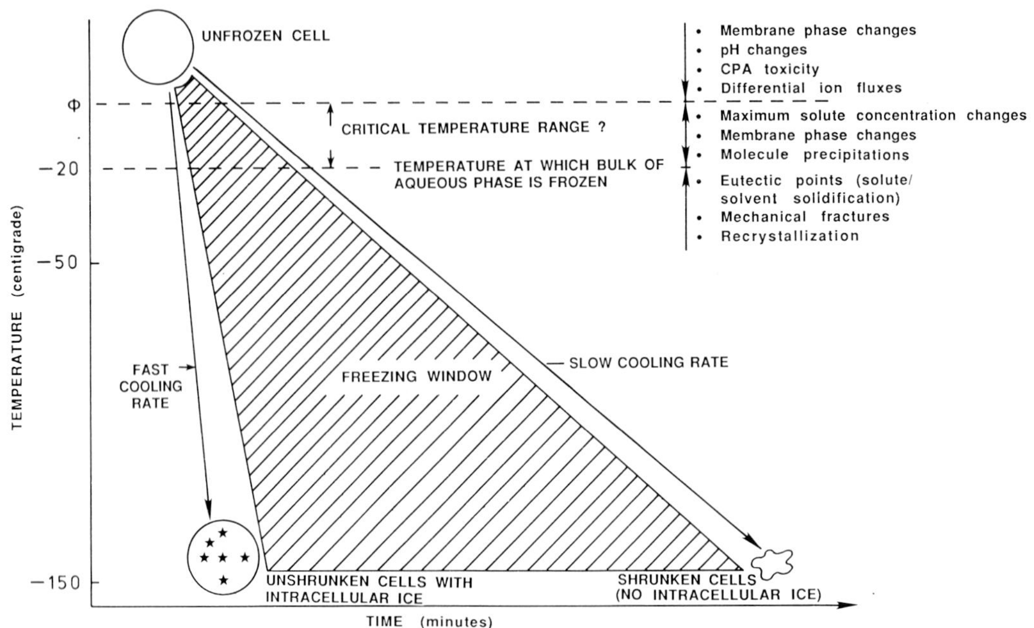

FIGURE 3.1. Effects of cooling rates during freezing on cell morphology and survival.

Alternatively, Schneider and Mazur[13] suggested that eight-cell embryos were not affected by the high concentrations of salts produced by freezing. They suggested that cellular survival may be determined by the fraction of extracellular solute that remains unfrozen, and that cellular distortion may cause significant damage to cells.

Studies on the survival of various cell types frozen at a variety of rates suggest that optimal survival occurs at a cooling rate somewhere between fast and slow. This optimal rate varies with different cell types (i.e., different volume-to-surface areas and different solvent permeabilities of membranes) and appears to correspond to those rates at which intracellular ice just begins to form. Indeed, Leibo and associates[14] and Rall[15] reported that the cooling rate that produces a reduction in survival of mouse embryos was the same rate that produces intracellular ice crystals in about 20 percent of cells.

In general terms, each cell type has a freezing "window" in which the change in temperature with time provides for optimal cell survival (Fig. 3.1). It is interesting that this proposed "window" is narrow at high temperatures and becomes increasingly wider as the temperature decreases, suggesting that deviation from a given freezing rate at high temperatures may be more critical to cell survival than deviations at low temperatures. The survival of cells frozen by what is termed a two-step cooling method further demonstrates the importance of controlling the freezing rate at high temperatures. With the two-step method, cells are frozen to a subzero temperature (usually −20°C, i.e., just above a critical eutectic point) and held at that temperature for a short period of time prior to resumption of cooling, which may now occur at a more rapid rate.[16] Presumably, extracellular ice crystals forming during what is designated the prefreeze (0° to −20°C) period causes a sufficiently large increase in external solute concentration to shrink the cells, reducing the probability of intracellular ice forming.

During cryopreservation of human heart valves, a consistent phenomenon in the cooling rate occurs at −18° to −19°C. At this point, the temperature of the freezing chamber must be rapidly increased in order to prevent a dramatic increase in the cooling rate of the valve tissue–solvent (Fig. 3.2). It is presumably at this temperature that the bulk of the extracellular

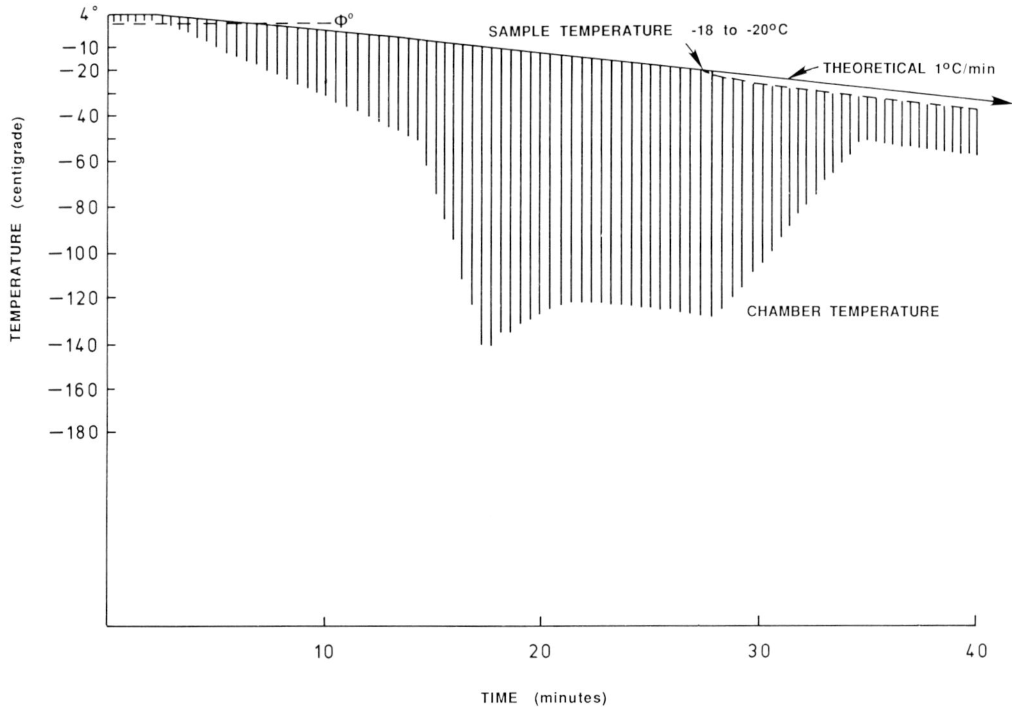

FIGURE 3.2. Portion of controlled-rate freezing curve. Note the deviation from the theoretical cooling rate, indicating the need to rapidly rewarm the freezing chamber when the sample temperature approaches −18° to −20°C.

water has frozen and the remaining solute–solvent mixture begins to solidify. Freezing programs presently in use by the Virginia Tissue Bank maintain a constant −1°C/minute decrease down to −40°C; however, it may be that a faster cooling rate at temperatures below −20°C will improve subsequent cell survival by restricting recrystallization.

Cryoprotective Agents

The value of cryoprotective agents (CPAs) to cell survival is presumably associated primarily with cells frozen by a slow cooling procedure. CPAs have several features in common, the most important of which is very high solubility in water. A second feature of an effective CPA is its limited toxicity toward the cells to be cryopreserved. Glycerol and DMSO are the most commonly employed CPAs, although salts such as magnesium chloride have been reported as well[17]; moreover, the dextrans, glycols, and starches as well as sucrose and polyvinyl pyrolidine appear to confer considerable cryoprotection to a variety of biologic systems.[18] According to Mazur,[19] cryoprotectants protect slowly frozen cells by one or more of the following mechanisms: suppression of salt concentrations; reduction of cell shrinkage at a given temperature; and reduction in the fraction of the solution frozen at a given temperature.

The phase rule may apply to the major function of CPAs for protecting cells. This rule states that the total concentration of solutes is fixed at a given temperature. In short, in a single solute system (i.e., NaCl) the required solute concentration must arise from that solute, whereas in a two-solute system, e.g., DMSO plus NaCl, the solute concentration obtained for a given temperature is the sum of the NaCl and DMSO concentrations. Inclusion of DMSO in the freezing solution effectively reduces the concentration of other solutes at each successive temperature in the freezing process.

Because the total solute concentration at any subzero temperature is fixed, the higher the CPA/salt ratio present at the beginning of cooling, the lower is the concentration of salt at a given subzero temperature. This reduction in non-CPA solute concentration is presumably the basis for the reduced solute damage to cells that occurs during slow freezing. However, studies to evaluate this assumption have found that replacement of ionic agents with an osmotically equivalent amount of nonelectrolyte (mannitol) still results in cellular damage—presumably due to the cryoprotectant.[20]

Although CPAs also reduce the amount of extracellular ice at each subzero temperature with a resultant increase in the volume of the unfrozen fraction, it is not known if fewer ice crystals are responsible for any of the reduction in cell damage.[13] The latter function of CPAs may also relate to their role in reducing membrane fusion during cryopreservation.[21] Consider, for example, that a decrease in the volume of the aqueous (unfrozen) component during freezing increases the density of cells within it (cell suspensions) and thus increases the potential for cell–cell interactions. Solutions of low osmolality would be expected to have a smaller percentage of the unfrozen fraction at each subzero temperature than a solution of high osmolality (i.e., presence of CPAs) and cell–cell interactions would be more pronounced. Pegg[22] reported increased hemolysis of human erythrocytes when they were frozen at high densities. Cellular fusion at low temperatures is less of a problem during cryopreservation of dilute cell suspensions but may well be of considerable significance during cryopreservation of a concentrated cell suspension or of complex tissues. The pharmacologic effects of CPAs such as DMSO and glycerol were reviewed by Shlafer.[18]

Thawing of Cryopreserved Tissues

It is generally accepted that rapid thawing of cells enhances survival. This observation is especially important for rapidly cooled cells and has been suggested to favor cell survival by suppressing the phenomenon known as recrystallization—the thawing and refreezing of water molecules that may occur during rewarming. Recrystallization is a phenomenon common to solutions that have been frozen under nonequilibrium conditions. Slow cooling (less than 1°C/minute) typically results in the formation of large crystals, whereas rapid cooling (more than 1°C/minute) produces smaller crystals. Small ice crystals are unstable because of their high surface energy, and they tend to re-form into large crystals to improve their thermodynamic stability. Such transitions readily occur during warming and may result in cell damage that was not present during the actual freezing event (although recrystallization could occur at the time of freezing). Cells frozen by a slow cooling process have fewer intracellular ice crystals and larger crystals, and thus are presumably less sensitive to the rate of thawing.

Rapid thawing is the preferred route for rewarming cryopreserved heart valves, as it restricts recrystallization. The process is normally accomplished by rapid immersion of the frozen valve in a large volume of water warmed to 42°C. Thawing is normally completed in less than 6 minutes; and so long as care is taken during packaging and when handling the valve during the thawing process, little mechanical damage occurs (see Chapter 4).

Slow thawing may better preserve the viability of certain cell types. Mammalian embryos and red blood cells appear to do better with a slow thawing rate.[23,24] This observation is probably explained by solute effects and solvent movements. Consider, for example, that during freezing a cell that is slowly cooled has minimal intracellular ice and is considerably shrunken in volume. During rapid thawing these cells experience considerable differences in solute concentrations and rapid rehydration by solvent (water).[25] Because red blood cells typically lack microvilli, the expandability of their surface area is limited, and they would be expected to be more sensitive to rapid osmotic changes (volume changes). A slower thawing rate would tend to minimize osmotic imbalances by providing time for the rehydrating solvent to enter the cell. Conversely, rapidly cooled cells would be expected to contain intracellular ice and not be shrunken in volume. During rapid or slow thawing, these cells would not be expected to experience dramatic osmotic imbalances or solute toxicity, and recrystallization would presumably be the major cause of cell damage.

Osmotic Imbalances

After thawing cryopreserved tissues, the CPAs must be removed. Although the mechanism for DMSO toxicity has not been determined, its ability to affect membrane fluidity[26] and cell structure through induced changes in cytoplasmic microtubules has been well documented.[27,28] It also forms stable coordination complexes with metals.[18] CPAs are generally removed by a stepwise dilution procedure. Measurements of cell volume changes during this process clearly demonstrate that the cells undergo dramatic volume changes at each dilution step.[1,19,29]

Cells embedded within a tissue matrix may survive step changes more readily than cell suspensions because of the restricted movement of solutes through the ion-exchange action of the macromolecular matrix or through a mechanism similar to that afforded by removal of the cryoprotectant in the presence of a nonpermeating solute such as sucrose. Both conditions may prevent cell swelling, as the cryoprotectant diffuses out of the cells along its concentration gradient. It might be informative to examine the effects of a continuous dilution of CPAs, using dialysis or gradient elution devices, on cell volume changes and subsequent survival. In addition, it has been reported[16,30] that many cell types tolerate CPA removal better at 37°C than at 0°C. This increased tolerance may be related to the ability of the cells to transport solute molecules more rapidly at 37°C than at 0°C. Thus the osmotic imbalances may be more quickly restored, and the cell(s) may more easily repair the damaging effects incurred by cryopreservation.

Effects of Temperature on Cell Membranes

Bilayer membranes are composed primarily of phospholipids, cholesterol, and proteins (glycoproteins). As the temperature decreases, the lipids tend to preferentially associate with other lipids, excluding membrane proteins, in a process called "lateral phase separation." As a result of this process, regions of the membrane contain high densities of membrane proteins floating like islands in a homogeneous "sea" of lipids. Many of these membrane proteins span the bilayer membrane, being exposed to the aqueous phase of the extracellular solvent and the cell cytoplasm; and they thus may now constitute a collection of aqueous channels more permeable to ions and perhaps ice crystal growth. As the temperature continues to decrease, the lipid components undergo a "fluid-to-gel" transition where the vibrational energy (and lateral movement) of the lipids decreases with decreasing temperature. The temperature at which this fluid-to-gel transition occurs depends on a number of factors, including but not restricted to: chain length of the fatty acids of the phospholipids (transition temperature increases with increasing chain length); degree of saturation/unsaturation of the fatty acids (unsaturated fatty acids decrease the tendency to form a "gel" at lower temperatures and thus lower the transition temperature); heterogeneity of fatty acid composition and charge distribution of the phosphatide group (e.g., choline, serine, inositol); and the presence of cholesterol (cholesterol tends to lower the phase transition temperature[21]).

Lipid modification, as a means of protecting bull spermatozoa during cryopreservation, has been studied with some success.[31] As an additional complication, in complex tissues cell-to-cell contacts are made through membrane glycoproteins, and thus different cell populations within the tissue may experience different reactions to temperature changes; moreover, the transmembrane junctions between cells may also be variable in terms of permitting solute movement. For a more thorough discussion of this subject, refer to the articles by Quinn[32] and Morris and Clarke.[33]

Biochemical and Histologic Characteristics of Allograft Heart Valves

An "average" adult heart valve processed for cryopreservation is typically 6 cm in length from the annulus to the distal aspect of the aortic conduit. The sums of the aortic valve cuspal areas, cuspal weight, and sinus of Valsalva volumes increase with age and with heart weight. In addition, in most valves examined (84%), the cusps within a given valve are of different sizes (area).[34] The valves are sized based on internal diameter, and the "average" thickness of the aortic wall is approximately 1.5 mm. A valve 6 cm in length with an inside diameter of 24 mm thus occupies a volume of approximately 7 $cm.^3$ Valves are typically frozen in a total volume of 100 ml, and the valve thus constitutes approximately 7–15% of the total volume to be frozen.

The valve leaflets consist of a cellular component and an acellular component. Within the cellular component, endothelial cells line the leaflet, forming a smooth boundary. Fibrocytes occur within the acellular matrix, which is composed primarily of collagen, elastin, and acid mucopolysaccharides (proteoglycans), as well as a variety of other low- and high-molecular-weight molecules.

Biochemical analyses of heart valve leaflet tissue have not been as extensive as the histologic studies. Collagen, consisting of a family of fibrous proteins, is the most abundant protein in the aortic valve cusp. There are five major types of collagen: I, II, III, IV, and V. Types I and III (composition [α1(III)]3) are found primarily in the cardiovascular system. Collagen represents an unusual protein in that approximately one-third of all the amino acid residues are glycine, with proline present in similarly high amounts. Proline and lysine residues in collagen are typically hydroxylated (4-hydroxyproline and 5-hydroxylysine), and carbohydrate residues (a disaccharide of glucose and galactose) are frequently covalently attached to the protein through hydroxylysine. The extent of glycosylation varies with the type of collagen and the tissue distribution. The basic structural component of fibrous collagen is called "tropocollagen," and it is with the formation of covalent crosslinks that tropocollagen is formed into the protein network that comprises the fibrous matrix of valve leaflet tissue.

Connective tissues are also rich in proteoglycans, which consist of polysaccharide (about 95%) and protein (about 5%) units. These very large polyanions bind water and cations, thereby forming the ground substance of connective tissue. The polysaccharide chains of proteoglycans are made up of disaccharide repeating units containing a derivative of an amino sugar (glucosamine or galactosamine), with at least one of the sugars in the disaccharide containing a negatively charged carboxylate or sulfate group. These carbohydrate units are attached to a core protein, and about 140 of these subunits are noncovalently bound at 300-Å intervals to a very long filament of hyaluronate. Human heart valves have been shown to have a high content of acid glycosaminoglycan (AGAG) proteoglycans, which are highest in the mitral and aortic valves and lowest in the tricuspid valve. The total amounts of AGAG are high at maturation and decrease with advancing age. The main AGAG is hyaluronic acid (HA), constituting approximately one-half of the total AGAG, with dermatan sulfate and chondroitin sulfate isomers each accounting for one-fourth to one-half of the total AGAG. Heparin sulfate is found to constitute a small percentage of the AGAG, and a minor amount of oversulfated dermatan sulfate is also present. With advancing age, the proportions of hyaluronic acid and chondroitin 4-sulfate tend to decrease, whereas those of chondroitin 6-sulfate, dermatan sulfate, and heparin sulfate tend to increase.[35,36]

Of interest to this review is the extent of covalent crosslinking of collagen and the proteoglycan composition of cryopreserved valve leaflet tissue. Collagenase, an enzyme that degrades collagen, may be released by damaged or dying matrix cells, and collagen crosslinking is dependent on aldol condensation (an enzyme-mediated process), which is in turn dependent on a viable matrix cell population. Campo and Ramono[37] have already clearly demonstrated that lysozymal modification of proteoglycans in cartilage may aid in the mineralization of bone, as proteoglycans in their native state typically inhibit mineralization.[38]

Hunter[39] proposed an ion-exchange mechanism for cartilage calcification in which calcium, bound to the anionic groups of proteoglycans, is displaced and rebound to phosphate ions when the concentration of phosphate increases.

Cryopreservation of heart valves results in cell damage and thus may increase enzymatic modifications to the noncellular matrix component. In addition, the observed loss of endothelial cells removes a permeability barrier to ions and hydrating solvent and may permit an increase in the concentration of phosphate ions in the valve matrix. That AGAG concentration becomes reduced in valves from older donors[36,40] may well correlate with their increased tendency to calcify, as less proteoglycan would be available to bind calcium, thereby enhancing calcium association with phosphate ions. The soluble nature of proteoglycans, as well as their tendency to bind cations (i.e., calcium) make them obvious candidates for biochemical studies on heart valve tissue as they relate to calcification and subsequent durability following transplantation. Little information is available describing the effects of cryopreservation on proteoglycan changes in heart valve tissues, and one might ask the question of whether loss of proteoglycans during valve processing results in valves that mimic valves from older donors in being more susceptible to subsequent calcification following transplantation.

The cellular composition of heart valve leaflets includes fibrocytes and endothelial cells. It is reasonable to assume a differential sensitivity of these two cell types to the cryopreservation process. Endothelial cells are exposed to the immediate solvent and appear to be easily dislodged during processing—perhaps as early as at the time of procurement. Hearts are typically washed in cold saline or lactated Ringer's solution to remove blood products and cool the valve tissue prior to transport in tissue culture medium. As discussed, a reduction in temperature differentially affects the sodium–potassium pump,[41] and cells typically swell because of the ionic imbalance.

In classic experiments, Collins and associates[42] reported that perfusion of dog kidneys with solutions containing 115 m*M* potassium, 30 m*M* $MgSO_4$, 57.5 m*M* phosphate, and 140 m*M* glucose resulted in functional kidneys. Acquatella and coworkers[43] suggested that such solutions tended to stabilize the water and ion content of tissues by mimicking the intracellular ion content and lessening cellular swelling.

Washing freshly procured heart valves in lactated Ringer's, rather than Acquatella's or Collins' solutions, probably results in swelling of the endothelial cells, enhancing their subsequent loss from the surface of the leaflet matrix during processing. Fibrocytes may be expected to be somewhat protected by the matrix from this swelling phenomenon, thereby increasing their chance of survival. It has been shown that solutions rich in impermeant ions and potassium provide for retention of cellular viability after subzero storage in the presence of DMSO, so it is suggested that Acquatella's or Collins' solution be used for washing freshly procured heart valves.

The work of Solberg and coworkers,[44] describing the greater loss of endothelial cells from saphenous veins exposed to 4°C temperatures than after exposure to 20°C tends to support the greater sensitivity of endothelial cells to ionic imbalances or, as the authors suggested, disruption of the cytoskeletal system.

Application of Cryopreservation to Heart Valves

Correlation of cellular viability, i.e., endothelial cells and fibroblasts (fibrocytes), with valve durability has not been adequately determined. Work by researchers such as Wheatley and McGregor[45] has suggested that following transplantation of "fresh" antibiotic-sterilized canine valves there is a rapid and apparently irreversible loss of viable cells from the valve leaflet tissues. Indeed, these researchers were unable to culture fibroblasts from valve tissue implanted for as short a time as 8 weeks. Concurrent histologic evaluation of transplanted tissues suggested a total absence of "donor" cells in the valve leaflets. O'Brien's group, however, were successful in isolating donor fibroblasts from a heart valve removed from a patient more than 9 years after operation.[2] Of interest to such studies were reports[46,47] describing the role of ABO blood group antigen incompatibility following valve transplantation.

Buch and associates[48] implanted unfixed-dog aortic valves (valves containing "viable" donor cells) from three sources: autograft, allograft, and xenograft. After 3 months of exposure to host factors, the autograft leaflets had a normal endothelium, were slightly thickened, and were hypercellular. The allograft leaflets had cellular infiltrates in the muscle tissue, denuded endothelium, and fibrin deposition over the bare collagen. The xenograft leaflets had sustained the most severe destruction and were acellular with attenuated and disrupted collagen fibers. These authors concluded that an immunologic response was the most plausible explanation for their findings.

Their studies were supported by other reports[49,50] describing the subcutaneous implantation of aortic valve allografts. Such allografts elicited mononuclear cell infiltrates in the grafts and both cytotoxic and hemagglutinating antibodies in the host serum. However, when irradiation-sterilized valves (no viable cells) were implanted in recipient hearts, ABO blood group incompatibilities appeared not to affect the final outcome of valve durability.[47] Indeed, Heslop and associates[47] suggested that rat valve leaflets are not antigenic, antigenicity appearing to reside primarily in the "rim of cardiac muscle."

From such studies one might conclude, with reservation, that the implantation of fresh donor valves (valves presumably retaining the greatest extent of cellular viability) should be immunologically matched to recipients, and that following a comparatively short period of implantation one should not expect to find viable donor cells in the leaflet tissue of the implanted valve. Alternatively, implantation of acellular valves would not require immunologic compatibility and would presumably result in the same absence of viable cells in the implanted valve. The question is thus: Is cellular viability important to valve durability, and can animal studies be related to work in humans?

Analyses of subgroups of patients receiving aortic valve allografts suggested that valves treated with antibiotics and stored in fresh nutrient media provided improved durability when the period between harvesting and storage was short and when the storage times were also brief, implying that cellular viability was an important feature.[2,51–54]

Cryopreservation techniques developed for single-cell suspensions and simple tissues were finally applied to valve tissues with encouraging findings,[53,55] and improved clinical results have been reported from a limited number of studies using cryopreserved valves. Studies by O'Brien's group reported actuarial data on 184 cryopreserved implants, demonstrating 95% patient and valve survival at 14 years. These data suggested that properly cryopreserved allograft valves may be vastly superior to any other prosthetic device[2,56–58] in terms of durability and performance.

Cryobiology[55,59] is a relatively young science with most techniques used being empirically derived. Human heart valve cryopreservation protocols can now be divided into five areas: (1) harvesting and transport of the donor heart; (2) valve preparation and antibiotic sterilization; (3) control-rate freezing with cryoprotectants; (4) storage of the processed valves; and (5) thawing/diluting and implantation methods.

From data now available[51–53,58,60–62] several general principles are emerging: (1) the shorter the warm ischemic time, the better is the cell viability; (2) the antibiotic concentrations should be nontoxic to valve cells yet effectively sterilize the allografts[62]; (3) certain antibiotics (e.g., penicillin) decrease cell viability[62]; (4) the duration of antibiotic incubation probably should not exceed 24 hours; (5) antibiotic incubation may be more effective at 37°C but results in increased cell damage versus incubation at 4°C; (6) optimal control-rate freezing, at present, appears to be 1°C/minute with 10% DMSO as a cryoprotectant; (7) valve allografts may be stored at liquid nitrogen vapor-phase temperatures (preferably below −130°C; see ref. 63 for a discussion on recrystallization) for indefinite periods of time; and (8) thawing methods appear to have significant effects on cell viability and mechanical integrity of the valves. The "best" procedures for each step have not yet been clearly elucidated, and valve preparation protocols currently in use while similar are rarely identical.

Effects of Loss of Cellular Viability in Cryopreserved Heart Valves

Histologic studies of valve allografts have been performed primarily on canine valves[64] or human valves recovered at autopsy or reoperation.[26,51,52,65–67] Preservation of donor fibroblast viability has been accepted as important to the short- and medium-term durability of transplanted valves. The degree of endothelial cell retention has been variable, and further study is needed to determine the role the endothelium plays in the success of allografts.[53,68] It may be suggested that endothelial cell retention or reendothelialization is a prime factor in the long-term survival of cryopreserved human heart valve allografts, being responsible for retention of proteoglycans in the valve leaflet matrix and reduction of calcification. Although traditional light microscopy represents the most widely utilized means of histologic evaluation of tissue sections, it is perhaps too subjective to represent an effective means of determining cellular viability or the condition of the noncellular matrix of valve leaflet tissue. Scanning electron microscopic examination of leaflet tissue has revealed that both the collagen bundles and endothelial cells lie in an axis perpendicular to the flow of blood across the tissue.[25] Although the endothelial cells are presumably not extensively involved in the synthesis of collagen or proteoglycan components of the leaflet, it may be suggested that the presence of a viable endothelial cell layer could be important in the reduction of loss of collagen fibers by the movement of blood across the valve leaflets. In addition, the electronegative charges of sulfate groups associated with proteoglycans would be expected to provide for the physical attraction and binding of divalent cations such as calcium. Calcification of transplanted heart valves represents a serious threat to the durability of valves, and research[35,69,70] has shown that such calcification begins quickly following transplantation and occurs primarily in areas immediately adjacent to fibroblasts (fibrocytes) within the collagen–proteoglycan matrix.[70] Because proteoglycans would be expected to occur in spaces just outside such cells, it seems appropriate to suggest a strong role for proteoglycans in the calcification of transplanted heart valve tissues. Such calcification processes spread rapidly throughout the leaflet and eventually appear as calcific deposits.[70]

These observations once again leave us with conflicting possibilities. The loss of endothelial cells on the surfaces of valve leaflets should result in the loss of proteoglycans and thus a reduction in the possible binding sites for calcium, i.e., reduction in total calcium concentration; yet this loss perhaps enhances calcium binding to phosphate ions, leading to calcification. Retention of a viable endothelial cell layer should limit the loss of proteoglycans with a presumptive reduced possibility of calcification. The reduction in passage of calcium or phosphate ions into the matrix by endothelial cells, however, may mitigate this process. Because it has already been suggested that following transplantation all cells are lost within a short period of time, the presence of a viable endothelial cell layer and matrix cell population at the time of implantation may only delay the process of calcification. Mineralization of implanted allograft valves may also be delayed through the systemic administration of, or cuspal treatment with,[71] diphosphonates such as are used in the treatment of certain metabolic bone diseases.[72,73] In short, direct correlation of cellular viability of transplanted valves with durability of these valves is not expected to be a simple matter. Histologic evaluation of valve leaflet tissues needs to consider both cellular and matrix components, and some effort is needed concerning quantification of such components. Scanning electron microscopy or use of *Ulex europaeus* (UEA-1) lectin as a marker for endothelial cells[74] gives a better estimate of the loss of endothelial cells from the surface of leaflet tissues, and transmission electron microscopy gives a more quantifiable estimate of the amount and distribution of proteoglycan and collagen and a closer look at the matrix cells.

Problems of Quantification of Cell Viability

The development of a quantifiable estimate of cellular viability is of immediate biochemical interest to valve cryopreservation efforts. Previous efforts at assessing cellular viability have focused on matrix cells (fibroblasts) and have primarily used autoradiography following radioactive amino acid or thymidine incorporation by individual cells[53,75] or glucose metabolism.[2] Early efforts by workers such as Khan and Gonzalez-Lavin[75] utilized methyl tritiated thymidine incorporation followed by autoradiography. One difficulty associated with the use of thymidine is the requirement for DNA synthesis (i.e., that cells be actively dividing). Also, autoradiography is not consistently quantifiable (i.e., it represents a subjective estimate of cellular viability based on the number of dividing cells as well as what constitutes a radiolabeled cell). A viable cell may not necessarily be a dividing cell.

O'Brien's group demonstrated the effectiveness of using glucose metabolism by pulmonary valves as a predicter of aortic valve "viability." Indeed, they use culturability of leaflet fibroblasts, histology, and whole-valve glucose utilization exceeding 16 mg/dl/24 hours as a test of valve "viability."[2] Other studies, such as those by Armiger and coworkers[76] relied on histologic studies with an effort at quantification of cell viability based on growth in cell culture.[76] Cell culture, as a means of assessing cell viability, is complicated by variable efficiencies of cell attachment and outgrowth as well as the observation that a viable cell may not necessarily be capable of proliferation. The ability to culture fibroblasts from cryopreserved valves may relate to whether fetal calf serum was included in the cryopreservation solution.

Better methods of cell viability assessment involve the measurement of incorporation rates of amino acids into the cellular components of valve leaflet tissues. These tests are quantifiable and measure transport rates of radiolabeled amino acids into viable cells and incorporation into proteins being synthesized by viable cells. Because cells must continually synthesize proteins de novo in order to remain viable and to maintain tissue structure and function, such tests should represent reliable indicators of cell viability.[53,77]

An excellent early study by van der Kamp and Nuata[77] described the incorporation of radiolabeled proline and methionine into proteins by rat valve fibroblasts. They clearly demonstrated that proline represented an ideal amino acid for measuring synthesis of matrix proteins in these valves, that proline incorporation was rapid (maximum at 3 hours), and that the synthesized proteins were distributed throughout the valve as a function of time. The radiolabeled methionine was incorporated more rapidly than proline, but radiolabeled methionine was quickly lost from the tissue (within 1 week) and was not incorporated into extracellular products.

Protein synthesis by mammalian cells includes proteins normally utilized for "housekeeping" purposes or for secretion to the extracellular environment (export). As a general statement, it may be said that two such populations of cells exist in the valve leaflet tissue of the heart. The fibroblast–fibrocyte population is involved in normal maintenance protein synthesis as well as export protein synthesis (collagen and proteoglycans). The endothelial cell population is involved primarily in maintenance protein synthesis (we may conveniently ignore export protein synthesis by this cell population as it relates to the transport assay), and we may therefore take advantage of these differences. In noncollagen protein the ratio of proline to leucine residues approximates 0.5, whereas in collagen protein this ratio typically exceeds 9.7.[78] Consequently, the matrix cell population should incorporate more proline into protein than leucine, and the nonmatrix cell population (endothelial cells) should incorporate more leucine than proline into protein. Therefore through this differential incorporation rate, one should be able to evaluate protein synthesis in the various cell populations, and the loss of the endothelial cell layer should dramatically reduce leucine incorporation compared to proline incorporation.

Complications to this procedure lie in the use of tissue sections rather that single-cell suspensions for the transport and incorporation assays. The work of Low and associates[78] has clearly demonstrated that the differential incorporation of two amino acids (proline and leucine) into different proteins affords a convenient method for estimating synthesis of the various kinds of protein. Leucine incorporation is generally preferred over methionine because proteins typically contain more leucine residues; hence more radiolabel may be incorporated for a given protein synthesis study. However, these researchers utilized free cell suspensions where all cells have equal access to radiolabeled compounds present in the incubation solution. With tissue sections the presence of the endothelial cell layer on the surface of the tissue section may partially exclude penetration of either, or both, radiolabeled amino acids into the matrix of the valve leaflet where they would be transportable by the matrix cells (fibroblasts). Loss of the endothelial cell layer during the cryopreservation process would presumably result in a reduction in accumulation of amino acids by the leaflet tissue, i.e., fewer total cells; but the ability of these same amino acids to more readily penetrate the valve matrix may compensate for this reduction by presenting a new population of cells that could transport and incorporate the radiolabeled amino acids. The differential incorporation of proline and leucine by the various cell populations should be important in this instance, in that it should permit resolution of this problem, as proline should be more strongly incorporated by the matrix cells than leucine. An additional approach to resolving this problem would be to determine the kinetic constants for amino acid transport by the various cell types. Proline is transported across intestinal brush borders via the "imino carrier."[79] The imino carrier is defined as the alanine-insensitive, Na^+-dependent proline transport system; it exhibits half-saturation at 1.0 m*M* proline at sodium concentrations of 30 m*M*. It is not known if the imino carrier in cardiovascular tissue mimics that in intestinal tissues.

Accumulation of radiolabeled amino acids by cells may be further complicated by the presence of intracellular pools of these same amino acids. As the radiolabeled amino acids are transported into the cells, the specific activities become smaller through a dilution effect, and significant delays may be encountered between the time an amino acid is transported across the plasma membrane and the time it becomes incorporated into cellular protein. The extent of the dilution effect also varies with the amount of nonradiolabeled (endogenously synthesized) amino acid present within different cell types. It is thus important that transport and incorporation be measured as a function of time and that the intracellular concentrations of "pooled" (endogenously synthesized) amino acids be determined. Ideally, the ability to block synthesis of the amino acid being transported would be of considerable advantage for assessing incorporation rates. At present, the transport and incorporation of radiolabeled proline appears to be used most frequently to assess cellular viability in postcryopreserved allograft valves.

Direction of Future Basic Research

As with much biomedical research, we have observed that a fresh and properly cryopreserved allograft heart valve functions much like a native valve. Its hemodynamic properties are superior to those of mechanical valves, and anticoagulation therapy is not required. It is clearly superior to mechanical valves, yet we do not know why. It is "foreign" tissue, yet seems to perform as if it were antigen-"neutral." It need not contain viable cells, yet it is durable for many years. In short, it works. We are thus left with the job of finding out why it works and perhaps how to improve its durability.

We often define a "viable" valve as one possessing viable cells and restrict our determination of viable cells to fibroblasts, ignoring endothelial cells.

One of the primary objectives of future research thus needs to be the establishment of a satisfactory test for cell viability. This test should be quantitative and preferably utilize a portion of the valve tissue that is not needed for implantation—it should be "nondestructive." The transport and incorporation of radiolabeled amino acids may serve this function, but we must first assure ourselves that accumulation rates are due to the cellular components and not to the noncellular components. To date, this aspect of the radiolabel incorporation has not been satisfactorily determined. We have also not developed incorporation methods that assess and differentiate the endothelial and fibroblast viabilities.

Future work must include a serious analysis of proteoglycan and AGAG changes with cryopreservation. The potential role of such molecules in calcification[80] nonspecific binding of radiolabeled amino acids, and protection of cellular components during valve processing suggest that they may have a direct effect on valve durability. It is fortunate that baseline studies delineating proteoglycan compositions of valves have been performed. These studies should make similar analyses on cryopreserved valves (and conduit tissues) easier. The fact that root/conduit tissues calcify before cuspal tissues should be of value in determining those factors responsible for calcification.

Much of the work to be performed is nonclinical. It has been clearly demonstrated that cryopreserved allograft heart valves work. The burden must now fall on the basic scientists to delineate why they work so well and how to improve the ultimate results.

References

1. Mazur, P, Miller RH: The use of permeability coefficients in predicting the osmotic response of human red blood cells during the removal of intracellular glycerol. *Cryobiology* 13:126, 1976.
2. O'Brien MF, Stafford EG, Gardner MAH, et al: A comparison of aortic valve replacement with viable cryopreserved and fresh allograft valves, with a note on chromosomal studies. *J Thorac Cardiovasc Surg* 94:812–823, 1987.
3. Smith AU, Polge C: Survival of spermatozoa at low temperatures. *Nature* 166:668, 1950.
4. Morris GJ: Direct chilling injury. In Grant BWW, Morris GJ (eds): *The Effects of Low Temperatures on Biological Systems*. London: Arnold Press, 1987, pp. 120–146.
5. Lovelock JE: The haemolysis of human red blood cells by freezing and thawing. *Biochim Biophys Acta* 10:414–426, 1953.
6. Morris GJ, Coulson GE, Meyer MA, et al: Cold shock: a wide-spread cellular reaction. *CryoLetters* 4:179–192, 1983.
7. Hobbs PV: *Ice Physics*. Oxford: Clarendon Press, 1974.
8. Fahy GM, MacFarlane DR, Angell CA, Merryman HT: Vitrification as an approach to cryopreservation. *Cryobiology* 21:407–426, 1984.
9. MacFarlane DR: Devitrification in glass-forming aqueous solutions. *Cryobiology* 23:230–244, 1986.
10. van der Berg L, Rose D: Effects of freezing on the pH and composition of sodium and potassium phosphate solutions: the reciprocal system KH_2PO_4-Na_2HPO_4-H_2O. *Arch Biochem Biophys* 81:319, 1959.
11. van der Berg L, Soliman FS: Composition and pH changes during freezing of solutions containing calcium and magnesium phosphates. *Cryobiology* 6:10, 1969.
12. Lovelock JE: The mechanism of the protective action of glycerol against haemolysis by freezing and thawing. *Biochim Biophys Acta* 11:28, 1953.
13. Schneider U, Mazur P: Relative influence of unfrozen fraction and salt concentration on the survival of slowly frozen eight-cell mouse embryos. *Cryobiology* 24:17–41, 1987.
14. Leibo SP, McGrath JJ, Cravalho EG: Microscopic observation of intracellular ice formation in mouse ova as a function of cooling rate. *Cryobiology* 15:257, 1978.
15. Rall WF: Physical chemical aspects of cryoprotection of human erythrocytes and mouse embryos. Ph.D. dissertation, University of Tennessee, 1979.
16. Farrant J: General observations on cell preservation. In Ashwood-Smith MJ, Farrant J (eds): *Low Temperature Preservation in Medicine and Biology*. London: Pitman, 1980, pp. 1–18.
17. Karow AM Jr, Carrier O Jr: Effects of cryoprotectant compounds on mammalian heart muscle. *Surg Gynecol Obstet* 128:571, 1969.
18. Shlafer M: Pharmacological considerations in cryopreservation. In Karow AM, Pegg DE (eds): *Organ Preservation for Transplantation*. 2nd Ed. New York: Marcel Dekker, 1981, pp. 177–212.
19. Mazur P: Fundamental cryobiology and the preservation of organs by freezing. In Karow AM Jr, Pegg DE (eds): *Organ Preservation for Transplantation*. 2nd Ed. New York: Marcel Dekker, 1981, pp. 143–175.
20. Fahy GM, Karow AM Jr: Posthypertonic osmotic shock and myocardial injury. *Cryobiology* 12:577, 1975.
21. Ladbrooke BD, Williams RM, Chapman D: Studies on lecithin-cholesterol-water interactions by differential scanning calorimetry and x-ray diffraction. *Biochim Biophys Acta* 150:333–340, 1968.
22. Pegg DE: The effect of cell concentration on the recovery of human erythrocytes after freezing and thawing in the presence of glycerol. *Cryobiology* 18:221–228, 1981.
23. Miller RH, Mazur P: Survival of frozen-thawed human red cells as a function of cooling and warming velocities. *Cryobiology* 13:404, 1976.
24. Whittingham DG, Leibo SP, Mazur P: Survival of mouse embryos frozen to −196 and −269°C. *Science* 178:411, 1972.
25. Deck JD: Endothelial cell orientation on aortic valve leaflets. *Cardiovasc Res* 20:760–767, 1986.
26. Barnett RE: The effects of dimethylsulfoxide and glycerol on Na^+, K^+-ATPase and membrane structure. *Cryobiology* 15:227, 1978.
27. Katsuda, S, Okada Y, Nakanishi I: Dimethyl sulfoxide induces microtubule formation in cultured

arterial smooth muscle cells. *Cell Biol Int Rep* 11:103–110, 1987.

28. Katsuda S, Okada Y, Nakanishi I, Tanaka J: The influence of dimethyl sulfoxide on cell growth and ultrastructural features of cultured smooth muscle cells. *J Electron Micros* 33:239–241, 1984.
29. Jackowski S, Leibo SP, Mazur P: Glycerol permeabilities of fertilized and unfertilized mouse ova. *J Exp Zool* 212:329, 1980.
30. Thorpe PE, Knight SC, Farrant J: Optimal conditions for the preservation of mouse lymph node cells in liquid nitrogen using cooling rate techniques. *Cryobiology* 13:126, 1976.
31. Graham JK, Foote RH: Effect of several lipids, fatty acyl chain length, and degree of unsaturation on the motility of bull spermatozoa after cold shock and freezing. *Cryobiology* 24:42–52, 1987.
32. Quinn PJ: A lipid-phase separation model of low temperature damage to biological membranes. *Cryobiology* 22:128–146, 1985.
33. Morris GJ, Clarke A: Effects of Low Temperatures on Biological Membranes. New York: Academic Press, 1981, pp. 241–377.
34. Silver MA, Roberts WC: Detailed anatomy of the normal functioning aortic valve in hearts of normal and increased weight. *Am J Cardiol* 55:454–461, 1985.
35. Schoen FJ, Tsao JW, Levy RJ: Calcification of bovine pericardium used in cardiac valve bioprostheses. *Am J Pathol* 123:134–145, 1986.
36. Murata K: Acidic glycosaminoglycans in human heart valves. *J Mol Cell Cardiol* 13:281–292, 1981.
37. Campo RD, Romano JG: Changes in cartilage proteoglycans associated with calcification. *Calcif Tissue Int* 39:175–184, 1986.
38. Tenenbaum HC, Hunter GK: Chondroitin sulfate inhibits calcification of bone formed in vitro. *Bone Mineral* 2:43–51, 1987.
39. Hunter GK: An ion-exchange mechanism of cartilage calcification. *Connect Tissue Res* 16:111–120, 1987.
40. Torii SR, Bashey I, Nakao K: Acid mucopolysaccharide composition of human heart valve. *Biochim Biophys Acta* 101:285–291, 1965.
41. Elford BC: Temperature dependence of cation permeability of dog red blood cells. *Nature* 248:522, 1974.
42. Collins GM, Bravo-Shugarman M, Terasaki PI: Kidney preservation for transplantation. *Lancet* 2:1219, 1969.
43. Acquatella H, Perez-Gonzalez M, Morales JM, Whittembury G: Ionic and histological changes in the kidney after perfusion and storage for transplantation. *Transplantation* 14:480, 1972.
44. Solberg S, Larsen T, Jorgensen L, Sorlie D: Cold induced endothelial cell detachment in human saphenous vein grafts. *J Cardiovasc Surg* 28:571–575, 1987.
45. Wheatley DJ, McGregor CGA: Post-implantation viability in canine allograft heart valves. *Cardiovasc Res* 11:78–85, 1977.
46. Balch CM, Karp RB: Blood group compatibility and aortic valve allotransplantation in man. *J Cardiovasc Surg* 70:256–259, 1975.
47. Heslop BF, Wilson SE, Hardy BE: Antigenicity of aortic valve allografts. *Ann Surg* 177:301–306, 1973.
48. Buch WS, Kosek JC, Angell WW: The role of rejection and mechanical trauma on valve graft viability. *J Thorac Cardiovasc Surg* 62:696–706, 1971.
49. Rossi MA, Braile DM, Teixeira DR, Carillo SV: Calcific degeneration of pericardial valvular xenografts implanted subcutaneously in rats. *Int J Cardiol* 12:331–339, 1986.
50. Levy RJ, Schoen FJ, Levy JT, et al: Biologic determinants of dystrophic calcification and osteocalcin deposition in glutaraldehyde-preserved porcine aortic valve leaflets implanted subcutaneously in rats. *Am J Pathol* 113:143–155, 1983.
51. Angell JD, Hawtrey O, Angell WM: A fresh, viable human heart valve bank: sterilization, sterility testing and cryogenic preservation. *Transplant Proc* 8(suppl 1), 1976.
52. Khanna SK, Ross JK, Monro JS: Homograft aortic valve replacement: seven years experience with antibiotic-treated valves. *Thorax* 36:330–337, 1981.
53. Van der Kamp AM, Visser WJ, Van Dongen JM, et al: Preservation of aortic heart valves with maintenance of cell viability. *J Surg Res* 30:47–56, 1981.
54. Wain WH, Pearch HM, Riddell RW, Ross DN: A reevaluation of the antibiotic sterilization of heart valve allografts. *Thorax* 32:740, 1977.
55. Ashwood-Smith MJ, Farrant J: *Low Temperature Preservation in Medicine and Biology*. London: Pitman, 1980.
56. Angell WW, Angell JD, Oury JH, et al: Long-term follow-up of viable frozen aortic homografts. *J Thorac Cardiovasc Surg* 93:815–822, 1987.
57. Kirklin JW, Blackstone EH, Maehara T, et al: Intermediate-term fate of cryopreserved allograft and xenograft valved conduits. *Ann Thorac Surg* 44:598–606, 1987.
58. O'Brien M: Comparison of fresh antibiotic sterilized and cryopreserved viable homografts: 15 year and 10 year clinical experience. Presented

at *Transplantation Techniques and Use of Cryopreserved Allograft Cardiac Valves: A Symposium and Laboratory for Surgeons.* Beaver Creek, Colorado, 18–20 September 1986.

59. Karow AM: Biophysical and chemical considerations in cryopreservation. In: *Organ Preservation for Transplantation.* New York: Marcel Dekker, Ed. Karow, Jr., AM & Pegg, DE 1981, pp. 13–30.
60. Magilligan DJ, Lewis JW, Tilley BL, Peterson E: The porcine bioprosthetic valve. *J Thorac Cardiovasc Surg* 89:499–507, 1985.
61. Ross DN, Martelli V, Wain WH: Allograft and autograft valves used for aortic valve replacement. In Ionescu MI (ed): *Tissue Heart Valves.* Boston: Butterworth, 1979, pp. 127–172.
62. Strickett MG, Barratt-Boyes BG, MacCulloch D: Disinfection of human heart valve allografts with antibiotics in low concentrations. *Pathology* 15:457–462, 1983.
63. Dowell LG, Rinfret AP: Low-temperature forms of ice as studied by x-ray diffraction. *Nature* 188:1144–1148, 1960.
64. Rajotte, RV, Shnitka TK, Liburd EM, et al: Histological studies on cultured canine heart valves recovered from −196°C. *Cryobiology* 14:15–22, 1977.
65. Arminger LC, Gavin JB, Barratt-Boyes BG: Histological assessment of orthotopic aortic valve leaflet allografts: its role in selecting graft pretreatment. *Pathology* 15:67–73, 1983.
66. Gavin JB, Herdson PB, Monro JJ, Barratt-Boyes BG: Pathology of antibiotic treated human heart valve allografts. *Thorax* 28:473–481, 1973.
67. Watts LK, Duffy P, Field RB, et al: Establishment of a viable homograft cardiac valve bank: a rapid method of determining homograft viability. *Ann Thorac Surg* 21:230–236, 1976.
68. Ishihara T, Ferrans VJ, Jones M, et al: Occurrence and significance of endothelial cells in implanted porcine bioprosthetic valves. *Am J Cardiol* 48:443–454, 1981.
69. Schoen FJ, Levy RJ, Nelson AC, et al: Onset and progression of experimental bioprosthetic heart valve calcification. *Lab Invest* 52:523–532, 1985.
70. Thubrikar MJ, Aouad J, Nolan SP: Patterns of calcific deposits in operatively excised stenotic or purely regurgitant aortic valves and their relation to mechanical stress. *Am J Cardiol* 58:304–308, 1986.
71. Levy RJ, Schoen FJ, Golomb G: Bioprosthetic heart valve calcification: clinical features, pathobiology and prospects for prevention: *Crit Rev Biocompat* 2:147–187, 1986.
72. Levy RJ, Hawley MA, Schoen FJ, et al: Inhibition by diphosphonate compounds of calcification of porcine bioprosthetic heart valve cusps implanted subcutaneously in rats. *Circulation* 71:349–356, 1985.
73. Levy RJ, Wolfrum J, Schoen FJ, et al: Inhibition of calcification of bioprosthetic heart valves by local controlled-released diphosphonate. *Science* 227:190–192, 1985.
74. Holthofer H: Vascularization of the embryonic kidney: detection of endothelial cells with Ulex europaeus I lectin. *Cell Differ* 20:27–31, 1987.
75. Khan AA, Gonzalez-Lavin L: Viability assessment of allograft values by autoradiography. *Yale J Biol Med* 49:347–350, 1976.
76. Armiger LC, Gavin JB, Barrat-Boyes BG: Histological assessment of orthotopic aortic valve leaflet allografts: its role in selecting graft pretreatment. *Pathology* 15:67–73, 1983.
77. Van der Kamp AWM, Nauta J: Fibroblast function and maintenance of aortic valve matrix. *Cardiovasc Res* 13:167–172, 1979.
78. Low RB, Hildebran JN, Absher PM, et al: Comparison of the use of isotopic proline vs. leucine to measure protein synthesis in cultured fibroblasts. *Connect Tissue Res* 14:179–185, 1986.
79. Stevens BR, Wright EM: Kinetics of the intestinal brush border proline (imino) carrier. *J Biol Chem* 262:6546–6551, 1987.
80. Dziewaitkowski DD: The role of sulfated proteinpolysaccharides in calcification. *Clin Orthop Rel Res* 35:189–201, 1964.

4—Allograft Valve Banking: Techniques and Technology

PERRY L. LANGE and RICHARD A. HOPKINS

The use of human allograft heart valves for replacement of congenitally defective or diseased heart valves has become clinically accepted in cardiothoracic surgery. From the early days of using wet-stored "nonviable" homografts to current methods of transplanting cryogenically preserved "viable" allografts, the superiority of human heart valve implants has been well documented.[1–7] However, as the clinical utilization of heart valve allografts increases, the availability of this human tissue will become a factor. With approximately 25,000 adult aortic valve replacements and 5000 pediatric reconstructions done annually in the United States,[8] ways to maximize the number of heart valves available for transplant must be sought.

This review is based on the methods of the Virginia Tissue Bank (VTB). The goal is to provide the highest quality allograft heart valve at the lowest possible cost to the recipient. Recipient safety must be ensured through strict heart donor screening criteria and stringent quality control measures encompassing the entire heart valve preparation protocol.

Heart valve preparation protocols are divided into seven areas: (1) donor selection and heart procurement; (2) heart valve dissection; (3) allograft sterilization/disinfection; (4) cryopreservation; (5) storage; (6) transportation and distribution; and (7) surgical preparation of the allograft. Each of the aforementioned areas is vital to the performance of the implanted allograft, and strict quality control standards must be adhered to such that the optimal replacement heart valve is provided for the patient population.

Donor Selection

Even though the production of allograft heart valves is not monitored by the United States Food and Drug Administration (FDA), the allograft tissue community has its own regulatory body, the American Association of Tissue Banks (AATB). The AATB has published guidelines that address donor selection and assure allograft tissue recipients of receiving disease- and contaminant- free implants.[9]

Each potential donor should be evaluated individually, reviewing the history and laboratory studies. When available, autopsy information may be valuable. Permission for heart donation should be obtained in writing from the donor's legal next-of-kin, even if a potential donor carries an organ donor card. Once permission is obtained, the donor must be screened to minimize any potential transfer of infectious or neoplastic processes. The AATB recommends the following guidelines[9] for sterile retrieval of donor tissue.

1. No infection or sepsis by history, physical examination, and laboratory testing
2. Sterile blood cultures
3. No history of intravenous drug use
4. No history of neoplasm other than basal cell carcinoma of the skin, carcinoma in situ of the uterus, or intracranial neoplasm
5. No history of hepatitis, syphilis, slow viral infections, Creutzfeldt-Jakob disease (CJD), acquired immume deficiency disease (AIDS), AIDS-related complex (ARC), or individuals at high risk for AIDS or ARC as specified by the U.S. Public Health Service

6. No history of autoimmune diseases
7. Negative serologic testing, if available
8. No toxic substances in potentially toxic amounts in the tissues to be collected
9. No evidence of serious illness of unknown etiology
10. No history of receiving pituitary-derived human growth hormone

Along with these AATB standards, the VTB recommends the following additional donor guidelines.

1. No evidence of viremia or systemic mycosis
2. No history or evidence of collagen vascular disease, diabetes, or tuberculosis
3. No history of prolonged steroid use

Accompanying these general donor guidelines, criteria specific for heart valve donors include the following.

1. No history of previous cardiac surgery, significant hypertension, significant murmurs, bacterial endocarditis, rheumatic fever, or untreated active pulmonary disease.
2. No history of cardiac injury, significant chest wall injury, resuscitation with prolonged closed chest massage or resuscitation with any open chest massage.
3. No history of valvular disease.
4. Adherence to age and size limits.
   a. Lower size limit: 10 pounds.
   b. Lower age limit: newborn.
   c. Upper age limit: 50 years.

   As discussed by several authors,[1,4] increasing heart donor age may yield a corresponding increase in calcification rates of transplanted allograft heart valves. Various age criteria of other programs[2,4,6] extend up to 65 years of age with good results, but the VTB has set a conservative upper age limit of 50, as suggested by several studies.[1,6,10] Because the largest possible allograft should be implanted that will not be distorted within the recipient's native annulus, the lower age and size limits were established with actual implantable allograft sizes in mind.
5. Adherence to time definitions.
   a. Multiple organ donor valves; eight hours time of death.
   b. "Postmortem" valves require that the heart be procured within 24 hours from cessation of heart action, if the donor is maintained in a cold room (4°C).

The VTB designates the time period of cessation of heart action until cardiac procurement as the "warm ischemic time." The allowable warm ischemic time differs from program to program. Cryolife[11] and the University of Chicago[7] allow 12 hours to elapse; the London National Heart Hospital (Ross and Bodnar) recovers hearts within 24 hours of death (E. Bodnar, at The First Workshop on Homologous and Autologous Heart Valves. Chicago: Deborah Heart and Lung Center, 5 April 1987), as does Angell[3]; the American Red Cross Tissue Bank of Los Angeles employs an 8-hour ischemic time limit (M. Almeida, American Red Cross Los Angeles—Tissue Services, personal communication, January 1987). The University of Alabama (Kirklin) attempts to limit the warm ischemic time as much as possible by recovering hearts from brain-dead organ donors at the time of removal of other organs for transplantation.[5] O'Brien agrees with limiting the heart ischemic time to an absolute minimum whenever possible M.F. O'Brien, personal communication, 7 March 1988).

Studies have shown that valve leaflets recovered past the 8–12-hour ischemic specification exhibit substantially decreased fibroblast viability; however, these "nonviable" heart valve allografts do have clinical applicability; but as presented by O'Brien, Kirklin, Barratt-Boyes, Ross, and others[4–6, 12–16] "nonviable" allograft heart valves may still out-perform other available prosthetic devices. With long-term durability being the only compromising factor, recipients with a shortened life expectancy (where the allograft would outlive the recipient) could still profit from the allograft's other inherent advantages. Thus hearts for heart valve transplantation may also be recovered from acceptable donors who are not vascular organ donors.

Before distributing any of the processed tissue, the following laboratory results should be obtained.

1. Blood cultures
2. HBsAg—non reactive
3. VDRL or RPR—negative

4. HTLV-III, HIV—negative
5. ABO (Rh)

Care should be taken to obtain blood specimens for hepatitis and AIDS screening analyses prior to any donor blood transfusions. This measure avoids the potential diluting effect of massive transfusions, which may result in a potentially false-negative test report.

A short synopsis of the heart donor's medical history should also be obtained. The following information should be available to surgeon at implantation.

1. Next-of-kin consent and donor permission form
2. Cause of death
3. Summary of donor's medical history
4. Time of cardiac cessation (aortic cross-clamp time, time of life support termination, or time of death)
5. Time of heart removal
6. Autopsy results, if performed
7. HLA typing, if available

AATB standards require donor records to be confidential, accurate, complete, and maintained for 7 years.

Procurement

Donor hearts for allograft heart valve transplantation should be obtained aseptically in an operating room or, alternatively, at autopsy in a clean fashion. The VTB processes only hearts that have been procured during an operative procedure under sterile conditions, which greatly reduces the opportunity of contaminant or pathogenic agents contacting the donor heart. Procurement techniques for the recovery of hearts in an autopsy setting is covered in other publications.[17a]

Recently, emphasis has been placed on the potential of using allograft valves recovered from explanted hearts of heart transplant recipients.[17b] The shortage of allograft heart valves is becoming increasingly acute with the growing acceptance of the procedure. These valves from explanted hearts would add to the number of valves available. These valves would also incorporate maximal viability with very short warm ischemic times of just a few minutes.

However, many questions arise concerning the utilization of such tissue. Donor screening needs to include donor myocardium biopsy testing, special consent from the living donor, and donor serologic retesting at specified intervals. The Virginia Tissue Bank recommends retesting at 3 and 6 month intervals. If the living donor should expire prior to allograft valve transplantation, an autopsy should be performed to rule out neoplastic processes.

All living donor tissue should be held in quarantine until results of donor screen retesting are obtained. Any positive findings would contra-indicate the tissue's usage.

When the heart is to be recovered immediately following vascular organ donation, the original surgical preparation should be extended to anticipate a median sternotomy. Although heart valve leaflets are relatively resistant to anoxia, removal of the heart within the first hour after cessation of heartbeat is ideal. If the cardiectomy is to be performed as a separate tissue donor procedure, the heart should be recovered first and as soon after death as possible.

The key aspects of the procurement of hearts for heart valves are aseptic technique, proper length of aorta and pulmonary (for future conduit usage in ventriculopulmonary artery reconstruction), and the avoidance of valve leaflet injury during the retrieval. During the procurement process, the absence of significant aortic/mitral valve regurgitation can be confirmed by palpation for thrills and so noted in the donor records. Detailed steps for sterile cardiectomy are as follows.

1. Shave and prepare the donor from chin to umbilicus to bilateral nipple line.
2. Drape the area (steri-drape coverage is recommended).
3. Make a median incision over the sternum.
4. Divide the subcutaneous tissue to expose the anterior surface of the sternum, xiphoid process to sternal notch.
5. Free the pericardium from the posterior sternum by blunt and sharp dissection. This procedure may need to be done intermittently during the sternotomy.
6. Perform median sternotomy with the Lebsche knife and mallet or sternal saw.

7. Install chest spreaders/rib retractors.
8. Incise pericardium to expose the heart and remove pericardial fluid.
9. For full exposure, secure the divided pericardium to the skin or a retractor.
10. Circumferentially dissect the ascending aorta to expose 2–3 cm of the brachiocephalic artery.
11. Circumferentially dissect the aortic arch to expose 2–3 cm of the left carotid and left subclavian arteries.
12. Expose and ligate the superior and inferior vena cava.
13. Evert the heart and transect the pulmonary veins. While incising the posterior pericardium, avoid entering the esophagus or trachea, as it would grossly contaminate the operative field.
14. Return the heart to normal position and expose the right and left pulmonary arteries.
15. Continue to dissect the pulmonary arteries to their first segment branch arteries, which requires dissection outside the pericardial cavity.
16. Transect the pulmonary arteries at their first segmental branches.
17. Transect the superior and inferior vena cava proximal to the ligatures.
18. Ligate the aorta beyond the left subclavian artery. *Do not* cross-clamp the aorta anywhere proximal to this ligature, as intimal damage may result that can render the aortic valve unusable.
19. Transect the brachiocephalic, left carotid, and left subclavian arteries. Transect the aortic arch distal to its ligature.
20. Safely divide any remaining connective tissue and remove the heart.
21. Place the heart in a large basin containing approximately 1 liter of cold (4°C) saline, Ringer's, Ringer's lactate, or Euro Collins solution, or tissue culture medium.
22. Rinse the heart free of blood and gently massage the ventricles to remove as much blood as possible.
23. The heart should be packaged in approximately 500 cc of cold saline, Ringer's lactate, Ringer's, or Euro Collins solution by any acceptable organ recovery system that utilizes double sterile bags or containers.
24. After packaging, the heart is handed off the sterile field, labeled appropriately, and placed in a shipping container at 4°C on wet ice for transport.

In order to maintain viability of heart valve leaflet cells prior to dissection procedures, all hearts should be received at the processing location within 24 hours of cardiectomy. This transportation time is termed "cold ischemic time" by the VTB. Our studies have shown that there is no significant effect on cellular viability between 16 and 30 hours of cold (4°C) ischemic transport time.[18a]

Recent studies involving whole vascular organ perfusion and enriched transport solutions have suggested that ischemic time limits may be increased.[18b] Transport medias utilizing adenosine and enriched with metabolic phosphates may "resuscitate" or preserve cellular viability.[18c]

All available donor information, heartbeat cessation time, and cardiectomy time should be included with the heart shipment to facilitate the valve dissection procedures.

Dissection

Dissection of the allograft is performed in an aseptic environment within the confines of a laminar flow hood. The working area should be sterile and draped according to normal surgical protocol. As well as using sterile instruments, ligatures, and graft sizers, the VTB utilizes a specifically designed "cold pan" to perform the heart dissection. This apparatus is a double-boiler type of system that externally circulates 4°C water and maintains these cold temperatures within the basin. The internal basin is filled with 1 liter of cold saline, Ringer's, Ringer's lactate, or Euro Collins solution, or tissue culture medium; and most of the heart dissection is performed in the 4°C bath. Maintaining the cardiac tissue in this cold state maximizes cellular viability.

The heart is removed from its sterile transport solution and placed onto the operative field within the cold pan. A sample of the transport medium is taken for culture to identify any potential contaminants or pathogens. Dissection is begun with the heart apex directed away from the person performing the procedure, with the anterior surface of the heart projected superiorly. The steps involved in the dissection procedures are as follows.

1. The anterior epicardium is incised over the entire length of the conduit and is dissected from the aorta to the aortic root. Arterial hemostats can be affixed to the most distal aspect of the conduit to provide countertraction. *Note:* Beware of the right and left coronary arteries and do not damage the ostia.
2. Once the anterior epicardium is removed from the aorta, turn to the posterior aspect of the heart. Repeat this procedure until the entire epicardium is circumferentially removed from the aorta to the aortic root. Return to the anterior aspect of the heart.
3. Incise the atrial adipose tissue covering the right coronary artery. *Do not cut the artery.* Dissect free the right coronary ostia and artery until 1 cm of artery is exposed. Ligate the artery with a 3–0 silk ligature 5 mm distal to the ostia and divide the artery another 5 mm distal to the ligature. Check this area of the aorta and the coronary artery itself for any nicks, holes, or abrasions and make note of such.
4. The left coronary artery is now dissected in a similar manner. The dissection is carried out just distal to the circumflex and left anterior descending (LAD) arteries. The left coronary artery is ligated with a single 3–0 silk ligature at the circumflex LAD bifurcation and divided. Again, make note of any problem areas.
5. The entire base of the aorta can now be fully exposed to the aortic root–myocardial junction.
6. Divide the pulmonary artery from the aortic arch, freeing both conduits.
7. Open the right ventricle just below the right coronary artery with a full-thickness incision. Holding the pulmonary artery in one hand, remove the right ventricle with a full-thickness cut in a circumferential manner. Leave a minimum of 1 cm of myocardium below the pulmonary valve leaflets. NOTE: Care must be taken when separating the base of the pulmonary artery from the aorta. The conus ligament/tendon, or the infundibulum, is often minute, and the aorta can easily be damaged during this step.
8. With the pulmonary artery dissected free, remove the epicardial adipose tissue and epicardium and maintain the pulmonary allograft in the cold pan solution until further dissection.
9. With a full-thickness cut, divide the aorta from the myocardium beginning at the previously made right ventricular incision. Continue posteriorly through the right atrium until the atrial septum is reached.
10. Return to the anterior aspect of the heart and transversely incise the ventricular septum. This full thickness incision through the septum should be approximately midway down the septum, below the left ventricular mitral cordae tendinae attachments.
11. Expose the entire left ventricle by making an incision to the heart apex. Care should be taken to stay well beyond the origins of the aortic valve leaflets in the Valsalva sinuses.
12. In the opened left ventricle, transect the chordae tendineae of the anterior mitral valve leaflets.
13. Make longitudinal incisions at both junctions of the anterior and posterior mitral valve leaflets. This maneuver divides the mitral valve.
14. Remove the entire left atrial myocardium and posterior mitral valve leaflet from the aortic base, leaving the anterior mitral valve leaflet attached to the aortic root.
15. Transversely divide the ventricular septum 1 cm below the aortic valve leaflets. Remove any remaining myocardium from the aorta and free the allograft from the heart with the anterior mitral leaflet still attached to the aortic conduit.
16. Trim excess myocardium, adipose, and connective tissue from the aortic base, leaving a uniform thickness of 2–3 mm of myocardium. Beware of the membranous portion of the septum near the aortic base and tricuspid valve junction. Avoid damaging any of the tissue in this area and leave at least 2 mm of myocardium attached.
17. Return to the pulmonary valve conduit and remove excess tissue. Avoid any unnecessary contact with the allograft leaflets.

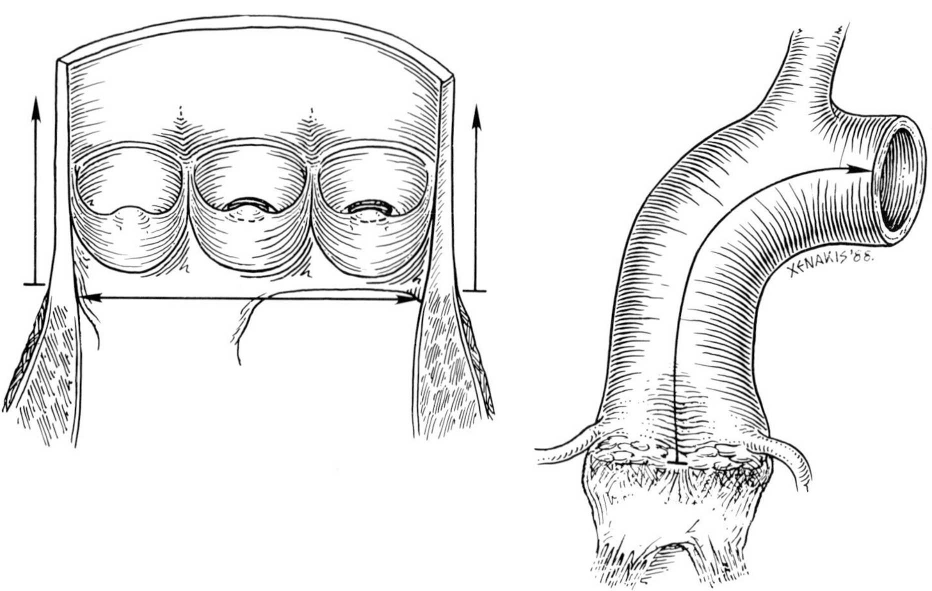

FIGURE 4.1. Valve diameter is measured as the internal diameter at the base of the aortic root. Length of conduit is as shown.

Sizing the allograft is a vital aspect of the processing procedures; consistency and accuracy are of the utmost importance. Incorrect sizing of the allograft aortic root diameter could require tailoring of the recipient's annulus and prolong the patient's aortic cross-clamp time. Adequate conduit length is also mandatory in ventriculo-pulmonary artery reconstructions. Proper communication between the implanting surgeon and the processing team is essential. All parties should be in agreement on the mechanics of sizing and know the parameters involved (Figs. 4.1 and 4.2).

The VTB uses specially designed sizing cones made of high-grade stainless steel, and Hegar dilators. The cone resembles a ring sizer and has diameter markings in millimeters imprinted on its smooth, polished surface. The cone sizer is able to indicate internal root diameters of 15–30 mm. For smaller pediatric valves, Hegar cervical dilators are utilized. Sizing cones made of smooth-surfaced Teflon have been employed by other allograft processors (M.F. O'Brien, at The First Workshop on Homologous and Autologous Heart Valves. Chicago: Deborah Heart and Lung Center, 5 April 1987). Valve root diameters may also be obtained by using standard cardiac valve sizing obturators. However, repeated obturator sizing of the valve has been found to damage the leaflets and should be avoided.[19] A single sliding of the allograft onto a moistened sizing cone to the appropriate diameter reading avoids this potential danger.

The internal diameter of the allograft root is determined and recorded. To obtain accurate sizing, the annulus must not be stretched or distorted. The lengths of the aortic conduit and main pulmonary artery are recorded along with the size of the right and left pulmonary artery remnants. It is important that the implanting surgical team know that valve sizes are determined by internal root diameters. Most allograft internal roots average 3 mm less than the recipient's annulus, as determined by preoperative echocardiogram. This 3-mm differentiation must be kept in mind when requesting a specific allograft. For the use of autologous heart valve reimplantation (pulmonary valve to aortic position), it has been reported that both pulmonary and aortic root diameters were similar (L. Gonzales-Lavin, at The First Workshop on Homologous and Autologous Heart Valves. Chicago: Deborah Heart and Lung Center, 5 April 1987). However, for our first 250 hearts processed, the pulmonary

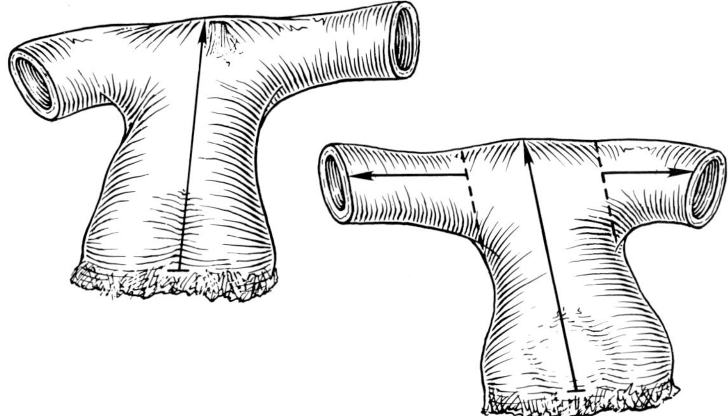

FIGURE 4.2. Pulmonary allograft dimensions: length of allograft and left and right pulmonary arteries.

valve root was consistently 2–4 mm larger than the aortic root, the differential increasing with the size of the heart.

During the sizing period the allograft should be kept cold and moist, and the leaflets should be carefully examined for any degenerative, traumatic, or congenital abnormalities. At the VTB, every allograft is assigned a quantifiable rating to assess its overall condition. The following is a list of the qualifications and conditions observed for a specific numerical rating.

0: Discarded valve due to any of the following reasons
- Bicuspid valve or other congenital defect
- Severe leaflet fenestrations
- Leaflets torn or abraded
- Intimal peel throughout the entire conduit length
- Leaflet atheroma observed
- Conduit cut short during procurement or commissural posts severely damaged
- Valve incompetent

1: Valve rarely retained for use
- Up to 30% of mitral valve covered with atheroma
- Significant atheroma on intimal surface of conduit
- Very fatty, soft, diseased myocardium
- Contusions of myocardium near valve root
- Slight commissural damage, calcification, etc.
- Evidence of significant cardiovascular (CV) disease noted
- Leaflet fenestrations noted

2: Abnormal valve
- Slight leaflet fenestrations
- Up to 15% atheroma coverage of mitral valve
- Small areas of contusions, but only on conduit well away from valve root area
- Myocardial tissue less than ideal
- No atheroma on semilunar leaflets
- Evidence of CV disease noted

3: Good valve
- Some small area of atheroma on mitral valve
- Semilunar leaflets free of damage, fenestrations, and atheroma
- No contusions
- Heart tissue good
- Conduit free of atheroma and damage
- Slight evidence of early-stage CV disease

4: Perfect valve
- Heart and all valves free of any problem area
- No evidence of CV disease
- You would want this valve transplanted into you!

Once the allograft condition is noted, all ratings, sizes, and comments are recorded in the donor chart along with the date and time of dissection. It is recommended that the manufacturers and lot numbers be recorded for all antibiotics and solutions used during processing. Each allograft should be assigned a separate identification number and all records maintained in a permanent donor chart.

Sterilization and Disinfection

In order to provide a sterile allograft for transplantation, identification and elimination of any potential contaminants is required. Sterilization involving incubation of the allograft in low-concentration broad-spectrum antibiotics is well documented.[20,21] Many antibiotic mixtures have been utilized with varying degrees of success regarding cellular viability, host ingrowth rate, disinfection efficiency, and valve survival rates.[3,16,22–27a]

It has been suggested that hearts recovered from multi-organ donors are microbiologically sterile and may be immediately transplanted or cryopreserved.[27b] However, Gonzalez-Lavin reports that 53% of his multi-organ donors' hearts yielded positive cultures (ibid). At the Virginia Tissue Bank, we found that approximately 32% of our homovital valves were contaminated. Like Gonzalez-Lavin, the Virginia Tissue Bank's primary contaminating bacteria have been staphylococcus aureus, s. epidermidis, and anaerobic diptheroids. It is therefore suggested that all allograft heart valves enter into a disinfection program.

Varying formulas using penicillin, gentamicin, kanamycin, azlocillin, metronidazol, flucloxacillin streptomycin, ticarcillin, methicillin, chloramphenicol, colistimethate, neomycin, erythromycin, and nystatin have been tried by several authors but have proved unsatisfactory for a variety of reasons, e.g., a decrease in cellular viability[12,28,29] and molecular cross-linkages with collagen and mucopolysaccharides inhibiting host ingrowth into the disinfected valve leaflets.[26,30] The VTB uses a modified version of the antibiotic treatment regimen recommended by Barratt-Boyes.[21] The following antibiotics are added to a sterile-filtered nutrient tissue culture medium to disinfect the allograft heart valves.

Cefoxitin	240 μg/ml medium
Lincomycin	120 μg/ml medium
Polymyxin B	100 μg/ml medium
Vancomycin	50 μg/ml medium

Several nutrient media have been used, including modified Hank's solution, TCM 199, MEM Eagle's, and RPMI 1640.[3,5,21,31a] The VTB utilizes sterile filtered RPMI 1640 as our disinfection medium, as recommended by Kirklin and associates[5] and Karp.[7]

The sterilization stage begins once the allograft is fully dissected. All antibiotics should be reconstituted with sterile bacteriostatic water and premixed with the appropriate nutrient medium. This antibiotic solution has a shelf life of 72 hours when stored at 4°C. Buffer may need to be added so that pH is maintained between 6.8 and 7.0. The allograft is placed in a suitable sterile container, and approximately 125 ml of the antibiotic solution is added. It is important that the solution completely submerge the tissue.

The container should be large enough that the entire allograft is freely movable within the interior and not contorted in any way. It has been found that distorting the tissue to fit a small container leaves weakened creases in the allograft conduit that will crack during the freezing/thawing process.

The allograft tissue is then stored at 4°C for 24 hours immersed in the antibiotic medium. Following the 24-hour incubation period, the heart valve is removed from cold storage, rinsed with tissue culture medium, and aseptically packaged for cryopreservative control-rate freezing.

Nearly all allograft heart valve programs advocate the use of antibiotics, but with widely varying allograft incubation parameters (Table 4.1). Many different antibiotics in various tissue culture medias are being employed, but all are in relatively low-doses, and with varying incubation times and temperatures.[31b]

O'Brien initially reported incubating allografts in a solution containing penicillin, streptomycin, and amphotericin B for 24 hours at 37°C.[6] More recently, however, he has changed to a sterilizing protocol of the gentler antibiotics with the complete avoidance of amphotericin B in the disinfecting solution. He now incubates the

TABLE 4.1.

Program	Antibiotics	Nutrient Medium
Yankah (et al, 1987):[31c] German Heart Center Berlin	Gentamycin, Azlocillin, Flucloxacillan, Metronidazd, Amphotericin B	RPMI 1640 & human serum
Kirklin (et al, 1987):[31d] University of Alabama	Streptomycin, Penicillin, Amphotericin B	RFMI 1640
Gonzalez-Lavin (et al, 1987):[31e] Deborah Heart and Lung Center New Jersey	Cefoxitin, Ticarcillin Neomycin, Polymixin Mycostatin	RPMI 1640 & fetal calf serum
Robert Karp (Watkins, 1988):[31f] University of Chicago & Virginia Tissue Bank	Cefoxitin, Lincomycin Polymixin B, Vancomycin	RPMI 1640
Angell (et al, 1987):[3] Scripp's Clinic San Diego	Colistimethate, Gentamicin Kanamycin, Lincomycin	TC199
Barratt-Boyes (et al, 1987):[6] Geen Lane Hospital Auckland	Cefoxitin, Lyncomycin Polymyxin B, Vancomycin Amphoterian B	TC199
Almeida (1988):[31g] American Red Cross Los Angeles	Cefoxitin, Lincomycin Vancomycin, Polymyxin B Amphotericin	RPMI 1640
O'Brien (et al, 1987; 1988):[4a,b] Charles Hospital Brisbane	Streptomycin, Penicillin	Eagle's MEM
Ross (Khanna, et al, 1981):[1] National Heart Hospital London	Gentamycin, Methicillin, Nystatin, Erythromycin Streptomycin	Modified Hank's

heart valve allografts for only 6 hours at 37°C, with these changes aimed at maximizing leaflet cell viability (M.F. O'Brien, personal communication, 7 March 1988).

The Virginia Tissue Bank has recently removed the Amphotericin B from the antibiotic incubation media. Even though the solution now omits any type of fungicide, it was felt that highly increased viability warranted the change. Our data suggest that the use of the antibiotic solution without Amphotericin B yields viability equivilant to that seen when valves are stored in nutrient media only.

However, the avoidance of Amphotericin B in the antibiotic solution does present a potential problem. There is a small percentage of fungi that can yield false negative culture reports.

Elimination of amphotericin B from the antibiotic regimen used to sterilize the grafts highlights the importance of thorough donor screening. Permission for autopsy and obtaining pertinent medical history, including detection of symptoms related to those found associated with systemic mycoses or infective endocarditis, are paramount to exclusion of fungal contaminants originating from the donor graft. Strict sterile technique during recovery, transport at 4 degrees centigrade, and cold, sterile processing are additional measures to prevent fungal proliferation. Approximately 15% of all cases of infective endocarditis are due primarily to two fungal agents, Candidiasis and Asperigillosis.[31h] Histoplasmosis has been implicated in rare numbers. Actinomycosis and Nocardiosis, fungal-like bacteria, have also often been implicated in myocarditis and endocarditis.[31i] The coexistence of a bacterial agent and an undetected yeast infection occurs in human endocarditis,[31j] so any donor history of endocarditis should be scrutinized. Fungal endocarditis is characterized by development of mycotic vegetations commonly attached to the aortic or mitral leaflets.[31j] It is apparent that fungal infections have a tendency to accumulate on leaflets of the left heart due to more optimal growth conditions for most fungi with to the increased oxygen tension found here. It has also been reported that the right heart offers a more effective host response to defend against infection.[31j] Most mycotic infections are acquired via airborne spores and ultimately manifest in the lungs making the left heart most susceptible to vegetation, especially on the surface of the leaflets. For these reasons the optimal tissue specimen for fungal and acid-fast bacillus cultures is the posterior mitral leaflet which is bisected as samples for each test. A sterile specimen, that is one that is void of bacterial contamination, is preferred as the presence of a fungus would not be inhibited by overgrowth of competitive bacterium. Grossly bacterially contaminated tissue sent for fungal culture may prove unsuitable for diagnostic procedures due to autolytic processes.[31k] This supports the practice of obtaining the tissue (post. mitral cusp) for AFB/ Fungal cultures after antibiotic treatment, just prior to packaging and cryopreservation of the allograft.

As noted by Wain and colleagues,[25] antibiotics cannot be expected to unfailingly disinfect every allograft. Originally, the VTB tried touch-culturing and tissue remnant sampling (aorta and mitral valve sections) as the mode of testing for sterility. Of the initial 300 hearts tested using these techniques, there was only one allograft that revealed a positive culture result following the antibiotic incubation period. However, it was determined that the touch culture and tissue sampling techniques could yield a high incidence of false-negative reports. It was found that approximately 0.14 ml of antibiotic/antimycotic agent was carried with the tissue sample or transported within the culture swab to the thioglycollate broth, and it was determined that this small amount of disinfecting solution transported during the sampling procedure was enough to restrict the growth of low concentrations of microorganisms during incubation at 37°C in the thioglycollate broth. This carryover of antibiotics would thus mask the presence of low-concentration microbial contaminants that may be present on the allograft tissue, resulting in the reporting of false-negative cultures. The carryover effect of the antibiotic solution has been substantiated by Waterworth and associates.[24]

The VTB currently utilizes a sterility control procedure similar to that of Angell and colleagues.[3] The final 24-hour antibiotic solution is filtered through a 0.45-μm Gelman Sciences filtration device (25-mm syringe filter holder; Gelman Sciences Inc., Ann Arbor, Michigan 48106). Using aseptic technique, the filter paper (with all trapped microorganisms) is incubated in thioglycollate broth at 37°C for 7 days and then plated aerobically onto trypticase soy agar with 5% sheep blood (trypticase soy agar II with 5% sheep blood; Becton Dickinson and Company—BBL Microbiology Systems, Cockeysville, Maryland 21030) and anaerobically in classic formula anaerobe blood agar (CDC anaerobic blood agar; Becton Dickinson and Company—BBL Microbiology Systems). The growth plates are incubated at 37°C and then read 2 days after plating. All isolated microorganisms are identified, and final disposition of the allograft is based on confirmation of tissue and packaging material sterility.

All allograft heart valves processed and disinfected by this protocol have thus far been rendered sterile by the 24-hour antibiotic incubation period, even after the heart procurement and transport media revealed multiple contaminants. Further reduction of the 24-hour incubation period, and thus increased cellular viability of the allograft, warrants further investigation.

Cryopreservation

Immediately following the antibiotic incubation period, cryopreservation of the allograft is begun. All packaging of the allograft should be done under strict aseptic conditions within a laminar flow unit. The allograft is removed from the antibiotic medium container, rinsed in fresh medium, and packaged with enough freezing solution to produce a total volume of 100 ml. At the time of packaging, cultures of all solutions, media, and packaging items are obtained. The allograft tissue is not released for transplantation until sterility of all tissue and packaging materials is confirmed.

The allograft and the appropriate amount of freezing solution is placed in a sterile pouch large enough to prevent distortions of the allograft. All air is removed from within the pouch, and it is heat-sealed. The allograft package is inserted into a slightly larger sterile pouch and again heat-sealed. This doubly packaged allograft is then taken to the freezing chamber for control-rate freezing.

The freezing medium is similar to the solution utilized by Kirklin and coworkers.[5] RPMI 1640 tissue culture medium is amended with dimethylsulfoxide (DMSO) to a 10% DMSO concentration and with fetal calf serum (FCS) to a concentration of 10% FCS. The RPMI 1640 and the FCS may be premixed and maintained at 4°C for up to 14 days (recommendation by Gibco Laboratories, Technical Service Department, Grand Island, New York 14072).

The DMSO is added to the cooled (4°C), premixed medium at the time of allograft packaging. DMSO is highly permeable to cell membranes and very soluble in aqueous solutions (see Chapter 3). The DMSO cryoprotectant may be added at either room temperature or 4°C. Although DMSO takes longer to reach osmotic equilibration at 4°C, it results in less stress to the affected cells and therefore yields higher cell viability than addition of the cryoprotectant at 37°C.[32,33] Our studies have shown that the added DMSO comes to equilibrium in the freezing medium within approximately 15 minutes.

The use of FCS in the freezing medium is still being debated. Most programs employ the use of 10–20% concentrations of FCS in the medium. The use of FCS or a high-molecular-weight colloid substitute, e.g., albumin or pasteurized plasma protein fraction (PPF), is well documented.[34] These large macromolecules affect the properties of the freezing solution to a greater extent than would be expected from their osmotic pressure and act directly on the cell membrane.[32] The colloid is thought to provide a necessary balance of oncotic pressure, thereby regulating the activity of the unfrozen water in the freezing solution and its movement into the tissue.[34] FCS is also believed to minimize the dilution shock to the allograft tissue during thawing by restricting cell swelling.[32] It is well established that serum is a valuable additive to nutrient media during cell culture growth, and the addition of serum to the freezing solution may also assist in cell preservation during the DMSO equilibration period just prior to cell freezing.

However, questions have been posed regarding the potential heterologous antigenicity induced in heart valve allografts by the FCS. Bodnar and colleagues have suggested that the calf serum content of the nutrient medium infiltrates the aortic wall during allograft preservation and induces a heavy second-set reaction.[35] They believe that FCS is not necessary during cryopreservation and have discontinued its use. Yankah also believes that the potential antigenicity of FCS may play a role in the rejection of allograft heart valves, and he is now using human-derived serum.[36] Some serum substitutes and plasma extenders are on the market, and the use of these agents may be warranted (Serum Plus; Hazleton Biologics, Inc., Lenexa, Kansas 66215). The Virginia Tissue Bank is currently undertaking viability and histological studies comparing the substitutes to calf serum.

Once the freezing medium is assembled and the allograft is packaged, the tissue is control-rate frozen with liquid nitrogen in a freezing chamber. The freezing chamber functions by monitoring a separate control heart valve placed in the chamber with the allograft. A temperature probe is embedded in the leaflets of the control valve. The freezing parameters of the control valve are assumed to mimic the freezing rate of the allograft being frozen. This assumption may be invalid, and new ways to monitor the temperature of the allograft as it freezes are being investigated.

Prior to allograft packaging, the control valve package must be assembled. A nontransplantable heart valve is used as the control valve. The freezing medium (RPMI + 10% FCS + 10% DMSO) is added to yield 100 ml total volume. The control pouch must be constructed with an absolutely watertight portal that allows a temperature probe to be inserted. The VTB utilizes a double O-ring heparin-lock system as the portal (Fig. 4.3). The system is capped with a latex injectable IV-bag port; the temperature probe may be inserted through this port, and freezing solution can be injected or withdrawn while maintaining the watertight integrity.

The control valve freezing medium should be changed every time a different allograft is frozen.

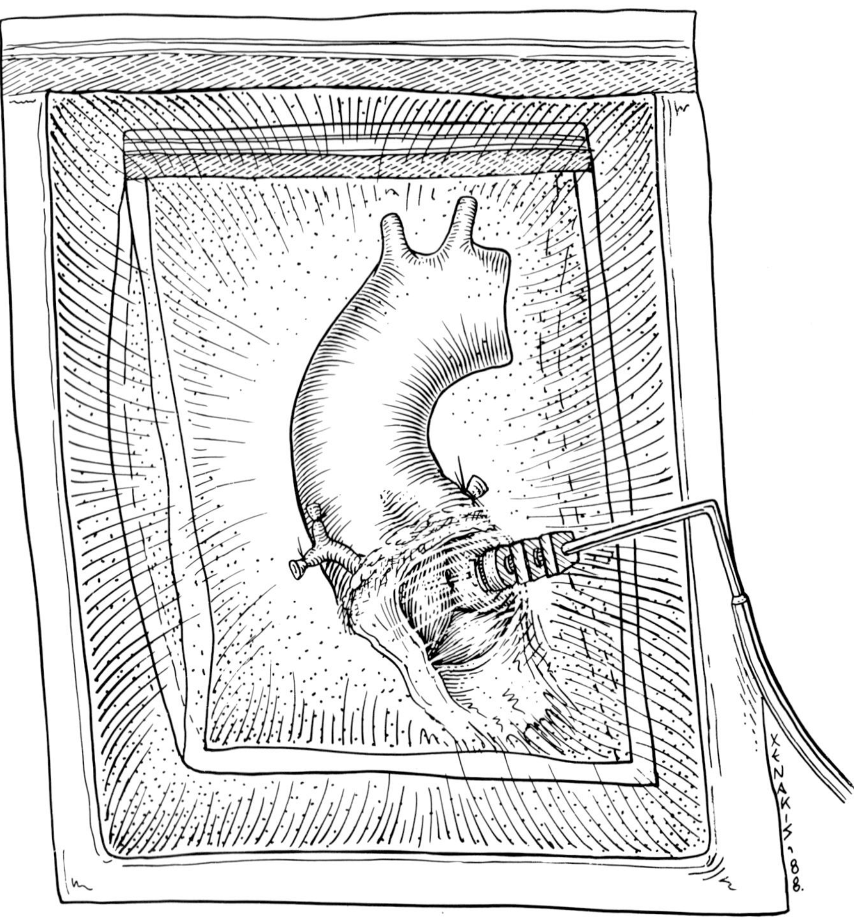

Figure 4.3. Control freezing pouch with temperature probe placed through a watertight portal.

As stated by Armiger and associates,[10] acid mucopolysaccharides are known to readily diffuse out of tissues held in aqueous solutions. The VTB has found consistent pH and osmolality changes within the control valve freezing medium with repeated freezing. Small-molecular-weight solutes continually leach from the sample tissue, altering the makeup of the freezing medium and thus changing the freezing program.

The control heart valve is kept frozen at liquid nitrogen vapor temperatures (−190° to −150°C) between allograft freeze runs. The control valve is thawed just prior to its use, and freezing solution is exchanged through the latex portal prior to its placement into the freezing chamber with the allograft tissue. Since every effort should be made to keep the physical makeup of the control sample as close as possible to the actual heart valve being cryopreserved, the freezing media of the control valve should be changed with each allograft freeze.

Allografts are frozen in a freezing chamber (Cryo Med Freezing Chamber 2700C; Cryo Med, Mount Clemens, Michigan 48045) at the controlled freezing rate of −1°C per minute utilizing a programmable microcomputer controller (Cryo Med Micro Controller 1010). Temperatures are continually monitored and recorded with a temperature chart recorder (Cryo Med Recorder 500). Controlled-rate freezing is terminated between −40° and −80°C, and the allograft is then transferred to permanent storage in vapor-phase liquid nitrogen (−190° to −150°C). The allograft valve may be stored indefinitely at these temperatures,[20] though Karow and Pegg postulated that nearly all biologic material can be stored at liquid nitrogen temperatures for approximately 10 years.[37]

Typical freezing curves are shown in Figures 4.4 and 4.5. Early in the freeze program the control valve and chamber temperatures are allowed to equilibrate at 4°C for approximately 10 minutes. From the time the allograft heart valve is placed in the cryopreservative medium during packaging until the end of the 10-minute chamber equilibration period, a total time of approximately 30 minutes has lapsed. During this 30-minute period the allograft should be prevented from warming above 10°C. It has been suggested that subjecting human fibroblasts to warm temperatures may adversely affect their post-thawing viability.[38] This 30-minute total equilibration period of the 10% DMSO freezing solution corresponds to that of Angell and colleagues, who include a 15-minute equilibration time in their protocol prior to packaging and control-rate freezing of the tissue.[3,39]

Once the allograft medium begins to freeze, adjustments in the freezing program must be made to compensate for the heat release, which occurs as the freezing solution begins to crystallize. To compensate for this heat of fusion, the freezing chamber must be quickly supercooled to temperatures below −100°C. Such supercooling allows the temperature of the allograft to decline at a steady −1°C per minute rate, avoiding the cellular damaging effects of inconsistent temperature fluctuations.

As the allograft temperature approaches −20°C, most of the extracellular water has frozen, and the remaining freezing medium has begun to solidify (see Chapter 3). The release of heat associated with water crystallization rapidly diminishes at this point. To maintain a consistent −1°C per minute freezing rate, the chamber must be rewarmed to temperatures just below that of the allograft's. From this point, temperature declines within the chamber are directly reflected in parallel temperature declines of the allograft tissue.

Differing rates of cryopreservative control-rate freezing have also been investigated. Merment and associates found −1°C per minute to yield a superior viability rate versus −0.1°C per minute or −5°C per minute.[39] VanderKamp and colleagues also theorized that −1°C per minute would be the best freezing rate to maximize fibroblast viability.[40] The VTB, University of Chicago Hospital,[7] University of Alabama,[5] and Prince Charles Hospital[41] are currently using −1°C per minute as their controlled freeze rate. However, Bodnar and Ross (E. Bodnar at The First Workshop on Homologous and Autologous Heart Valves. Chicago: Deborah Heart and Lung Center, 5 April 1987) and Armiger and colleagues[10] use −1.5°C per minute as their freezing standard.

Although most facilities utilize a microcomputer and freezing chamber[17] to control the freezing rate, Barratt-Boyes cryopreserves allografts using insulated heat sink boxes (B.G. Barratt-Boyes, personal communication, 5 April 1987). The heat sink method of cryopreservation has been shown to produce a variable rate cooling between −1° and −2°C per minute,[42] which corresponds to the cooling rate of −1.5°C per minute Barratt-Boyes has described. However, control-rate freezing by the use of heat sink boxes does not compensate for the latent heat release as ice crystals form within the freezing medium. Without the previously discussed chamber supercooling, intracellular ice may be forming that would decrease cellular viability[43] (refer to Chapter 3).

There are many factors that can affect the freezing rate of an allograft. Many of the biochemical aspects have been discussed previously (see Chapter 3). The constituents of the freezing medium have a profound effect on the rate of freezing. Glycerol, DMSO, and ethylene glycol have all been tried as cryoprotective agents for allograft heart valves. Comparing DMSO, glycerol, and ethylene glycol, VanderKamp and associates found that DMSO at a 10% concentration yielded the highest number of viable fibroblasts.[40] They investigated varying concentrations of DMSO (5%, 10%, 15%, 20%) and found a 10% concentration to yield superior cell survival. Kirklin and associates,[5] Karp,[7] and O'Brien and coworkers[41] use a 10% DMSO freezing medium, whereas Angell's group[3] employs a 7.5% concentration. Most programs now utilize DMSO as the cryoprotectant, except Bodnar and Ross who use a 15% glycerol formula (E. Bodnar, at The First Workshop on Homologous and Autologous Heart Valves. Chicago:

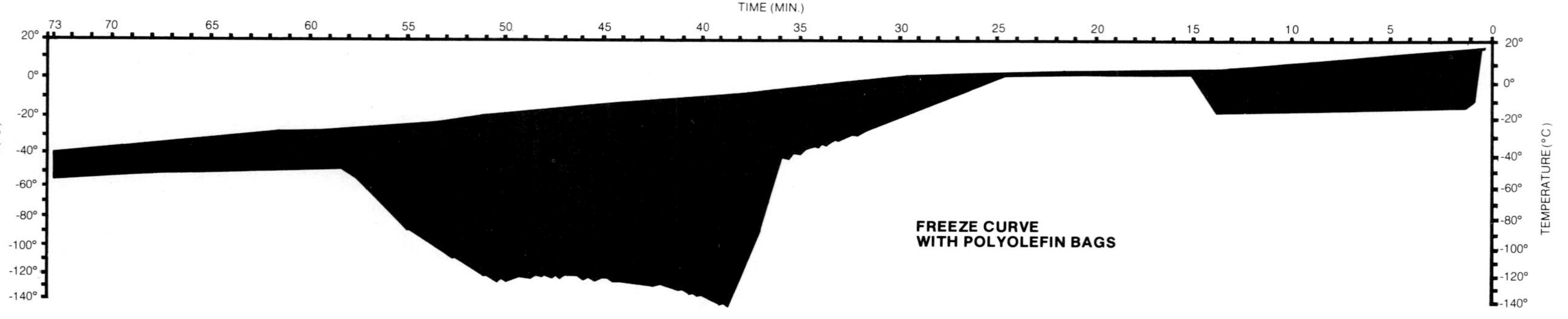

FIGURE 4.4. Computer-controlled freezing curve. Time is from right to left. This curve is for a valve inside two polyolefin bags. The upper straight line is the 1°C/minute drop in tissue temperature; the lower curve described by the vertical lines is the chamber temperature.

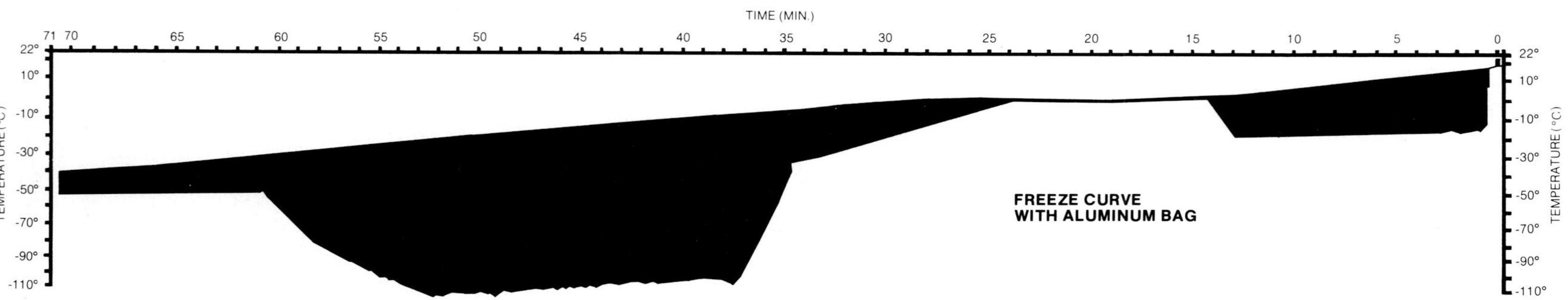

FIGURE 4.5. Freezing curve for a heart valve in an aluminum bag. Note the different chamber temperatures required to maintain the steady 1°C/minute linear freeze compared to Figure 4.4.

Deborah Heart and Lung Center, 5 April 1987).[13]

Another element in the cryopreservation freezing solution is the variability of nutrient media into which the DMSO is added. Angell and associates use TC199 with HEPES amended with a 20% concentration of fetal calf serum.[3] Kirklin and colleagues,[5] Karp,[7] and the VTB utilize RPMI 1640 tissue culture medium with a 10% FCS concentration, whereas Bodnar, Ross, and Yankah use human serum to guard against the potential antigenicity of the calf sera (Presented at The First Workshop on Homologous and Autologous Heart Valves. Chicago: Deborah Heart and Lung Center, 5 April 1987).

Along with these differentiations in the freezing medium, other technical variances have been observed to affect the freezing rate of a heart valve allograft.

1. There are several probes on the market that indicate the temperature of the control valve as it freezes. Blunt-tip probes (Cryo Med Thermocouple Temperature Probes) can be inserted through the control package portal and situated with the tip of the probe either in the supraleaflet area of the control valve aorta or in the subleaflet area by entering through the proximal aortic root. A needle probe (Brymill Temperature Probe; Brymill Corporation—Cryosurgical Equipment, Vernon, Connecticut 06066) may be embedded in the aortic wall of the control valve or through one of the control leaflets. Altering probe placement affects temperature readings.

2. Control valve packaging bags can be of several varieties. Allografts with conduits up to 7 cm in length and 100 ml total volume easily fit in a 4 × 6 inch pouch. This internal pouch is then placed in a larger 5 × 8 inch pouch. The VTB utilizes clear polyester-polyolefin modified bags as the internal pouch (Kapak Corporation, St. Louis Park, Minnesota 55416) and trilaminate aluminum-polypropylene bags as the external pouch (Kapak Corporation). Originally, a 5 × 8 inch clear polyolefin bag was used as the external pouch, but the aluminum foil bag was found to have superior durability in a wider range of temperatures. However, use of the foil pouch drastically altered the freezing curve; can be seen by comparing figures 4.4 and 4.5. Approximately 30% less chamber temperature was required to overcome the heat release of crystallization as the allograft was freezing. The polyolefin bag required the chamber to drop to about −140°C, whereas the aluminum foil bag required a maximal low temperature of only −105°C. The metallic content of the foil pouch serves as a superior temperature conductor and insulator.

3. The total volume of the control valve package should be maintained at 100 ml. When replenishing freezing medium, a calibrated syringe should be used to exactly measure the amount of medium withdrawn. Alterations in the freezing curve have been observed when volume changes of as little as 5% are made.

4. The number of allograft packages placed in the freezing chamber can also affect the control valve freezing curve. A pulmonary and an aortic allograft can be frozen simultaneously, but more than two allograft packages liberate too much heat into the freezing chamber. The heat release of three or more allograft packages causes a rise in the control valve package temperature, altering the freezing curve. A completely different freeze program must be developed when multiple allografts are frozen simultaneously.

5. It was also found that freezing programs were altered by using different freezing chambers from the manufacturer. Slight variations in door sealant moldings, liquid nitrogen fan speeds, and other chamber components yielded varying freezing results; the program should be recalibrated when equipment changes are made.

6. Package placement within the freezing chamber is also important. The control valve and the allograft package should be placed equidistant from the liquid nitrogen source. Both packages should be situated at the same angle with equal package surface area exposed to the liquid nitrogen vapor. Allowing different freezing conditions to exist between the control and allograft package does not alter the control valve freezing rate, but the actual freezing curve of the allograft may not parallel that of the monitored control valve.

7. The ratio of tissue versus medium within the allograft package is also a variable that affects the overall freezing program. It has been found

that the smaller pediatric-size allografts (less tissue mass) freeze at a slightly slower rate than adult allografts (more tissue mass) using the same freeze program. The pediatric valve has a larger proportion of fluid within the total 100-ml volume, thus liberating more latent heat of crystallization as the larger amount of fluid freezes. It is suggested that different freeze programs and control valves be used for pediatric and adult allografts owing to differing amounts of tissue mass.

8. Altering the volume/surface ratio of the allograft package also affects the freezing rate. By increasing the total volume of the allograft package, more heat is liberated, thereby increasing the amount of liquid nitrogen that must be injected into the freezing chamber to compensate. The VTB utilizes 150 ml total volume to freeze aortic valves with conduits up to 14 cm in length. It was found that the freezing chamber had to be cooled an additional 25–30% with the 150-ml package than when a 100-ml package was frozen.

Storage

Upon termination of the freezing program at −40°C, the allograft is immediately removed from the freezing chamber. An identifying label should be stapled to the external pouch, affixed superior to the heat seal line such that pouch sterility is uncompromised. The label should include the individual allograft identification number and the valve size. The allograft package is then placed in a precooled, prelabeled, specially designed cardboard storage box (Heart Valve Box; Dillard Paper Company, Greensboro, North Carolina 27407). The storage box is placed in liquid nitrogen vapor-phase temperature (−150° to −190°C) storage. The time interval of allograft removal from the freezing chamber to liquid nitrogen vapor storage should be kept to a minimum in order to avoid thermal fluctuations of the tissue.

The key to long-term allograft storage is maintenance of the frozen tissue below the glass transition point of the freezing solution, approximately −130°C. At temperatures above −130°C, several changes in frozen tissue structure may occur that can affect cellular viability. Cells frozen at the relatively rapid rate of −1°C per minute yield small ice crystals. As the unstable small ice crystals coalesce to form larger ones, any tissue caught between the merging ice is damaged, and cellular viability is compromised.[32] As the frozen allograft tissue temperature rises above −130°C, the rate of ice recrystallization accelerates.[44]

Macrocrystallization is the general phenomenon of small ice crystals coalescing to form larger crystals. Thermodynamically, small crystals are less stable than large ones because of their higher surface energy.[44] The small crystals naturally fuse in an effort to minimize their surface energies. Macrorecrystallization is of three types.[45]

1. Irruptive recrystallization: the method by which ice crystals rapidly resume their growth within a specific temperature range during slow rewarming and change from transparent to opaque under normal light conditions
2. Migratory recrystallization: the growth of large ice crystals at the expense of small ones during gradual rewarming until the melting point is reached
3. Spontaneous recrystallization: occurs during rapid cooling as the latent heat released during freezing is not dissipated enough to prevent a localized rise in temperature, thus giving rise to recrystallization within the local affected area

It has also been postulated that any intracellular ice may recrystallize with existing extracellular iced through pores in the cell membrane,[46] thereby compromising cellular viability. Intracellular ice recrystallization has been detected at temperatures as low as −130°C,[47] so temperature fluctuations above this level are to be avoided.

Below the glass transitional temperature of approximately −130°C, molecules still vibrate but do not move from one position to another, thus preventing chemical reactions.[48] Storage times of 10 years[49] to 32,000[50] years have been speculated. Even though some physical[51] and chemical[52] changes have been reported in cultured cells at −130°C, maintenance of the allograft below −130°C should ensure long-term allograft cell viability.

Allowing the temperature of the frozen allograft to warm to temperatures of −100°C during storage or transportation can affect the long-term storage potential. At −100°C many cell types have been observed to age appreciably owing to enzymatic activity[53a] and physical reactions,[49] thereby reducing viability.

Damage to the crypreserved allograft has also been seen when the frozen tissue was allowed to become immersed within the liquid nitrogen pool. In the early days of the University of Alabama's program, the frozen tissue was routinely stored in liquid nitrogen.[53b] (Watkins, 1988). Upon thawing, tissue fractures of the allograft were discovered, primarily affecting the aortic conduit. This same phenomena has been seen by us and others following accidental immersion of aortic allografts in liquid nitrogen.

Several models of liquid nitrogen vapor-phase storage units are available (Cryo Med, Mount Clemens, Michigan 48045; Minnesota Valley Engineering Inc., New Prague, Minnesota 56071; Taylor-Wharton, Indianapolis, Indiana 46224). Regardless of the size unit employed, temperature gradients exist within the storage area dependent on the distance above the liquid nitrogen pool of −196°C.

In an in-house report published by Minnesota Valley Engineering (MVE),[54] it was determined that a maximum temperature of −150°C is attained at 15 inches above the liquid nitrogen level. This study utilized an MVE VPS-80 storage unit (current model XLC-440) with a storage cavity of 27 inches depth and 18 inches diameter and a reservoir of 4 inches of liquid nitrogen at the bottom. In a VTB study using the Cryo Med CMS-328 freezer, a maximum temperature of −142°C was obtained at 12 inches above the liquid nitrogen level. The storage unit measured 27 inches depth and 31 inches diameter, and it contained 6 inches of liquid nitrogen. Thus tissue temperatures under −130°C can easily be maintained using several types and sizes of liquid nitrogen storage freezer.

To increase the allograft storage capacity of the freezer unit, the liquid nitrogen vapor temperatures (−190° to −150°C) in the lower levels of the storage cavity must also be maintained in the upper cavity. For holding limited quantities of a heart valve inventory, single-layer storage on the freezer platform just above the liquid nitrogen level is recommended. Approximately 60 heart valves fit into a single storage layer of a freezer unit with a 30-inch diameter, and about 16 allografts can be held in an 18-inch diameter freezer unit.

However, for larger inventories, stacking the allografts (in rigid cardboard retaining boxes) into two layers on the freezer platform is possible—if liquid nitrogen vapor temperatures can be maintained throughout the entire storage cavity. Several items are available that can easily increase the storage capacity of any unit (Minnesota Valley Engineering Inc.).

Aluminum bars (0.25 × 1.25 × 24 inches) can be affixed to the storage platform, with the proximal 4 inches immersed in the liquid nitrogen pool and the distal 20 inches rising to the top of the storage cavity. Aluminum is an excellent thermal conductor. The VTB found a decrease of 8°C in temperatures at the top of the storage cavity with the use of these rods.

Also, various thicknesses of the styrofoam sublids are available. These inserts fit tightly within the diameter of the freezer unit and can be designed to rest within the storage cavity on top of the added aluminum bars. With a combination of these items, temperatures within the upper region of the liquid nitrogen storage freezer can be lowered an additional 10°C. This lowering of the entire freezer cavity below −130°C may double the storage capacity of the unit.

Transportation and Distribution

The goal of any cryogenic transportation system is to provide the cryopreserved tissue without shipping damage and without subjecting the frozen allograft to injurious thermal fluctuations. Maintaining the tissue below −130°C is imperative. Several systems of cryogenic transportation have been devised, dependent on the distance of travel and the length of time the tissue is subject to transfer.

In situations where the allograft processing and storage facility is in the same complex as the surgical suite, several options are available. The tissue can be thawed in warm saline while it is in transit to the surgical suite and then aseptically delivered to the sterile field for successive rinsing and further warming.[17] The allograft can also be transported to the operating room in insulated containers containing liquid nitrogen (FreezSafe Insulated Container; Polyfoam Packers Corporated, Wheeling, Illinois 60090). The frozen tissue is placed on retaining racks situated just above 4 inches of liquid nitrogen. At room temperature transport (20°–25°C), the entire pool of liquid nitrogen vaporizes in approximately 30 minutes but maintains temperatures below −130°C for only 10 minutes (In-house report: Virginia Tissue Bank, Virginia Beach, Virginia 23455). Thus the allowable distance from the liquid nitrogen storage unit to the surgical suite is limited.

Most commercial airlines do not accept containers containing spillable liquid nitrogen or closed pressurized systems of liquid nitrogen. To address the issue of transporting cryopreserved tissues over long distances, new methods of maintaining liquid nitrogen vapor temperatures (below −130°C) had to be developed. Several options of long distance cryogenic transport are available. A patented design[55] utilizing solid carbon dioxide impregnated with liquid nitrogen has been used to transport cryopreserved tissues. This system maintains temperatures of −120°C for up to 10 hours.[56] However, this design leaves room for potential thermal damage to the tissue as the temperature warms above −130°C or if the transportation is delayed longer than the 8- to 10-hour limit.

To guard against possible thermal damage to the frozen allografts, the VTB, in conjunction with MVE, has developed a cryogenic dry shipper that maintains temperatures below −150°C for up to 4 days. A large 40-liter bulk cryoflask was converted to a dry-shipping unit and carries three or four allografts per shipment. A calcium-based porous material was added to the flask cavity, and liquid nitrogen is poured directly into this material. With several fillings, the porous material is saturated with liquid nitrogen. The excess liquid nitrogen is poured off, and the absorbed liquid nitrogen is held in a nonspillable fashion by the calcium-based material. A loose-fitting, well-ventilated lid is attached, yielding a nonpressurized cryogenic shipper that optimizes transportation of cryopreserved tissues. This shipper, called the Bulk dry-shipper XLC-140T, is available from MVE.

When shipping the allografts, care must be taken to avoid damaging the tissue. The allograft packages are brittle at liquid nitrogen vapor temperatures, and damage to these packages has been seen. Packing cotton balls, surgical sponges, or other shock-absorbent materials around the packages within the retaining cardboard storage boxes provides some measure of protection. Also, packing the internal cavity of the shipping container with soft towels or other such material offers further resistance to shipping damage. Use of the aluminum foil external pouch has proved to be superior to the transparent polyolefin bag in withstanding shipping damage.

The AATB has published specific guidelines concerning tissue distribution for allograft implantation.[9]

1. *Package label:* Packages should have following accompanying information:
   - Name of product
   - Name and address of tissue bank
   - Tissue identification number
   - Expiration date, if applicable
   - Sterilization procedure used, if applicable
   - Preservative used and its concentration; or if no preservation is used and the absence of a preservative is a safety factor, the words "no preservative"
   - Number of containers, if more than one
   - Amount of product in the container expressed as volume or weight, or such combination of the foregoing as needed for an accurate description of the contents, whichever is applicable
   - Recommended storage temperature
   - Special instructions indicated by the particular product
   - Presence of known sensitizing substances or reference to an enclosed package insert containing appropriate information
   - Type and calculated amount of antibiotics added during processing
   - Source of the product, when it is a factor in safe administration
   - Statement that the tissue was prepared from a donor who was nonreactive when tested for HIV antibody and hepatitis B surface antigen (HBsAG), using a test required by the U.S. Food and Drug Administration

(FDA). In lieu of inclusion on the package label, such information may be included in the package insert

2. *Contents sterility:* Packaging shall ensure integrity and maintain sterility of the contents.
3. *Package insert:* All tissues shall be accompanied by a package insert which contains instructions for proper storage and reconstitution when appropriate. Specific instructions shall be enclosed with tissues requiring special handling.
4. *Recall procedures:* A written procedure shall exist for recall of tissues or notification of recipient centers of the possibility of tissue contamination, defects in processing, preparation, or distribution, or other factors affecting suitability of the tissues for their intended application.
5. *Report of adverse reactions:* Every effort shall be made to obtain information on adverse reactions.

Expedient transport of the allograft heart valve is obvious. Several overnight carriers and courier services handle nonspillable liquid nitrogen containers. However, a prearranged service agreement and some preplanning is recommended in order to avoid possible delays in allograft delivery to the transplanting facility.

Thawing and Dilution

Preparing the frozen allograft for transplantation involves thawing the tissue at a specific rate, removing the cryoprotective agents, and restoring the cryopreserved tissue to osmotic isotonicity. Careful handling of the allograft and strict adherence to protocols are imperative. To maximize cellular viability, heart valve leaflet manipulation should be kept to a minimum. After thawing and dilution, the "recovering" heart valve should be kept moist and bathed in a physiologic solution at all times during implantation.

Heart valve allografts frozen at a rate of −1°C per minute are considered to be rapidly cooled and should also be thawed at a rapid rate to enhance cell survival.[50,57] As discussed in Chapter 3, rapid warming serves to protect the cells that may have any intracellular ice formation by limiting the amount of small ice recrystallization. Farrant and Woolgar suggested that the injury to biologic tissue associated with intracellular ice formation occurs primarily during the rewarming phase and not during the initial crystallization of cooling.[50] Not only is cell damage seen during rewarming (as a function of ice recrystallization), but it has also been suggested that the melting of intracellular ice and the resultant restoration of osmotic gradients may also cause cellular injury.[50] Refer to Chapter 3 for a further discussion of osmotic/solute concentration cellular damage.

It is generally accepted that thawing the frozen allograft in a 37°–42°C bath produces a rapid enough warming rate to inhibit macrorecrystallization and enhance cell survival.[17,32,33] As can be seen in Figure 4.6, when an allograft is thawed in a constantly maintained 40°C bath, the heart valve rapidly warms to approximately −60°C after 1 minute from an initial prethaw temperature of −170°C. This process yields an initial warming rate of 110°C per minute. The frozen tissue then warms to −30°C after 2 minutes (30°C per minute), to −14°C after 3 minutes (16°C per minute), and is completely thawed in approximately 5 minutes. It is important to maintain the warming bath at a constant 40°C by continually monitoring its temperature and adding additional warm fluid to the bath as heat is transferred to the frozen allograft. Allowing the bath to cool further decreases an already declining thaw rate, exposing the tissue to the recrystallization effects of a slow rewarming process.

The VTB investigated the thawing of nontransplantable heart valve allografts in baths of 60°–80°C. Though the thawing rate was much faster, several problems were noted: The extra-allograft freezing medium warmed to temperatures above 10°C while intraconduit ice was still present; and a small percentage of the conduits developed full-thickness cracks during the thawing process. Therefore thawing the allograft in a bath above 42°C is not recommended.

The allograft should be thawed within the surgical suite under aseptic conditions just prior to its use in surgery. An alternative method was presented by Kirklin and Barratt-Boyes[17] in which the frozen tissue is thawed during its transport from the storage freezer to the operating room. Once the allograft is fully thawed under these nonsterile conditions, the heart valve is aseptically removed from its sterile pouch,

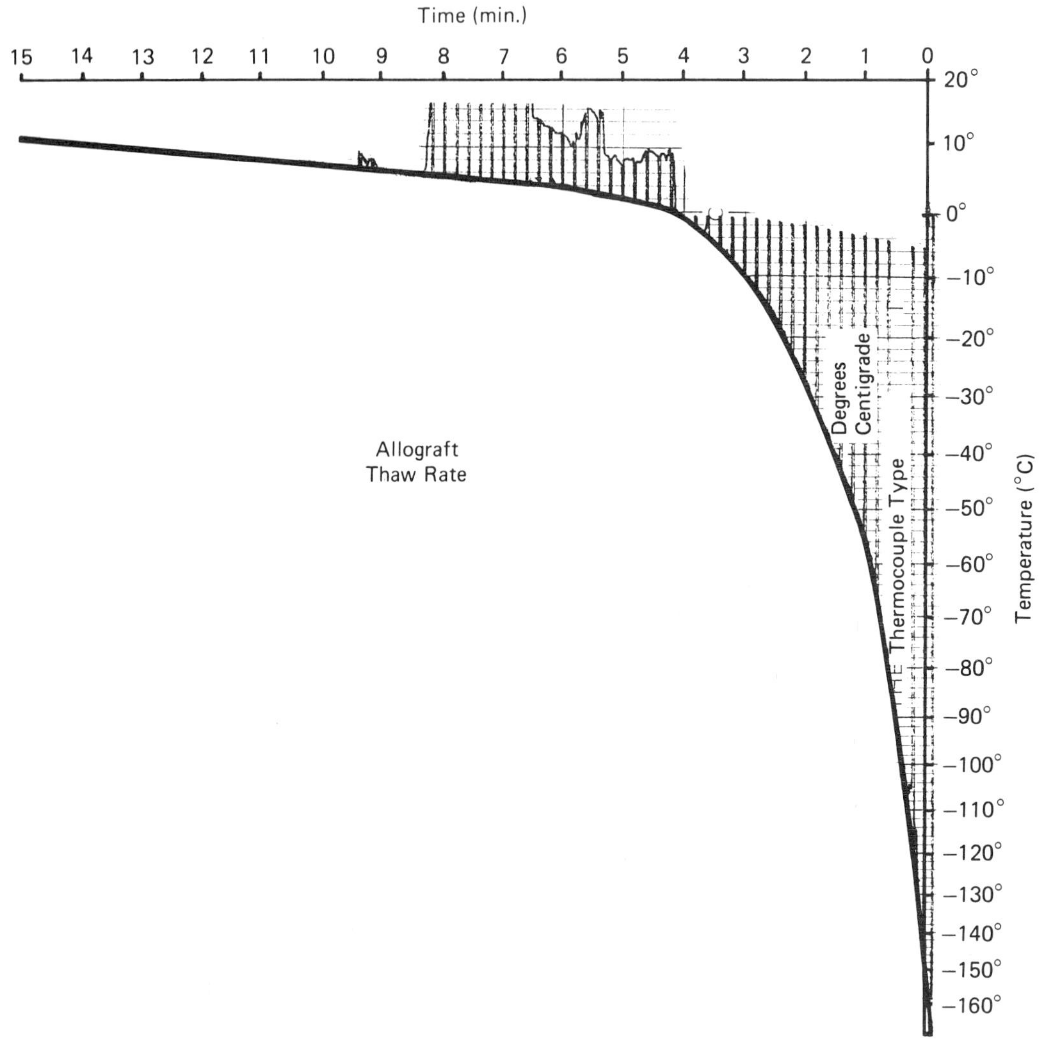

FIGURE 4.6. Allograft thaw rate in a constantly maintained 40°C bath.

and the freezing medium dilution process is performed under sterile conditions within the operating suite. Though this technique solves the problem of how to transfer the allograft from liquid nitrogen vapor storage to the operating room, there is a high risk of possible microbial contamination by subjecting the sterile tissue pouch to a nonsterile bath.

Several protocols for thawing the allograft and diluting the cryoprotectant have been developed by Karp,[7] Angell and associates,[13] Kirklin and associates,[5] and others. These techniques involve immersion of the frozen allograft (or the entire allograft pouch) in a 37°–42°C bath and then stepwise reequilibration of the allograft to isotonicity over a 10- to 15-minute period. The gradual stepwise rinses employ an isotonic physiologic solution that gradually allows the dehydrated cryopreserved cells to establish osmotic equilibrium and to rehydrate. This step-by-step protocol also increasingly dilutes the cryoprotectant (DMSO) employed in the freezing solution.

The procedure followed for the preparation of VTB allograft heart valves is performed entirely within the operating room and is as follows.

Upon arrival at the operating room assemble all needed equipment on a sterile back table.

The *person doing the thawing should double-glove.*

1. Two sterile 500-ml basins and one large 5000-ml basin are needed.
2. Pour approximately 3000 ml 40°C sterile saline into the large basin.
3. Pour 400 ml 4°C RPMI tissue culture medium with 10% fetal calf serum (FCS) into one of the 500-ml basins. Leave the other small basin empty.
4. Place sterile Mayo scissors, DeBakey forceps, Kocher clamp, two 50-cc syringes, and a small 100-cc basin on the back table.
5. Remove cryopreserved valve pouch from cryotransport container. CAUTION: *It is extremely cold; use insulated gloves.*
6. Dry the outer pouch thoroughly.
7. Circulating nurse then opens the pouch with sterile scissors, being careful not to contaminate the inner, sterile pouch.
8. Contents are presented to the scrub nurse who retrieves the inner sterile pouch with a Kocher clamp. NOTE: *Do not puncture inner pouch.*
9. Place inner pouch in the large basin and gently agitate the pouch for 3–4 minutes.
10. Add the remaining 1000 ml of warmed saline to the large basin and gently agitate the pouch an additional 2–3 minutes.
11. When ice turns to slush (do not allow medium to completely thaw), open the pouch with sterile Mayo scissors and pour its contents into the empty small basin. Discard outer gloves.
12. Add 33 ml of RPMI tissue culture medium with 10% FCS from its basin to the homograft-containing basin. Gently agitate for 1 minute.
13. Add another 66 ml of the medium and gently agitate for 1 minute.
14. Add 200 ml more of solution to the allograft and agitate for an additional minute.
15. Transfer the valve using sterile DeBakey forceps to the remaining 100 ml of fluid in the solution basin. *Handle valve gently by the distal aspect only.*
16. Obtain approximately 50 cc of the recipient's heparinized blood. Transfer the homograft to a small 100-ml basin containing the anticoagulated blood.
17. Maintain the *completely immersed* homograft within the recipient's blood until needed for implantation.
18. If the prepared homograft is not soon implanted, place the small basin of tissue and blood on ice until needed.
19. A sample of the cryopreserved valve may be obtained for culturing, at the surgeon's discretion, to ensure sterility.

Once the allograft is thawed, the cryoprotectant must be diluted and the tissue restored to isotonicity. Whereas Karp[7] and others perform all the thawing and dilution aspect in medium at 42°C, the VTB advocates medium dilution at 4°–10°C. As previously discussed, DMSO may be toxic to human cells above 10°C, so the entire gradual dilution of the cryoprotectant is done in cooled medium. Once the DMSO residual is reduced to near 0%, the allograft is placed in recipient blood at 20°–25°C and allowed to return to isotonicity at the warmer temperatures.

The dilution medium is RPMI 1640 amended with 10% FCS. As the original freezing medium (RPMI 1640 + 10% FCS + 10% DMSO) is initially diluted with 33 ml of the dilution medium, the cryoprotectant concentration is reduced to 7.5%. The addition of 66 ml more of the dilution medium then cuts the DMSO concentration to 5%. By adding another 200 ml of the medium, the DMSO is lowered to a 2.5% concentration, and the allograft is then transferred to a nutrient solution without DMSO.

Between each of these successive dilutions, a 1-minute incubation period is called for. During this 1-minute interval, the DMSO is allowed to diffuse out of the cell, and the cell is rehydrated as gradual isotonicity is reached. As discussed in Chapter 3, the dilution shock and the process of cellular rehydration are potential areas of cellular damage. An abruptly rapid dilution process can lead to the cells being subjected to damaging osmotic stress and resultant cell swelling. When the extracellular solution is hypotonic (following freezing) to the intracellular area, the resulting osmotic stresses are due to changes in concentration of soluble ionic solutes, pH changes, and fluid viscosity alternations.[58] A return to normal isotonic conditions during gradual dilution is crucial to cell survival.

The dilution process may be carried out at either 4° or 37°C.[32] Several cryobiologists believe that dilution at 37°C enables the cell to tolerate osmotic stress better than dilution at the colder temperatures.[59] However, prolonged exposure of the heart valve to the cryoprotectant at the warmer temperatures may prove to be toxic. It has been suggested that cellular preservation can be maximized by diluting the freezing medium at 4°C.[32]

The VTB advocates a combination of these protocols. Performing the initial dilutions at 4°–10°C avoids the toxic effects of DMSO. By transferring the allograft valve to recipient blood (at 20°–25°C) prior to graft implantation (at 37°C), the tissue is thus allowed to gradually rewarm from 4° to 37°C over the entire dilution process and to reach full osmotic equilibrium.

Some programs advocate avoidance of fetal calf serum in the dilution medium because of its potential antigenicity[35] (C. Watkins, University of Chicago Hospital, personal communication, April 1988). However, the presence of some type of serum or extracellular colloid has been advocated by Bank and Brockbank[32] and Ashwood-Smith and Farrant.[59] The serum helps reduce the trauma to the rehydrating cell and minimizes the dilution shock. The use of human serum[36] or a serum substitute in the dilution medium warrants further investigation.

During the thawing and dilution aspects of allograft heart valve preparation, several safety precautions are suggested to avoid damaging the tissue.

1. Do not allow the allograft package to become immersed in liquid nitrogen. Not only would it crack the polyolefin pouch, but these extremely low temperatures may cause cracking in the allograft conduit when thawed.
2. Do not allow the frozen allograft to be removed from liquid nitrogen vapor storage until it is to be thawed for surgery. From VTB in-house studies, it was found that a frozen allograft at −180°C warms to −130°C in approximately 3–4 minutes when exposed to room air.
3. If the most external sterile pouch cracks or sterility is compromised, the allograft can still be thawed under sterile conditions and used for transplantation. However, thawing should be done on a table separate from the one used for the dilution steps. All gowns and gloves should also be changed to avoid possible contamination of the sterile inner pouch.
4. Do not allow the freezing medium to warm above 10°C when thawing. As discussed, DMSO may be toxic to human cells at warm temperatures. Remove the thawing allograft and solution from the warming bath once the medium has turned to slush but is not completely thawed.
5. Keep the allograft fully immersed at all times. Allograft exposure to air at the time of surgical implantation has been suspected to damage endothelial cells.[60a] Allowing the entire tissue graft to dry out during its 45 minutes of surgical implantation greatly reduces cellular viability. Judicious, constant wetting of the heart valve during insertion is strongly suggested.
6. Careful handling of the allograft is paramount. Avoid any contact with the leaflet structures, and handle the heart valve from the most distal aspect of the conduit only. It has been suggested by several authors that a major percentage of a cryopreserved heart valve's damage occurs during rough handling by the transplanting surgical team.[60b]

Quality Assurance and Quality Control

Quality assurance/quality control within the allograft tissue field cannot be overemphasized. Providing an absolutely sterile heart valve for surgical transplantation should be the goal of any cardiac valve processing facility. The AATB has published guidelines that discuss the various aspects of allograft tissue pursuits. The *Standards for Tissue Banking*[61] encompass organizational requirements of a tissue bank, acquisition of tissues, and retrieval, processing, preservation, storage, and distribution of human tissues. Adherence to these standards is intended to ensure the safety of allograft tissue.

Strict donor screening is vital and was discussed earlier in the chapter. During the first 2 years of the VTB's heart valve program, approximately 3% of the heart valve donors were found to have unacceptable laboratory analysis results, rendering the tissue nontransplantable (positive hepatitis, syphilis, or AIDS screen; viremia; septicemia). Several donors were declined for various reasons, e.g., a positive medical history, toxic substance exposure, serious illness of unknown etiology, death by unknown causes, prolonged steroid use, or mitigating cardiac specific etiologies. Autopsy reports on all donors are not required but are suggested, especially for heart valve donors who were not vascular organ donors (kidneys, liver, pancreas) and fall within the upper age limit for cardiac donation. Ruling out possibly undetected systemic carcinomas or other neoplastic processes is a must. Refer to Donor Selection, above, for further details.

Once an acceptable donor heart is procured, identification of any contaminating organisms begins. Procurement and transport cultures are obtained by utilizing touch culture swabs, filtration of media, or actual tissue sampling. These cultures are incubated in thioglycollate medium at 37°C for 7 days. After 1 week a representative inoculation is plated aerobically and anaerobically and read 48 hours after plating. Definitive identification of all isolates should be performed by an accredited microbiology or reference laboratory. Among the VTB samples, approximately 10% of all hearts (recovered by sterile procurement techniques only) yielded some type of contaminating organism that had been present at recovery.

The allograft heart valve is then subjected to disinfection by antibiotics for varying lengths of time (refer to Sterilization and Disinfection, above). Following sterilization the allograft is packaged for control-rate freezing, and prior to packaging samples (for culturing) are obtained of all solutions and materials that come into contact with the tissue. The freezing bags are touch-cultured, as are samples of the premixed medium (RPMI 1640 + 10% FCS), DMSO, and antibiotic sterilization solutions. These cultures are incubated and plated in the same manner as the procurement cultures. Any positive growth from these end-stage cultures renders the heart valve nontransplantable.

To date, 3.6% of all VTB processed heart valves have produced positive cultures at packaging as follows:

Item	*Percent of total hearts processed*
Antibiotic medium	0.45
Packaging bags	0.89
DMSO	1.78
RPMI-FCS medium	0.45
Total positive cultures (%)	3.57

Of this 3.6%, all isolated contaminating organisms were of the diphtheroid variety or the *Staphylococcus* coagulase-negative species (*S. epidermidis*). Although these contaminants are common laboratory organisms and can be attributed to culture technique error, any positive culture result at this stage yields the allograft nontransplantable.

To guard against possible false-negative antibiotic solution results (see Sterilization and Disinfection, above), the entire disinfecting solution is filtered and the filter paper incubated and plated. To date, there have been no positive cultures obtained from the sterilizing solution when employing the filtration method. Any positive result would render the valve nontransplantable.

At the time of processing, two tissue samples (mitral leaflet) are removed from the antibiotic incubation solution, incubated temporarily in 3 ml of thioglycollate, and transported at room temperature to a reference laboratory. The tissue samples are cultured for the presence of fungal or acid-fast organisms (for tuberculosis). These tests require 4–10 weeks of incubation. All cryopreserved allografts should be held from release until negative results for fungal and acid-fast organisms are obtained. For detailed descriptions of the culture technique, references are available.[62] Again, any positive results yield a nontransplantable allograft.

Quality assurance does not encompass donor selection and processing cultures alone. The sterility and maintenance of all equipment used during the preparation of an allograft heart valve is necessary. Systematic assurance of sterile instruments and laminar flow hoods must be maintained. The general dissection area must be of operating room quality. Also, strict guidelines should be followed for discarding potentially hazardous human tissue and waste products; refer to the local health code for details.

All heart valve dissections should be performed by qualified experienced medical personnel. At the VTB, all heart valve processing is done by VTB-certified tissue bank technicians after undergoing extensive training in surgical dissection techniques. The VTB's heart discard rate due to technical error is less than 4%.

Once the allografts are removed from the heart, all remaining cardiac tissue is kept in −80°C storage for 60 days. Requests by medical examiners for heart tissue to investigate at autopsy occur infrequently.

As the allograft is undergoing control-rate freezing, deviations from an exact −1°C per minute linear rate do occur. The effect on cell survival rates as a result of these deviations still need to be investigated. Each heart valve program must set its own acceptable deviation limits. As discussed in Chapter 3, a cryopreservation "freezing window" exists. Within a given range of temperature (0° to −20°C) large deviations from a linear rate of decline in tissue temperature may compromise cellular viability. The VTB recommends the following limits of deviations for all VTB process heart valve allografts.

Tissue/medium temperature (°C)	*Degree of variance allowed* (°C)
0–5	1
5–10	2
10–15	4
15–20	8

As seen in Figure 3.1, the freezing curve windows expand as the tissue temperature declines, leaving larger allowable limits of error.

Quality control of the actual allograft heart valves must be ensured. Though some programs perform viability testing on every heart valve processed, the VTB performs tritiated proline radioisotope uptake studies on approximately 10% of the transplantable valves (see Chapter 3 for a discussion of viability testing). Gonzales-Lavin (The First Workshop on Homologous and Autologous Heart Valves. Chicago: Deborah Heart and Lung Center, 5 April 1987) performs radioisotope uptake studies with the tricuspid leaflets of all processed hearts. He believes that the viability of a processed tricuspid valve mimics the cell survival rate of the aortic and pulmonary valves. Viability testing of every processed heart valve is ideal but may not be cost-effective.

Once an allograft is determined to be acceptable for transplant, all donor and processing records are examined and approved by the medical director of the program, who should be a physician knowledgeable in allograft tissue banking.

Quality control does not end with the implantation of the allograft heart valve. The VTB executes an extensive follow-up program of all recipients. Before a valve is released to an implanting surgeon, agreements are signed stating that all follow-up forms sent to them will be completed and returned. Follow-up forms are sent out every 6 months postoperatively, and the compilation of clinical data is maintained on computerized data management systems.

References

1. Khanna SK, Ross JK, Monro JL: Homograft aortic valve replacement—seven years' experience with antibiotic-treated valves. *Thorax* 36:330–337, 1981.
2. Wain WH, Greco R, Ignegeri A, et al: 15 Years experience with 615 homograft and autograft aortic valve replacements. *Int J Artif Organs* 3:169–172, 1980.
3. Angell WW, Angell JD, Oury JH, et al: Long-term follow-up of viable frozen aortic homografts. *J Thorac Cardiovasc Surg* 93:815–822, 1987.

4a. O'Brien MF, Stafford EG, Gardner AH, et al: A comparison of aortic valve replacement with viable cryopreserved and fresh allograft valves, with a note on chromosomal studies. *J Thorac Cardiovasc Surg* 94:812–823, 1987.

4b. O'Brien MF, personal communication, 7 March, 1988.

5. Kirklin JW, Blackstone EH, Maehara T, et al: Intermediate-term fate of cryopreserved allograft and xenograft valved conduits. *Ann Thorac Surg* 44:598–606, 1987.
6. Barratt-Boyes BG, Roche AHG, Subramanyan R, et al: Long-term follow-up of the antibiotic sterilized aortic homograft valve inserted freehand in the aortic position. *Circulation* 75:768–777, 1987.
7. Karp RB: The use of free-hand unstented aortic valve allografts for replacement of the aortic valve. *J Cardiac Surg* 1:23–32, 1986.
8. *American Heart Association Annual Report, 1985:* Dallas: AHA National Center.
9. The American Association of Tissue Banks: *Tech-*

nical Manual for Tissue Banking. Arlington, VA: AATB, 1987.

10. Armiger LC, Thomson RW, Strickett MG, Barratt-Boyes BG: Morphology of heart valves preserved by liquid nitrogen freezing. *Thorax* 40:778–786, 1985.
11. *Clinical Program 101—Homograft Heart Valves*. Marietta, GA: Cryolife, Inc., 1985, p. 12.
12. Angell JD, Christopher BS, Hawtrey O, Angell WM: A fresh viable human heart valve bank—sterilization, sterility testing and cryogenic preservation. *Transplant Proc* 8(suppl 1):127–141, 1976.
13. Kay PH, Ross DN: 15 Years' experience with the aortic homograft: the conduit of choice for right ventricular outflow tract reconstruction. *Ann Thorac Surg* 40:360–364, 1985.
14. Allwork SP, Pucci JJ, Cleland WP, Bentall HH: The longevity of sterilized aortic valve homografts 1966–1972. *J Cardiovasc Surg* 27:213–216, 1986.
15. Fontan F, Chaussat A, Deville C, et al: Aortic valve homografts in the surgical treatment of complex cardiac malformations. *J Thorac Cardiovasc Surg* 87:649–657, 1984.
16. Barratt-Boyes GB, Roche ABG, Whitlock RML: 6 Year review of the results of freehand aortic valve replacement using an antibiotic sterilized homograft valve. *Circulation* 55:353–361, 1977.
17a. Kirklin JW, Barratt-Boyes BG: *Cardiac Surgery*. New York: Wiley, 1986, p. 421.
17b. A. Schuler S, Yankah AC, Hetzer R: Allogenic valve procurement in cardiac transplantation. *Cardiac Valve Allografts 1962–1987*. New York: Springer-Verlag 1987, pp. 13–16.
18a. Wolfinbarger L, Weintraub B: *Technical Program Report: Heart Valve Cryopreservation*. Virginia Beach, VA: Virginia Tissue Bank, 1987.
18b. Belzer FO, Sollinger HW, Glass NR, et al: Beneficial effects of adenosine and phosphate in kidney preservation. *Transplantation*. 36:633–636, 1983.
18c. Henry ML, Sommer BG, Ferguson RM. Improved immediate function of renal allografts with Belzer perfusate. *Transplantation*. 45:73–75, 1988.
19. Mohri H, Reichenbach DD, Merendino KA: Biology of homologous and heterologous aortic valves. In: *Biological Tissue in Heart Valve Replacement*. London: Butterworth, 1979, p. 144.
20. Ross DN, Martelli V, Wain WH: Allograft and autograft valves used for aortic valve replacement. In Ignescu MI (ed): *Tissue Heart Valves*. Boston: Butterworth, 1979, pp. 127–172.
21. Strickett MG, Barratt-Boyes BG, MacCulloch D: Disinfection of human heart valve allografts with antibiotics in low concentration. *Pathology* 15:457–462, 1983.
22. Yacoub M, Kittle CF: Sterilization of valve homografts by antibiotic solutions. *Circulation* 41(suppl):29–31, 1970.
23. Lockey E, Al-Janabi N, Gonzales-Lavin L, Ross DN: A method of sterilizing and preserving fresh allograft heart valves. *Thorax* 27:398–400, 1972.
24. Waterworth PM, Lockey E, Berry EM, Pearce HM: A critical investigation into the antibiotic sterilization of heart valve homografts. *Thorax* 29:432–436, 1974.
25. Wain WH, Pearce HM, Riddell RW, Ross DN: A re-evaluation of antibiotic sterilization of heart valve allografts. *Thorax* 32:740–742, 1977.
26. Gavin JB, Herdson PB, Monro JL, Barratt-Boyes BG: Pathology of antibiotic-treated human heart valve allografts. *Thorax* 28:473–481, 1973.
27a. Gavin JB, Barratt-Boyes BG, Hitchcock GC, Herdson PB: Histopathology of fresh human aortic valve allografts. *Thorax* 28:482–487, 1973.
27b. Gonzalez-Lavin L, McGrath L, Alvarez M, Graf D: Antibiotic sterilization in the preparation of homovital homograft valves: Is it necessary? *Cardiac Valve Allografts 1962–1987*. New York: Springer-Verlag 1987, pp. 17–21.
28. Girinath MR, Gavin JB, Strickett MG, Barratt-Boyes BG: The effects of antibiotics and storage on the viability and ultrastructure of fibroblasts in canine heart valves prepared for grafting. *Aust NZ J Surg* 44:170, 1974.
29. Armiger LC, Gavin JB, Barratt-Boyes BG: Histological assessment of orthotopic aortic valve leaflet allografts: its role in selecting graft pre-treatment. *Pathology* 15:67–73, 1983.
30. Gavin JB, Monro JL: The pathology of pulmonary and aortic valve allografts used as mitral replacements in dogs. *Pathology* 6:119–127, 1974.
31a. Watts LK, Duffy P, Field RB, et al: Establishment of a viable homograft cardiac valve bank—a rapid method of determining homograft viability. *Ann Thorac Surg* 21:230–236, 1976.
31b. Yankah AC, Hetzer R: *Cardiac Valve Allografts 1962–1987*. New York: Springer-Verlag, 1987, pp. 23–26.
31c. Yankah AC, Hetzer JR: Procurement and viability of cardiac valve allografts. *Cardiac Valve Allografts 1962–1987*. New York: Springer-Verlag, 1987, pp. 23–26.
31d. Kirklin JK, Kirklin JW, Pacifico JAD, Phillips S: Cryopreservation of aortic valve homografts. *Cardiac Valve Allografts 1962–1987*. New York: Springer-Verlag, 1987, pp. 35–36.
31e. Gonzalez-Lavin L, Bianchi J, Graf D, Amini S, Gordon CI: Homograft valve calcification—

Evidence for an immunological influence. *Cardiac Valve Allografts 1962–1987*. New York: Springer-Verlag, 1987, pp. 69–74.
31f. Watkins C: University of Chicago Hospital Heart Valve Program, personal communication, October 1988.
31g. Almeida M: American Red Cross, Los Angeles, Heart Valve Program, personal communication, October 1988.
31h. Robbins, SL: *Pathologic Basis of Disease*, 3rd edition, Philadelphia: WB Saunders Co., 1984, pp. 581, 593.
31i. Morehead, RP: *Human Pathology*, New York: McGraw-Hill, Inc., 1965, pp. 420–423.
31j. McGinnis, MR: *Current Topics in Medical Mycology*, Volume 1, Chapter 3, New York: Springer-Verlag, 1985.
31k. Sommerwith, AC, Jarett, L: *Gradwohl's Clinical Laboratory Methods and Diagnosis*, Volume 2, 8th Edition. St. Louis: C.V. Mosby Co., 1980, p. 2205.
32. Bank HL, Brockbank K: Basic principles of cryobiology. *J Cardiac Surg* 2(suppl):137–143, 1987.
33. Ashwood-Smith MJ, Farrant J: *Low Temperature Preservation in Medicine and Biology*. Tunbridge Wells, Kent: Pitman, 1980, p. 12.
34. Karow AM, Pegg DE: *Organ Preservation for Transplantation* New York: Marcel Dekker, 1981, p. 480.
35. Bodnar E, Olsen EGJ, Florio R, et al: Heterologous antigenicity induced in human aortic homografts during preservation. *Eur J Cardiothorac Surg* 2:43–47, 1988.
36. Yankah AC: At The First Workshop on Homologous and Autologous Heart Valves. Chicago: Deborah Heart and Lung Center, 5 April 1987.
37. Karow AM, Pegg DE: *Organ Preservation for Transplantation* New York: Marcel Dekker, 1981, p. 122.
38. *Clinical Program 101—Homograft Heart Valves*. Marietta, GA: Cryolife, Inc., August 1985, p. 17.
39. Mermet B, Buch W, Angell W: Viable heart valve graft—preservation in the frozen state. *Surg Forum* 21:156, 1970.
40. VanderKamp AWM, Visser WJ, VanDongen JM, et al: Preservation of aortic heart valves with maintenance of cell viability. *J Surg Res* 30:47–56, 1981.
41. O'Brien MF, Stafford G, Gardner M, et al: The viable cryopreserved allograft aortic valve. *J Cardiac Surg* 2(suppl):153–167, 1987.
42. May SR, Guttman RM, Wainwright JF: Cryopreservation of skin using an insulated heat sink box stored at −70 degrees C. *Cryobiology* 22:205–214, 1985.
43. Grout BWW, Morris GJ: Freezing and cellular organization. In: *The Effect of Low Temperatures on Biological Systems*. London: Edward Arnold, 1987, pp. 147–173.
44. Karow AM, Pegg DE: *Organ Preservation for Transplantation*. New York: Marcel Dekker, 1981, p. 118.
45. Grout BWW, Morris GJ: *The Effects of Low Temperatures on Biological Systems*. London: Edward Arnold, 1987, pp. 45–46.
46. Mazur P: The role of cell membranes in the freezing of yeast and other single cells. *Ann NY Acad Sci* 125:658, 1965.
47. Dowell LG, Rinfret AP: Low temperature forms of ice as studied by x-ray diffraction. *Nature* 188:1144, 1960.
48. Ashwood-Smith MJ, Farrant J: *Low Temperature Preservation in Medicine and Biology*. Tunbridge Wells, Kent: Pitman, 1980, p. 291.
49. Luyet BJ: On various phase transitions occurring in aqueous solutions at low temperatures. *Ann NY Acad Sci* 85:549, 1960.
50. Ashwood-Smith MJ, Farrant J: *Low Temperature Preservation in Medicine and Biology*. Tunbridge Wells, Kent: Pitman, 1980, p. 22.
51. Farrant J, Woolgar AE: Possible relationships between the physical properties of solutions and cell damage during freezing. In: *The Frozen Cell*. London: Churchill, 1979, p. 97.
52. Peterson WD, Stulbert CS: Freeze preservation of cultured animal cells. *Cryobiology* 1:80, 1964.
53a. Josylyn MA: The action of enzymes in the dried state and in concentrated solutions. In: *Proceedings of the Eighth International Congress of Refrigeration*. 1952, p. 331.
53b. Watkins C: University of Chicago Hospital Heart Valve Program, personal communication, 1988.
54. *Test Report 212: Temperature Profile*. New Pague, MN: MVE Engineering, 18 February 1985.
55. Cryolife Inc.: U.S. Patent 4,597,266: Freezing agent and container. 1 July 1986.
56. Cryolife Inc.: Thermal cycling during transport of homograft tissue may compromise cell viability. *Cryolife Techn Memorandum* 2(1):July 1987.
57. Grout BWW, Morris GJ: *The Effects of Low Temperatures on Biological Systems*. London: Edward Arnold, 1987, pp. 162–166.
58. Grout BWW, Morris GJ: *The Effects of Low Tem-*

peratures on Biological Systems. London: Edward Arnold, 1987, p. 148.

59. Ashwood-Smith MJ, Farrant J: *Low Temperature Preservation in Medicine and Biology*. Tunbridge Wells, Kent: Pitman, 1980, p. 15.

60a. O'Brien MF: (*Panel Discussion #1*) *J Cardiac Surg* 2(suppl):169, 1987.

60b. O'Brien MF: Discussion. *Cardiac Valve Allografts 1967–1987*. New York: Springer-Verlag, 1987, p. 50.

61. American Association of Tissue Banks: *Standards for Tissue Banking*, Arlington, VA: AATB, 1984.

62. Finegold SM, Martin WJ, Scott EG: *Bailey and Scott's Diagnostic Microbiology*. 5th Ed., St. Louis: Mosby, 1978.

5—Effects of Preimplantation Processing on Bioprosthetic and Biologic CardiacValve Morphology

STEPHEN L. HILBERT, VICTOR J. FERRANS, and MICHAEL JONES

The evolution of cardiac valve substitutes for the management of valvular heart disease has been taking place for approximately a quarter-century. A heterogeneous group of components, including pyrolytic carbon, polymeric, and tissue-derived materials, have been configured into mechanical, polymeric, bioprosthetic, and biologic valve designs.[1–11] For the purpose of this review, however, only tissue-derived xenograft and allograft cardiac valves are discussed.

Xenografts are frequently referred to as bioprosthetic heart valves (BPs). Historically, a variety of tissue-derived materials, ranging from nontreated fascia lata and glycerol-treated dura mater to aldehyde-treated porcine aortic valves and bovine parietal pericardial tissue, have been configured into trileaflet, bileaflet, and monoleaflet valves.[12–16] The long-term results of autologous fascia lata valves have not been satisfactory, and the use of glycerol-treated dura mater valves has declined.[17–20] Thus most BPs in clinical use are porcine aortic valve and bovine pericardial trileaflet prostheses.

Preimplantation processing of BPs is necessary to reduce the antigenicity of xenograft tissues, increase their durability, ensure sterility, and reduce the rate of calcification. In contrast to xenografts, human pulmonary and aortic valve allografts are not routinely treated with aldehydes, although they also undergo preimplantation processing, e.g., disinfection and sterilization, storage in antibiotics or nutrient media, cryopreservation, and freezing. This chapter presents a review of bioprosthetic and biologic valve preimplantation processing, followed by a discussion of the resultant alterations of native tissue morphology and valvular function.

Preimplantation Processing and Sterilization

Bioprosthetic Valves

Aldehyde Fixation

Preimplantation chemical treatment of the procine aortic valve (PAV) and bovine pericardial tissue involves fixation using low concentrations (<1%) of glutaraldehyde. The conditions of fixation (e.g., glutaraldehyde purity and concentration, temperature, pH, time) determine the extent and type of protein crosslinking (intra- and intermolecular) that occurs.

Glutaraldehyde reacts with primary amine groups (e.g., those in lysine, hydroxylysine, and *N*-terminal amino acid residues in collagen) to form Schiff base, unsaturated addition reaction, and pyridinium-type products (crosslinks). The precise mechanism involved in the formation of glutaraldehyde-induced collagen crosslinking is unknown.[21–23] As a result of glutaraldehyde-induced crosslinking, BP collagen is altered in comparison to that in the native aortic valve or pericardial tissue, as demonstrated by a reduction in tissue compliance, increased thermal stability (shrinkage temperature), and increased resistance to proteolytic enzyme digestion.[20–25] The shrinkage temperature of pericardial tissue

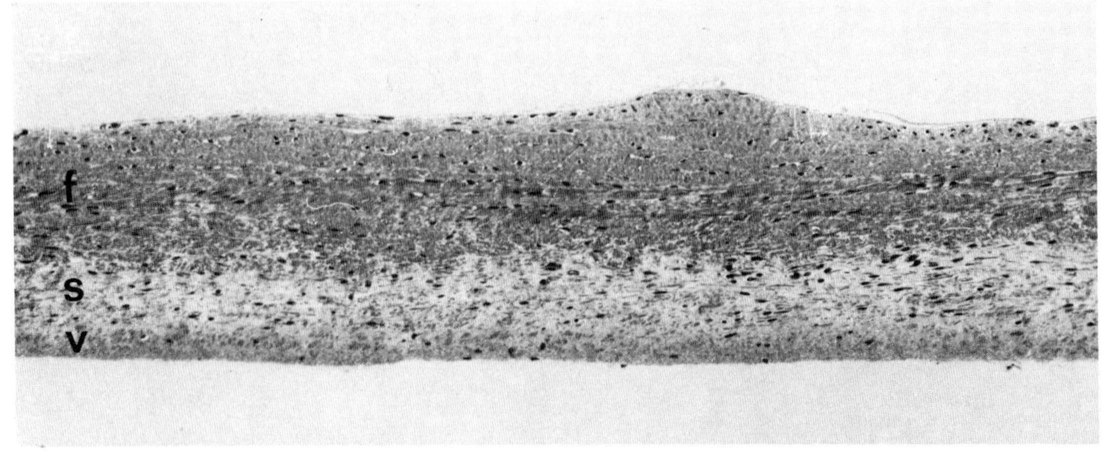

Figure 5.1. Histologic section of unimplanted, high-pressure-fixed PAV xenograft. Note the flat or compressed appearance of the cusp. (V) ventricularis; (S) spongiosa; (F) fibrosa. Glycol methacrylate-embedded tissue; hematoxylin/eosin stain. ×150.

is reduced by extraction of proteoglycans but not by extraction of lipids.[26]

Glutaraldehyde is more effective as a crosslinking agent than formaldehyde, which reacts with primary amines in proteins to form hydroxymethyl secondary amines. These agents can react with free amides to form crosslinks that are unstable.[21] In PAVs, formaldehyde-induced crosslinks are initially stable but steadily dissociate following storage at 37°C in normal saline over a period of 10 months; however, glutaraldehyde-induced crosslinks remain stable.[21] This stability may account for the increased durability of glutaraldehyde-treated BPs compared to formaldehyde-treated BPs.[27–34]

Fixation of PAVs may be accomplished under either high pressure (e.g., 70–80 mm Hg) or low pressure (i.e., < 2 mm Hg), producing a noticeable difference in valve morphology, particularly in the crimping or waviness of collagen (Figs. 5.1 and 5.2). Pericardial tissues fabricated into BPs are fixed by immersion, without pressure or stretching. It has been suggested[35] that maintenance of the crimped (nonstretched) collagen morphology in the native aortic valve and pericardium results in improved accommodation of the mechanical forces associated with leaflet opening and closure.[35–40] Whether low-pressure fixation increases the durability of glutaraldehyde-treated xenografts remains to be demonstrated. Variations in fixation conditions could result in increased biodegradation and antigenicity as well as in inconsistent physicochemical and mechanical properties of the BPs.

Glycerol Treatment

Valves fabricated of gycerol-treated human dura mater have been used extensively as cardiac valve substitutes, mostly in Latin America.[15] For valve fabrication, the dura mater tissue is removed at necropsy, using sterile technique, up to 20 hours after death; it is then washed in water for 1–2 hours, placed in 98% glycerol at room temperature for 10–20 days, rehydrated in sterile saline, and cut into leaflets. These leaflets are mounted on the stent, and the valve is stored in glycerol. One day before use, the valves are placed in a physiologic electrolyte solution containing cephalothin, rifampin, and amphotericin B at 4°C.[41]

Dura mater is composed mostly of dense collagen. Glycerol treatment probably involves a combination of effects, including dehydration, extraction of tissue components, chemical denaturation by glycerol, and fixation by aldehydes present as impurities. Glycerol-treated dura mater valves can have a long durability, in contrast to untreated dura mater valves.[41,42] Nevertheless, implanted dura mater valves develop tears

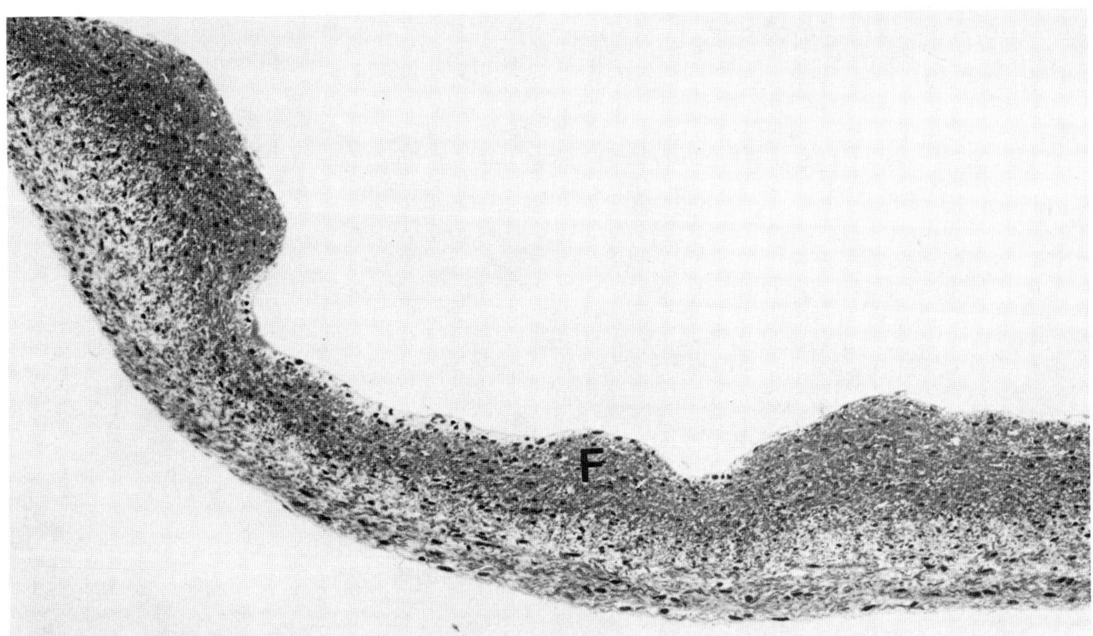

FIGURE 5.2. Histologic section of unimplanted, low-pressure-fixed PAV xenograft. More of the native collagen morphology is retained by this fixation process. Note the convoluted appearance of the fibrosa (F). (Compare to Fig. 5.1.) Glycol methacrylate-embedded tissue; hematoxylin-eosin stain. ×150.

and calcific deposits[41] that resemble those observed in PAVs and pericardial BPs, and their use has decreased sharply.[19] The transmission of Creutzfeldt-Jakob disease (CJD) has been associated with the use of cardaveric human dura mater.[43] The potential for the transmission of CJD and other virus-related neurologic disorders may further limit the use of dura mater BPs.

Anticalcification Treatments

Calcification frequently occurs in BPs implanted as substitute cardiac valves in animals[44–49] and patients[33,50–52] and is the most important single cause of BP dysfunction.[53,54] Calcification mainly involves collagen fibrils (Figs. 5.3 and 5.4) and microthrombi (Fig. 5.5).[48,55] These calcific deposits may increase in size, eventually forming larger nodules that cause stenosis and contribute to the formation of tears and perforations.

Ultrastructural studies reveal three distinct patterns of collagen fibril calcification: complete calcification of the fibrils, calcification restricted to the surfaces of the fibrils, and calcification limited to the space between the fibrils (Figs. 5.3 and 5.4).[55] The calcification of BPs seems to be initiated in organelles (e.g., mitochondria (Fig. 5.6) and nuclei) of devitalized connective tissue cells.[56] The phospholipids present in the membranes of these structures may serve as nucleation sites for calcification.

Patient populations with high risk of BP calcification include children and young adults, patients with chronic renal disease or hyperparathyroidism, and patients with infected BPs.[57–68] The relation of glutaraldehyde cross-linking to calcification of collagen remains unclear.[69–71] Subcutaneous implantation studies suggest that glutaraldehyde-treated PAVs and pericardium calcify more readily than untreated tissues; however, glutaraldehyde fixation did not increase the amount of calcification of pieces of human dura mater implanted subcutaneously in rats.[71]

Calcium-binding proteins have been reported to occur within BPs and other calcified tissues.[47,48,72–77] The high content of carboxyl-

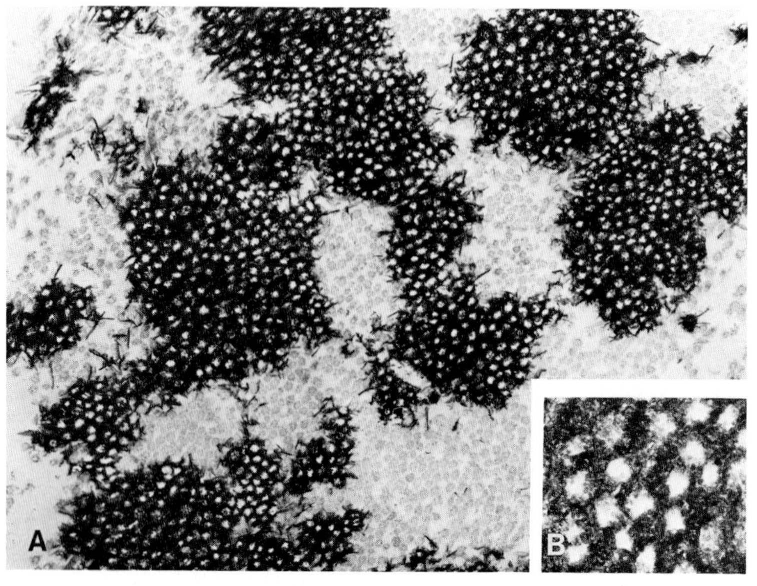

Figure 5.3. Calcification of collagen fibrils may involve entire fibrils (see Fig. 5.4), be localized on the fibril surfaces, or be present between individual collagen fibrils. Uranyl acetate/lead citrate stain. **A**, ×25,500; **B**, ×75,000.

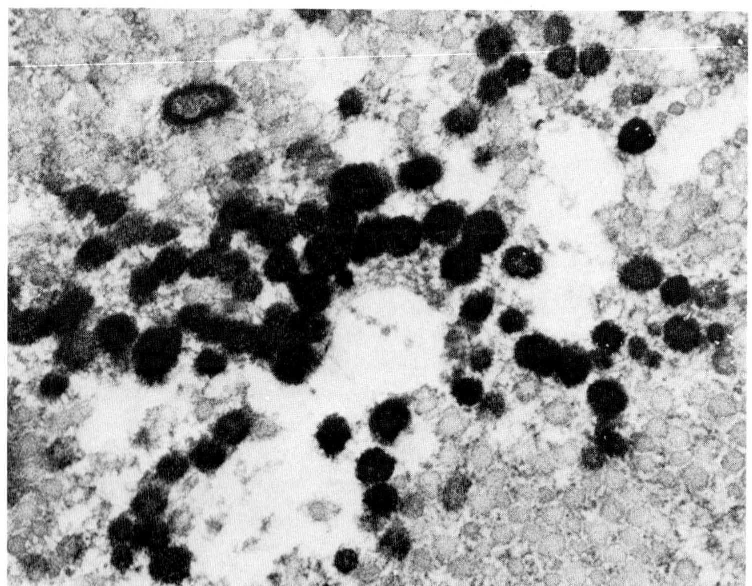

Figure 5.4. Transmission electron micrograph showing calcification involving entire collagen fibrils in an explanted bovine pericardial BP. Uranyl acetate/lead citrate stain. ×56,000.

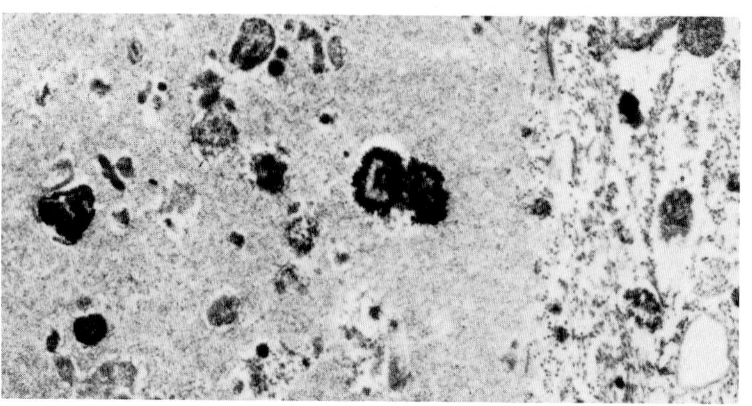

Figure 5.5. Transmission electron micrograph showing the calcification of devitalized cells within thrombotic material on the surface of an explanted PAV xenograft. Uranyl acetate/lead citrate stain. ×15,000.

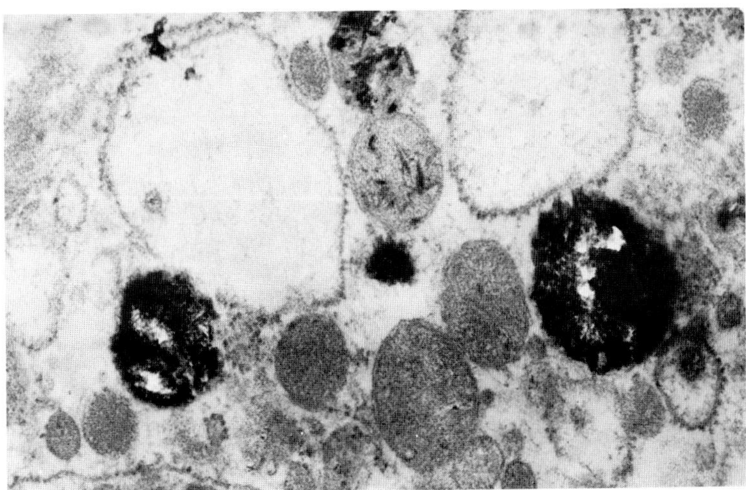

FIGURE 5.6. Electron micrograph depicting the calcification of mitochondria within a devitalized PAV xenograft cell. Uranyl acetate/lead citrate stain. ×60,000.

ated amino acids (e.g., γ-carboxyglutamic acid and aminomalonic acid) determines the affinity of these proteins for calcium. It has been proposed that the administration of vitamin K antagonists (i.e., coumarin anticoagulants), which inhibit the carboxylation of amino acids,[78] may decrease BP calcification.[79,80]

Subcutaneous and intramuscular implantation studies of surfactant-treated PAVs and pericardial tissues indicate that the following agents mitigate calcification: Triton X-100 plus *N*-lauryl sarcosine, sodium dodecyl sulfate (SDS), polysorbate, and deoxycholic acid.[80,81] In valves implanted in sheep for 20–52 weeks, the polysorbate and SDS processes reduce the calcification that develops in PAVs but not in pericardial BPs[45,46,82] (Table 5.1). The reason for this selectivity is unknown.

The mechanism by which preimplantation surfactant treatment of PAVs reduces calcification is unclear. It has been suggested that these treatments affect the membrane surface charge, the ground substance, the collagen fibrils, or phospholipids.[81,83] Morphologic studies have shown that calcification of collagen fibrils is decreased in explanted PAVs that had undergone preimplantation surfactant treatments.[45,46]

Diphosphonates (pyrophosphate analogues) form complexes with calcium, resulting in a localized reduction in extracellular calcium; they also interfere with the formation of hydroxyapatite crystals.[84–86] The systemic administration of diphosphonates reduces the calcification of BP leaflets implanted subcutaneously in animals.[87,88] However, diphosphonates have severe adverse effects on growth and calcification of bone.[87,89] These effects have been minimized by the local administration of diphosphonates in close proximity to the subcutaneously implanted BP tissue.[89–91] Valves containing diphosphonates incorporated into the sewing ring have been implanted with encouraging initial results.[92] No anticalcification benefit could be demonstrated when pericardial valves containing covalently bound aminohydroxypropane diphosphonic acid were implanted in the mitral position in sheep.[82]

A number of other anticalcification treatments have been developed, including collagen modification by blocking potential calcium-binding sites with compounds such as magnesium chloride, toluidine blue, and leucotoluidine blue;[80,81,93,94] chemical modification by means of esterification;[95] charge modification utilizing protamine sulfate;[96] prevention of phospholipid penetration by the formation of a hydrogel (polyacrylamide) within the PAV cusp;[80] decreasing the available calcium by local administration of phosphocitrate;[97] and decreasing the available phosphate in the valvular tissue by using an organic buffer such as HEPES.[94] These treatments are effective in subcutaneous or intramuscular implantation models in small animals. Significant discrepancies have been found when BP anticalcification treatments have been evaluated by subcutaneous or intramuscular implanta-

Table 5.1 Calcium content of valves treated with anticalcification agents.

Valve type[a]	No.	Calcium (mean ± SEM) (mg/g tissue dry weight)
Standard PAVs (controls for polysorbate-80 and Triton X-100 + *N*-lauryl sarcosine)	22	99.8 ± 11.1
Polysorbate-80-treated PAVs	15	7.6 ± 2.6 ($p < 0.001$)
Triton X-100 and *N*-lauryl sarcosine-treated PVAs	14	12.7 ± 3.8 ($p < 0.001$)
Standard BPVs (controls for polysorbate-80)	18	73.1 ± 10.3
Polysorbate-80-treated BPVs	11	55.2 ± 12.7
Standard BPVs (polyacrylamide controls)[b]	10	66.1 ± 15.5
Polyacrylamide-treated BPVs[b]	8	112.9 ± 15.3 ($p < 0.05$)
Standard PAVs (SDS controls)	28	64.7 ± 9.6
SDS treated PVAs	17	17.7 ± 4.2 ($p < 0.001$)
Standard BPVs (SDS controls)	12	136.2 ± 3.6
SDS treated BPVs	24	117.7 ± 5.3
Standard BPVs (diphosphonate controls)	17	104.3 ± 9.1
Diphosphonate (ADP)-treated BVPs	12	126.6 ± 7.3 ($p < 0.07$)
Standard PAVs (toluidine blue controls)	17	139.3 ± 14.7
Toluidine blue-treated PAVs	21	81.6 ± 12.0 ($p < 0.05$)

[a] PAVs = porcine aortic valves. BPVs = bovine pericardial valves. SDS = sodium dodecyl sulfate. ADP = aminohydroxypropane diphosphonic acid.
[b] Implanted in the tricuspid position; all other valves implanted in the mitral position.
From Jones et al.[82]

tion in small animal models and by implantation in the tricuspid or mitral position in sheep. Treatment with surfactants, toluidine blue, and polyacrylamide decreased calcification of both pericardial and PAV cusps in subcutaneous implantation models but not of BPs implanted in sheep. Such differences may be related to the long-term physicochemical stability of the interaction between glutaraldehyde-treated tissue and the anticalcification agent, and to the physiological and mechanical differences associated with intracardiac versus subcutaneous or intramuscular implantation.

Polyacrylamide incorporation into leaflets was found to mitigate BP calcification after subcutaneous implantation in rabbits; however, this effect was lost if the treated BPs were first mechanically cycled in a pulse duplicator.[80] A protective effect of polyacrylamide could not be demonstrated after intracardiac implantation in calves or sheep.[80,82] Similarly, toluidine blue-treated BPs showed a reduction in calcification following intramuscular implantation in rats[81] but not after intracardiac implantation in calves[81] or sheep.[82] Toluidine blue treatment lost its effectiveness after 12 weeks of intramuscular implantation, implying that its interaction with glutaraldehyde-treated tissue is reversible.[81]

The stability of BP glutaraldehyde-treated tissue crosslinking was questioned following the observation that PAVs stored in 0.2% glutaraldehyde for periods ranging from 12 to 40 months showed a reduction in leaflet calcification after subcutaneous implantation in rats.[98] The results of this study imply that the time elapsed between tissue fixation and BP implantation influences the extent of leaflet calcification; however, the results of intracardiac implantation in sheep suggest that the degree of calcification of PAVs and pericardial BPs is not influenced by the "shelf-life" of the BP.[46] Thus the extrapolation of small animal subcutaneous or intramuscular implantation data to predict the effectiveness of anticalcification treatments following cardiac valve replacement is not advised.

In addition to the evaluation of the effectiveness of BP anticalcification treatments, studies must also be conducted to ensure that BP durability (i.e., resistance to mechanical wear) is not compromised. In our experience, polysorbate and SDS treatments do not alter the short-term durability of BPs following mitral valve replace-

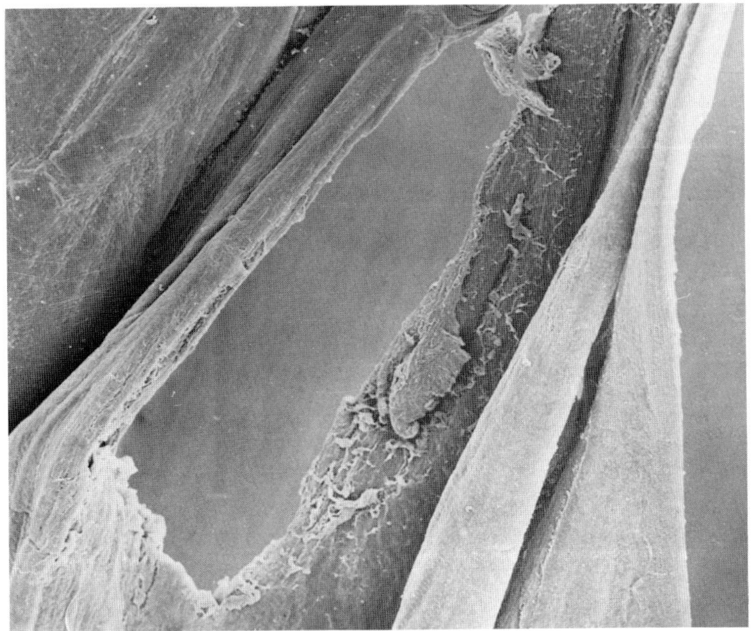

FIGURE 5.7. Scanning electron micrograph of a cuspal perforation occurring in an explanted PAV xenograft that had undergone Triton X-100 plus *N*-lauryl sarcosine anticalcification treatment and was implanted for 20 weeks in the mitral position in a sheep. ×75.

ment in sheep for a period of 20 weeks; however, preliminary studies of PAVs treated with Triton X-100 plus *N*-lauryl sarcosine indicate that the durability of these valves is reduced[82] as a result of cuspal perforations and tears (Fig. 5.7).

Sterilization

Glutaraldehyde and formaldehyde are frequently referred to as sterilants, although they are ineffective against slow viruses.[43] In this context, aldehyde-containing sterilants may be more accurately described as high-level disinfectants. The effectiveness of glutaraldehyde as a sterilant for bacteria, fungi, and enteroviruses is dependent on conditions (concentration, pH, temperature, exposure time) similar to those needed for tissue fixation.[21] The optimal sterilization conditions may be determined by comparing calculated *D* values, or the time required (in hours) to kill 90% of the microbes present. Studies of this type (death kinetic curves and calculated *D* values) indicate that glutaraldehyde and formaldehyde are effective sterilants; however, low concentrations of glutaraldehyde (e.g., those used for BP processing) are less effective against mycobacteria and spores of bacteria (*Bacillus subtilis*, *Clostridium sporogenes*) and fungi (*Chaetomium globosum*).[21,99] These findings were substantiated by the report of contamination by *Mycobacterium chelonii* of a limited number of PAVs implanted in patients.[100,101] Formaldehyde 4% is a more effective antifungal and antimicrobial agent than are low concentrations (0.2% and 0.625%) of glutaraldehyde. Thus following glutaraldehyde fixation xenografts are now routinely sterilized using formaldehyde-containing solutions.

Mounting

To facilitate their implantation, BPs in current use are mounted on stents; in contrast, most allografts are implanted directly without stents. There are two basic types of stents: rigid (Fig. 5.8) and flexible (Figs. 5.9 and 5.10). The degree of flexibility of the different types of "flexible" stents varies considerably. Stents are composed of an outer sewing ring; a ring-like structural frame with three stent posts or struts, which provide structural support to the commissures; and a covering layer of cloth (usually Dacron or Teflon). In rigid stents the frame is composed of metal; in flexible stents it is made of plastic or thin metal wire that allows a slight bending motion of the stent posts during BP opening

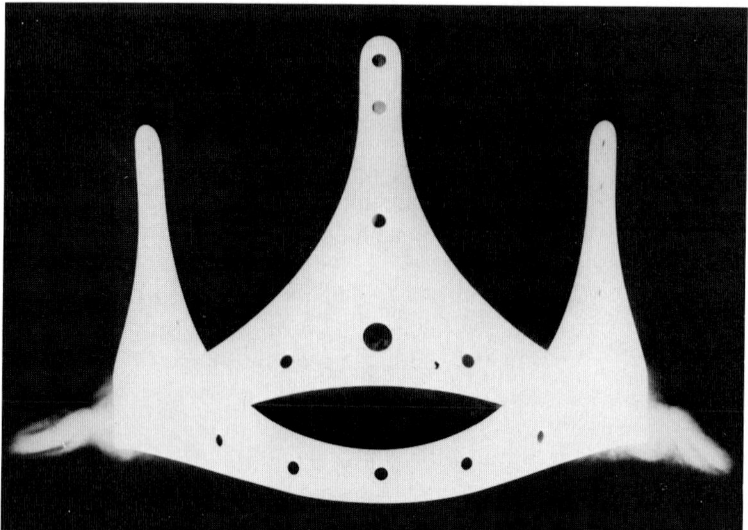

Figure 5.8. Radiograph of an unimplanted bovine pericardial BP mounted on a rigid metallic stent. ×3.

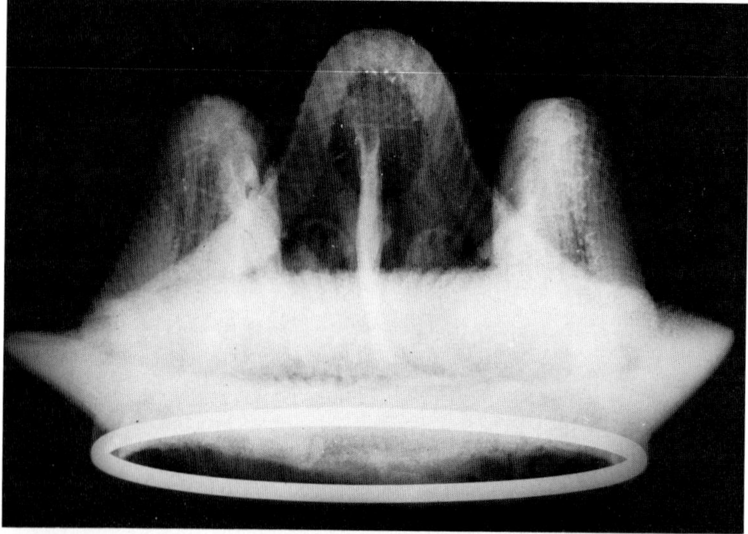

Figure 5.9. Radiograph of an unimplanted PAV xenograft mounted on a flexible polymeric stent with a radiopaque ring incorporated into the inflow aspect of the sewing ring. ×3.

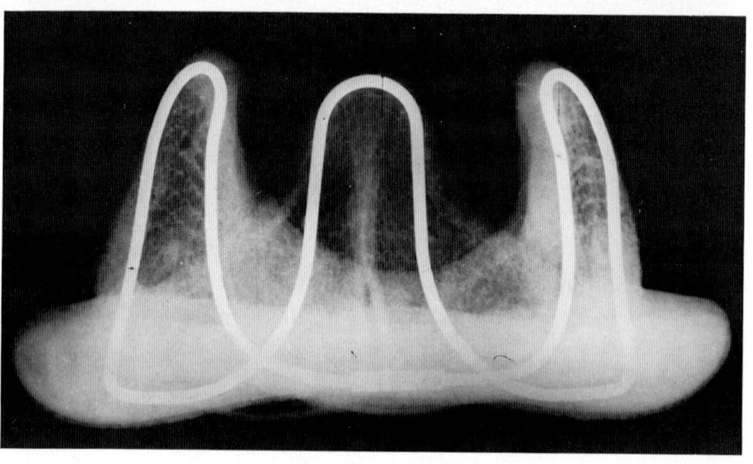

Figure 5.10. Radiograph of an unimplanted PAV xenograft showing a flexible stent consisting of a wireform that also serves as a radiopaque marker. ×3.

and closing. With many types of BPs the sewing rings vary in configuration according to whether the BP is to be implanted in the semilunar or the atrioventricular position in order to conform to the differences in surgical implantation technique (i.e., from the outflow or the inflow side, respectively) in these two positions. However, practically all BPs are configured as trileaflet valves, regardless of the position of implantation. Although stents have been designed to duplicate some of the features of the native aortic valve annulus, stented BPs do not undergo the same changes in dimensions and geometry (systolic expansion, diastolic contraction, and systolic outward deflection of the commissures) as do the annulus and cusps of native valves during the cardiac cycle. The main reason is that the stents of BPs are not expansile, as are the native valve annuli. For this reason the mechanical forces to which BP leaflets are subjected during opening and closing are higher and less evenly distributed than those acting on native valve leaflets.[35,102–108]

When the native aortic valve is completely open the cusps are flat, under tension, and at constant length.[104] When PAVs open, the shape of the orifice may be circular or some variation of a circular form, depending on specific conditions of pressure and flow.[104] These shapes result from a reversal of curvature of the cusps in a nonexpansile stent.[103] The compressive forces associated with this cuspal motion are thought to be important causes of tissue dehiscence and tears because they lead to fracture of the leaflet collagen bundles.[39] These failure modes were relatively frequent in early models of PAVs, which were mounted on rigid stents[30–32,109]; thus flexible stents have been developed to reduce the occurrence of primary tissue failure by dissipating the stresses associated with leaflet motion, particularly with leaflet closure.[109] To further reduce the incidence of PAV xenograft leaflet dehiscence, a cloth bias strip (buttress) is sewn over the PAV–stent interface to reduce the stresses that otherwise would be applied to the sutures that attach the tissue to the stent.[110]

Two general approaches to flexible stent design have been selected to minimize the stresses on BP leaflet tissue during opening and closure: (1) a stent that has a rigid inlet and in which the stent posts undergo some degree of outward motion during valve opening and inward motion during valve closure[109,111] (Fig. 5.9); and (2) a newly designed stent made of thin wire configured such that it allows expansion and contraction of the inflow orifice as well as radial deflections of the stent posts[112] (Fig. 5.10). The long-term durability of BPs with this stent design has not been assessed.

The materials used to fabricate flexible stents range from polypropylene and polyacetal resin to metal wire.[109,111,112] Ideally, the materials selected for stent fabrication should have a high resistance to fatigue induced by cyclic bending (i.e., to avoid stent fracture) and should undergo minimal plastic deformation (creep). Progressive inward deflection of polypropylene stent posts has been attributed to creep, external compression of oversized valves, and tissue ingrowth into the stent cloth.[113–116]

Continuing modifications that have been made in the design of stents for PAVs include changes in the technique of mounting tissue on the stent (i.e., mounting the PAV higher on the stent increases the effective orifice size), the configuration of the metal or plastic structural core, the height of the stent posts, and the materials contained within the sewing ring[111,112]; reducing the muscle shelf to a minimum; and development of a "modified orifice valve" in which the right coronary cusp (which contains the "muscle shelf") has been replaced by a nonmuscle shelf cusp from another aortic valve[117] and a "supraannular valve" in which the sewing ring has a scalloped configuration resembling that of the native aortic root.[118]

Rigid (Fig. 5.8) and flexible stents have been used to fabricate bovine pericardial BPs.[119] The attachment of the tissue to the stent posts has presented continuing problems in the design of pericardial BPs. The use of an attachment or alignment suture placed near the top of the stent posts (Fig. 5.11) creates an area of localized high mechanical stress that can lead to cuspal tears near the commissures.[120–122] This important complication limits the durability of pericardial BPs.[123–128] These valves also have developed perforations secondary to abrasions caused by contact, during leaflet opening, between peri-

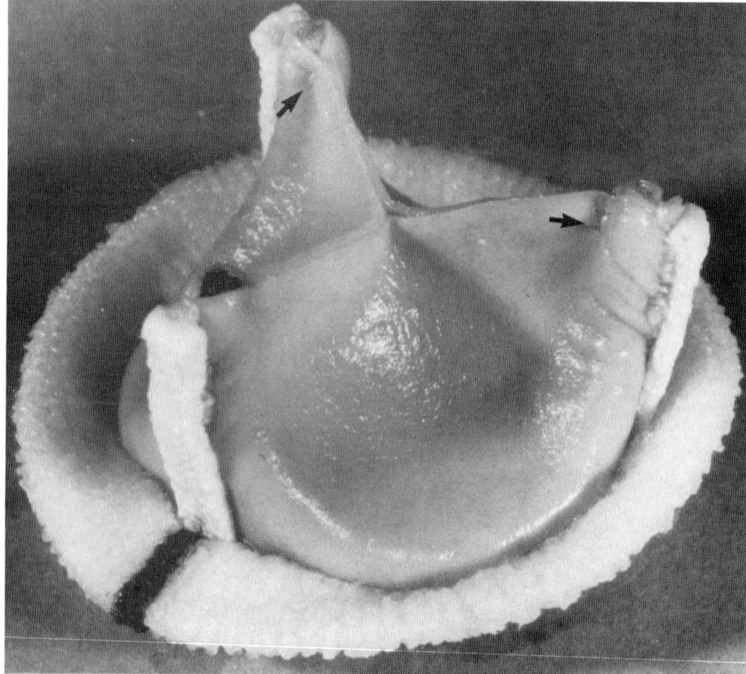

Figure 5.11. Unimplanted bovine pericardial BP illustrating an alignment suture (arrow) to facilitate leaflet coaptation. Bias strips also have been applied to the outside of the stent posts. ×4.

cardial tissue and either the cloth covering the portion of the stent between two stent posts or the fabric buttress on the outside of the stent post.[121]

One innovation involves the use of "low profile" stents with short stent posts to reduce the bulk of the BP and to increase its effective orifice area.[119,129] A few prototype designs of low profile stents for pericardial valves have utilized sharply pointed stent posts, and they have been recently reported to induce myocardial damage, ventricular aneurysms, and ventricular ruptures because of contact with the left ventricular wall either during or after implantation in the mitral position.[130] Nevertheless, such complications also have been reported in association with both pericardial and porcine BPs having the usual, blunter types of stent posts.[130]

Cuspal dehiscence in antibiotic-treated allografts mounted on rigid stents has been reported to occur to a greater extent than in similarly prepared but unstented allografts.[131] The development of a flexible stent and the use of a bias strip for mounting aortic valve allografts were reported not to reduce the incidence of tissue dehiscence.[132]

Allografts

A renewed interest in the use of pulmonary and aortic valve allografts (homografts) has occurred, as the long-term durability expectations of BPs have not been realized, particularly in children and young adults.[59,66] Use of the aortic valve allograft began approximately 30 years ago[133] and the first subcoronary artery implantation of an aortic valve allograft was performed in 1962.[134,135] In 1966 reconstruction of the right ventricular outflow tract was accomplished using an aortic valve allograft.[136] The primary limitation of the use of allografts as cardiac valve substitutes centers about the logistical problems of collecting, processing, testing for infectious diseases, and maintaining an adequate inventory of various sizes of allograft valves. A variety of preimplantation processing techniques have been reported, ranging from treatment by chemicals, antibiotics, and irradiation to freezing, lyophilization, and cryopreservation.[137–152] The long-term clinical performance of allografts is influenced by the method of preimplantation processing as well as by the mode of storage.[137–152]

Sterilization

Allograft disinfection or sterilization has been accomplished by a variety of techniques, including exposure to ethylene oxide gas; immersion in solutions containing glutaraldehyde, formaldehyde, β-propiolactone, or antibiotics; and gamma or electron beam irradiation. Ideally, the method of sterilization should not alter the morphology or the mechanical properties of the allograft. Sterilants such as aldehydes, ethylene oxide, and β-propiolactone do alter the mechanical properties of the valve, whereas sterilization by means of exposure to low levels (e.g., 2 megarads) of gamma or electron beam irradiation or disinfection using antibiotics does not.[146,153] An increased rate of cusp rupture has been reported to occur in allografts that were sterilized using ethylene oxide or β-propiolactone.[154,155] In addition to a reduction in tensile strength, β-propiolactone sterilization induces cuspal thickening with a concomitant decrease in surface area (i.e., tissue shrinkage).[153] The resultant alteration of cuspal geometry may affect leaflet coaptation, thereby predisposing allografts to regurgitation. It should be noted that β-propiolactone and ethylene oxide are carcinogenic.[156,157]

Sterilization methods utilizing low doses of radiation and disinfection by exposure to high concentrations of antibiotics do not alter the mechanical properties or geometry of allograft cusps; however, these methods do result in the loss of cell viability. Most allografts currently implanted worldwide are treated with combinations of antibiotics such as gentamicin, lincomycin, colistimethate, kanamycin, cefoxitin, vancomycin, polymyxin B, and amphotericin B[142] (personal communication, Virginia Tissue Bank).

Storage

Lyophilization (freeze-drying), immersion in antibiotics, and freezing have all been employed as methods of allograft storage.[138,150,151,158–160] Most of the allografts currently in clinical use are either stored in nutrient solutions with antibiotics at 4°C or are cryopreserved, frozen, and subsequently stored in liquid nitrogen vapor.[145,148,149,151,161] Lyophilization is a convenient method of storage. The results of short-term implantation in animals suggest that the performance of lyophilized valves is comparable to that of fresh allografts.[138,162] However, the tensile strength is decreased as a result of the lyophilization process. This decrease may account for the cuspal ruptures that have been reported to occur in lyophilized allografts implanted in patients.[153,163] Primary cuspal ruptures occur either at the cusp–aortic wall junction or in the free edge in close proximity to a commissure.[138] Both of these rupture sites are in regions of high compressive and tensile stress, implying that lyophilization has altered the allograft collagen by reducing its mechanical durability. In addition to altered mechanical properties, lyophilized allografts have been reported to be more susceptible to calcification, although there is great variability among individual valves stored in this manner.[164]

Storage in antibiotics has proved to be effective.[143,161,165] Neither the mechanical properties nor the morphology of the principal connective tissue components (i.e., collagen and elastin) are altered; however, the number of viable cells in the allograft is gradually reduced. Studies of allografts stored (4°C) in Hanks' balanced salt solution or nutrient medium indicate that cellular viability can be maintained for short periods of time (0.5–1 week) followed by a marked reduction (2–4 weeks) and loss of viability (1 month).[142,161] Thus whether the allograft is stored in antibiotics, Hanks' balanced salt solution, or nutrient medium, there is a marked reduction in the number of viable cells as the storage time increases. Most of the allografts currently implanted clinically have adequately preserved collagen and elastin but have undergone a marked reduction in the number of viable cells.[161]

The contribution of the maintenance of the viability of valvular endothelial and connective tissue cells to the long-term durability of allografts is unknown. Morphologic studies of explanted allografts indicate that primary valve failure results from tissue deterioration (stretching, thinning, perforation, tearing) that occurs in nonviable allografts and in acellular regions of viable allografts.[142] As a result of these findings, cryogenic technology is being used to enhance the preservation of allograft cell viability during

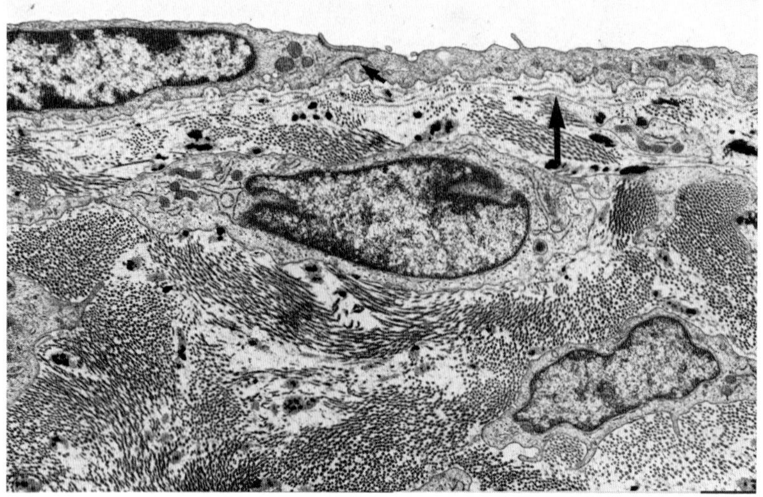

Figure 5.12. Transmission electron micograph of the outflow surface of a native PAV. Note the presence of an intact endothelial cell layer, a cell–cell junctional complex (arrowhead), and reduplication of basement membrane (arrow) material. Fibroblasts, collagen fibrils, and elastic fibers (stained black) are seen in the fibrosa. Kajikawa stain. ×9000.

storage.[148,149] Contemporary cryopreservation protocols include pulmonary and aortic valve allograft collection, usually at multiple organ harvesting within 6 hours (category 1), but no longer than 24 hours (category 2), after death. Following antibiotic sterilization (24 hours at 37°C or 48 hours at 4°C) the allograft is placed in nutrient medium containing 10% dimethylsulfoxide (DMSO), control-rate-frozen (1°C/min) to −40°C, and stored in liquid nitrogen vapor (−150° to −190°C) (personal communication, Virginia Tissue Bank).

Morphology of Unimplanted Heart Valve Substitutes

Porcine Aortic Valve Bioprostheses

The PAV consists of three asymmetric cusps and the adjacent portion of the aortic ring and aortic root. The right coronary cusp of the PAV is larger than the other two cusps; its basal region contains a layer of cardiac myocytes (muscle shelf) that is an extension of the ventricular septum. Because of the presence of this muscle shelf, the opening of the right coronary cusp is delayed or incomplete compared to that of the other two cusps. The devitalized myocytes in the muscle shelf frequently calcify after PAV implantation.

Histologically, three regions are apparent when the PAV is cut from the free edge to the base, flat-embedded, and sectioned: the ventricularis (inflow side), the spongiosa (central portion), and the fibrosa (outflow side)[31] (Figs. 5.1 and 5.2). The native PAV is covered by a layer of endothelial cells; however, most of these cells are lost as a result of preimplantation handling and processing (Figs. 5.12 and 5.13). Scanning electron microscopic studies show that few endothelial cells are present on the surfaces of the processed PAVs, the cusps of which are typically covered by basement membrane. Reduplication of the basement membrane is frequently observed in the outflow surface (Fig. 5.12). The prominence of elastic fibers in the ventricularis is a useful means of identifying this region of the PAV cusp (Fig. 5.13). The spongiosa consists of loosely arranged collagen fibers, elastic fibers, and an abundance of proteoglycans (Fig. 5.14). A marked reduction in proteoglycan content in the spongiosa is observed following preimplantation processing of PAVs. Collagen is the principal structural component of the fibrosa. The collagen is arranged in wavy or crimped bundles oriented parallel to the free edge of the cusp. The collagen bundles progressively thicken as they converge on and become an integral part of the commissure. These prominent collagen bundles or cords present within the fibrosa are a convenient means of identifying the outflow side of the PAV. The morphology of these bundles indicates whether the valve was fixed at high or low pres-

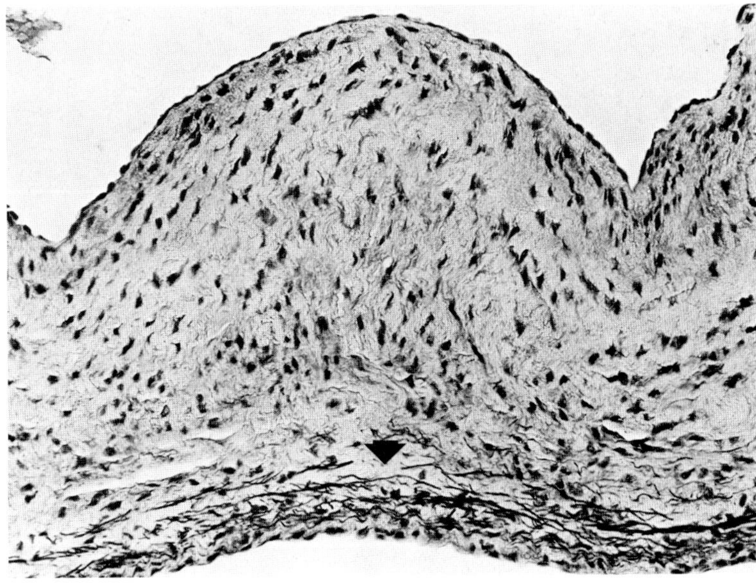

FIGURE 5.13. Representative histologic section of a freshly harvested native PAV showing an endothelial cell lining on both inflow (bottom) and outflow (top) surfaces. Elastic fibers (arrowhead) are abundant within the ventricularis. Movat pentachrome stain. ×240.

sure (Figs. 5.1 and 5.2). The prominence of the collagen cords and the cuspal thickness are reduced if the PAV has undergone high-pressure fixation. The degree of autolysis of the cellular components (fibroblasts, myofibroblasts, mesenchymal cells, cardiac myocytes) of the valve is variable in commercially available PAVs. The staining characteristics with hematoxylin and eosin are altered by glutaraldehyde fixation, resulting in a decrease in basophilia and an increase in eosinophila.[31,166]

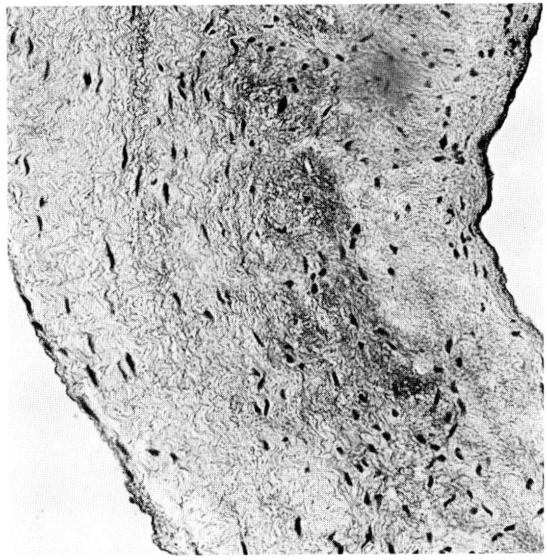

FIGURE 5.14. Representative histologic section of a native PAV demonstrating the presence of proteoglycans in the spongiosa. Alcian blue/PAS stain. ×240.

A variety of nondestructive optical techniques, such as differential interference contrast (Nomarski), darkfield, and polarized light microscopy were evaluated to determine their utility for studying BP collagen morphology.[40] Polarized light microscopy (incident and transmitted) is the preferred optical method for evaluating the extent of collagen waviness and orientation (with respect to the valvular free edge) of the collagen bundles in wet, intact BP cusps (Figs. 5.15 and 5.16).

Collagen configuration and orientation differs in various regions of the PAV. Collagen bundles in the fibrosa and collagen cords are wavy and are oriented parallel to the free edge (Figs. 5.15B and 5.16B), whereas those present in the ventricularis are straight and multidirectional. Other variations (e.g., bends or kinks in the paracommissural cords) have also been observed,[40] although their significance is uncertain. Similar bends were observed in motion pictures of valvular opening and closure in high-pressure-fixed PAVs but not in low-pressure-fixed PAVs; these bends or kinks were present in the leaflet free edges in close proximity to the valve commissures.[25]

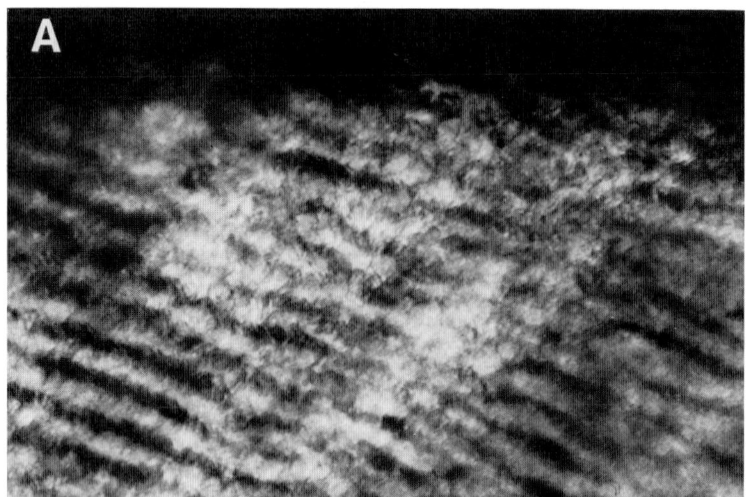

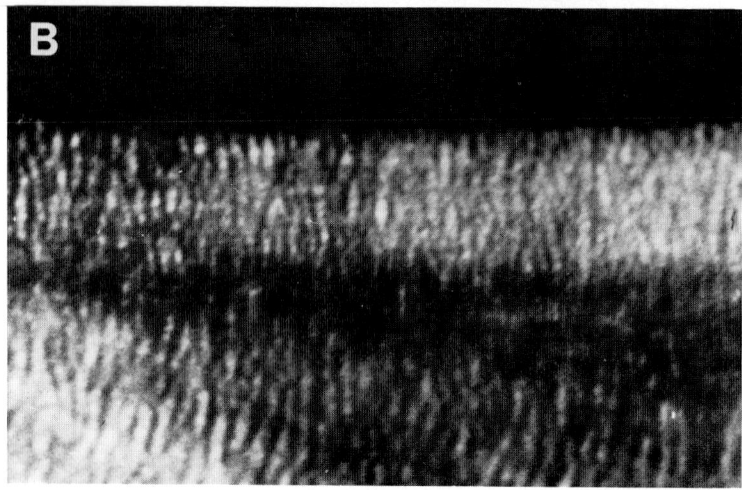

Figure 5.15. Transmitted polarized light micrographs demonstrating the orientation of collagen bundles with respect to the free edge (top) in a bovine pericardial BP (**A**) and a PAV xenograft (**B**). The collagen bundles in (**A**) transect the free edge, whereas in (**B**) they course parallel to the free edge. **A**, ×150; **B**, ×45.

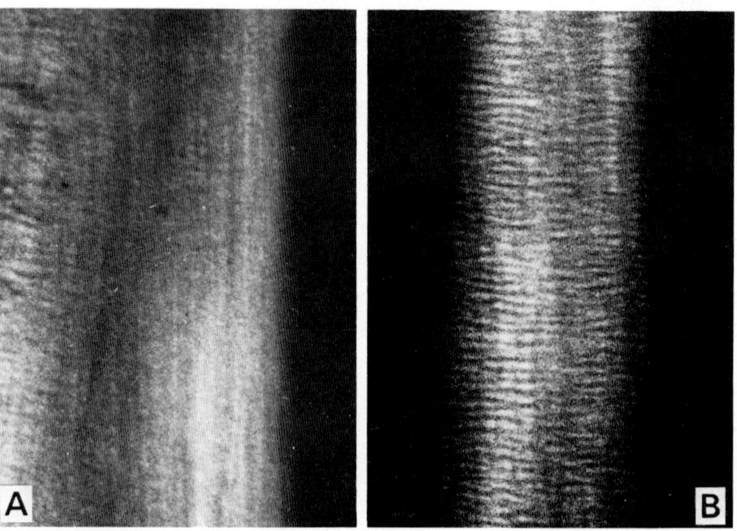

Figure 5.16. Polarized light micrographs depicting the differences seen in collagen bundle crimp in collagen cords present on the outflow surface of high-pressure-fixed (**A**) and low-pressure-fixed (**B**) PAV xenografts. The collagen bundles are straightened as a result of high-pressure fixation (**A**), whereas the native wavy collagen morphology is retained following low-pressure fixation (**B**). **A**, ×75; **B**, ×45.

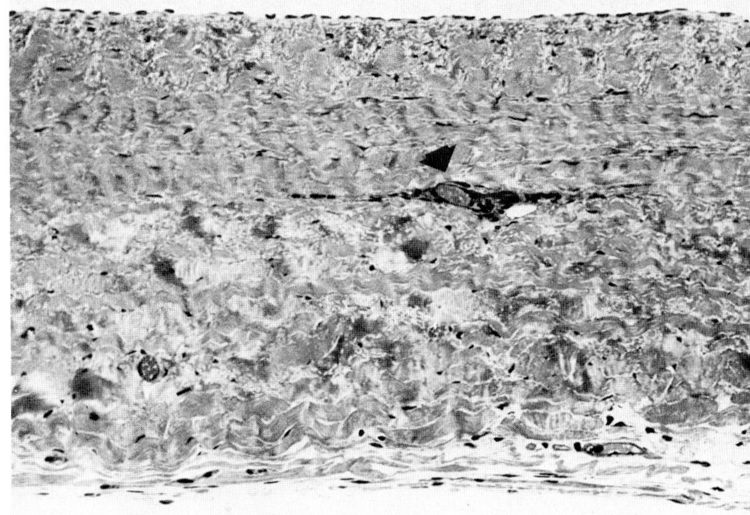

FIGURE 5.17. Histologic section of bovine parietal pericardium that has not undergone preimplantation processing. Note the mesothelial cells on the serosal surface (top) and a blood vessel (arrowhead). Glycol methacrylate-embedded tissue; alkaline toluidine blue stain. ×150.

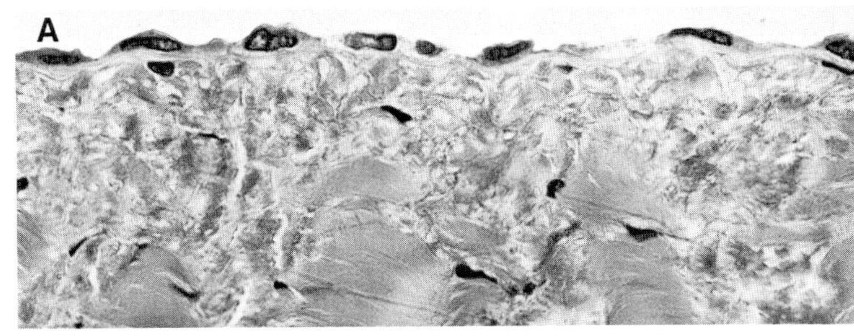

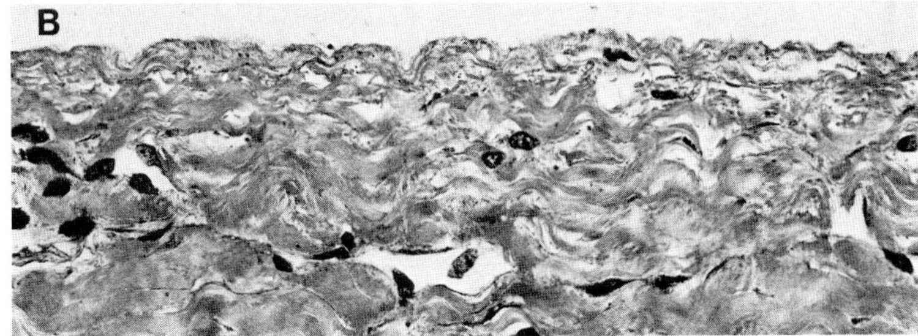

FIGURE 5.18. Histologic sections comparing the outflow (serosal) surface of native bovine parietal pericardium (**A**) and an unimplanted bovine pericardial BP (**B**). Glycol methacrylate-embedded tissue; alkaline toluidine blue stain. ×700.

Pericardial Bioprostheses

Most of the pericardial BPs are fabricated from bovine parietal pericardium, with the exception of the Polystan valve, in which porcine parietal pericardium is used.[167] Pericardial BPs are most frequently configured into trileaflet valves; however, monocusp and bicuspid valves also have been designed.[1,3,5,12–14]

Parietal pericardium is composed of three layers; a serosal layer, consisting of mesothelial cells; the fibrosa, containing collagen bundles, elastic fibers, nerves, blood vessels, and lymphatics; and epipericardial connective tissue, composed of loosely arranged collagen and elastic fibers (Fig. 5.17). Fibroblasts are present in the fibrosa and epipericardial connective tissue; occasionally, adipose tissue, histiocytes, and mast cells are also seen. Preimplantation processing results in loss of the mesothelial cell layer (Fig. 5.18). Noticeable differences are evident on macroscopic examination of the inflow

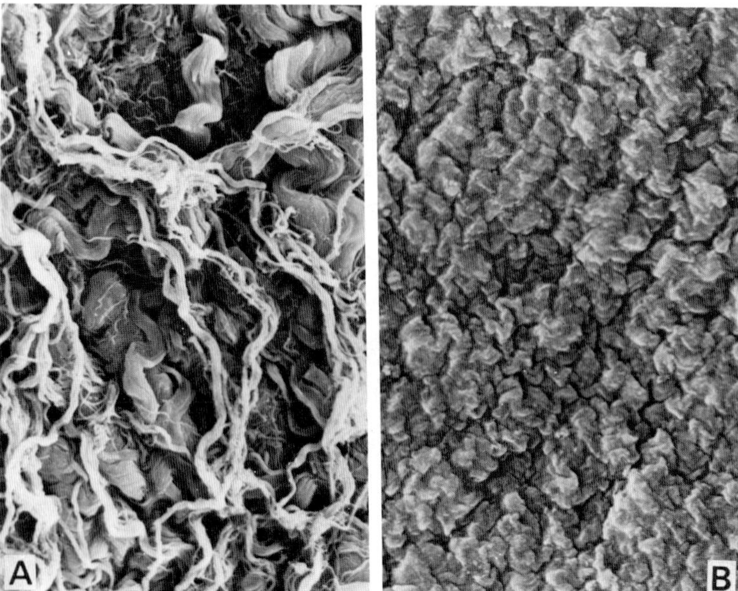

Figure 5.19. Representative scanning electron micrographs of the inflow (**A**) and outflow (**B**) surfaces of an unimplanted bovine pericardial BP. Note the contrasting appearance of the rough inflow side (**A**) and the smoother outflow side (**B**). ×900.

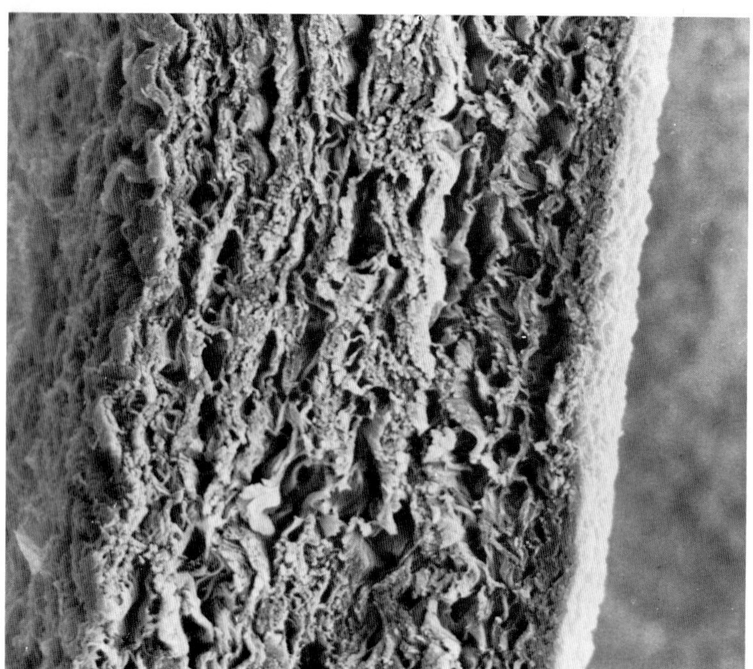

Figure 5.20. Scanning electron micrograph of the free edge of an unimplanted bovine pericardial BP. The inflow surface is on the left and the outflow surface on the right. Note the stratified, wavy, slightly separated appearance of the collagen bundles within the out surface at the free edge. Compare to Figure 5.17, which shows a histologic section of the same biomaterial. ×1000.

(epipericardial) and outflow (serosal) surfaces. The inflow side of the pericardial BP is rough. Whereas the outflow side is smooth. This difference is striking when observed by means of scanning electron microscopy (Fig. 5.19). The serosal surface is covered by basement membrane with underlying collagen fibrils; in contrast, coarse collagen bundles are present on the epipericardial surface.[168] Nondestructive optical methods utilizing polarized light microscopy have revealed that the collagen bundles in parietal pericardium are overlapping and multidirectional rather than highly oriented and layered. The waviness or crimp of collagen bundles is more pronounced than that seen in PAVs, and the collagen bundles are not always oriented parallel to the free edge, as they are in aortic valves (Fig. 5.15).[40,166]

Pulmonary and Aortic Valve Allografts

The morphologic descriptions of pulmonary and aortic valve allografts are discussed together, as the histologic differences between the two semilunar valves are minimal. When grossly compared to the aortic valve, however, the pulmonary valve is thinner and more delicate.

Human semilunar valves consist of the same three distinct histologic layers (ventricularis, spongiosa, fibrosa) found in porcine aortic valves. The ventricularis (inflow side), which may be regarded as an extension of the ventricular endocardium, has prominent elastic fibers oriented perpendicular to the free edge of the cusp. It is thickened along the coaptation surface, forming a fibroelastic nodule in the center of the free edge (nodulus Arantii and nodulus Morgagni, aortic and pulmonary valves, respectively). The central portion, or spongiosa, consists of loosely organized collagen fibers, fibroblasts, myofibroblasts, poorly differentiated mesenchymal cells, and proteoglycans. The fibrosa is composed of collagen bundles oriented parallel to the free edge, fibroblasts, and a small number of elastic fibers. These elastic fibers may appear as a distinct layer known as the arterialis near the outflow surface in the basal region of the cusp. Lastly, the cuspal surface is covered by a layer of endothelial cells. The human aortic and pulmonic valves do not contain a "muscle shelf" such as that present in the right coronary cusp of the porcine aortic valve.[169,170]

Progressive morphologic changes occur in human aortic valves with increasing age. These changes are more common in men and include degeneration of collagen fibers, formation of a fibroelastic "spur" along the coaptation surface, a decrease in the number of fibroblasts and in proteoglycan content, and accumulation of lipid and calcific deposits.[138,155,171] Thus donor criteria for allograft heart valves usually include an age restriction (e.g., 2 months to 50 years) and lack of a medical history of previous cardiac surgery, uncontrolled hypertension, significant murmurs, rheumatic fever, malignant disease, and autoimmune or vascular diseases[149,172] (personal communication, Virginia Tissue Bank).

Allograft preimplantation processing developed out of the need to maintain an inventory or bank of allografts of various sizes for use as cardiac valve substitutes. The spectrum of allograft preimplantation processing ranges from none to treatment with aldehydes, antibiotics, β-propiolactone, ethylene oxide, irradiation, lyophilization, and freezing. The effects of these various processes on allograft morphology may be generally placed in one of the following categories: a nonviable allograft retaining the characteristic semilunar valve morphology (e.g., long-term antibiotic storage, aldehyde-treated, irradiation-sterilized); a nonviable allograft with disrupted valvular morphology (e.g., β-propiolactone-treated and lyophilized); and an allograft with reduced cellularity and retention of semilunar valve morphology (e.g., stored for short times in antibiotic-containing solutions, cryopreserved, frozen, and thawed). Allografts processed by lyophilization have a "honeycomb" histologic appearance, indicating that the connective tissue components have been disrupted by ice crystal formation.[155]

The unstented aortic valve allograft is most frequently used for aortic valve replacement and reconstruction of the right ventricular outflow tract (RVOT).[173,174] The availability of aortic valve allografts is limited, which has reduced their use in RVOT reconstruction, although favorable long-term results have been obtained with aortic valve allografts compared to conduits bearing xenograft valves.[175–179] The pulmonary allograft has been suggested as an alternative to the aortic valve allograft for RVOT reconstruction. Pulmonary valves may be harvested from donors in which the aortic valve would routinely be discarded owing to the presence of atherosclerotic and calcific lesions. The harvesting of pulmonary valves would increase the availability of valvular allografts for use in RVOT reconstruction. It has also been suggested that the pulmonary valve may have a better hemodynamic performance and may be less prone to calcification,

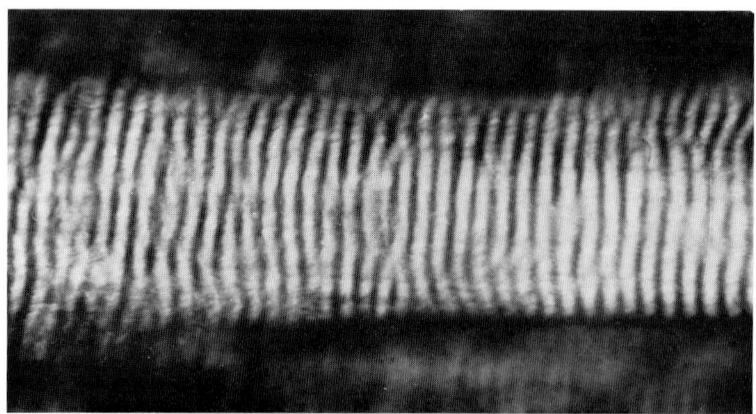

Figure 5.21. Transmitted polarized light micrograph of a cryopreserved pulmonary valve allograft depicting retention of collagen waviness (crimp) in collagen cords on the outflow surface. This repeating birefringent banding pattern is indicative of crimped collagen morphology. ×120.

which typically occurs in the aortic wall of aortic valve allografts.[161]

We have evaluated the effects of a contemporary method of allograft collection (which involves antibiotic treatment, cryopreservation, and freezing and thawing) on valvular morphology. This preliminary study included the collection of human pulmonary valves (mean donor age 32 years, range 12–46 years; six male patients, four female patients with documented warm times (i.e., time elapsed from death to excision of the heart; mean 3.3 ± 4 hours, range 0.20–8.75 hours) and cold times (length of time the heart is stored at 4°C before the initiation of allograft dissection and treatment with antibiotics; mean 15.7 ± 6.6 hours, range 6.5–18.0 hours). The valves were disinfected, cryopreserved, frozen, and thawed; they were: disinfected by immersion for 48 hours at 4°C in nutrient medium (RPMI 1640) containing polymyxin B (100 μg/ml), cefoxitin (240 μg/ml), vancomycin (50 μg/ml), lincomycin (120 μg/ml), and amphotericin B (100 μg/ml); transferred to fresh nutrient medium supplemented with 10% fetal calf serum (heat-inactivated) and 10% DMSO; control-rate-frozen (1°C/minute) to −40°C; stored in liquid nitrogen vapor (−150° to −190°C) for up to 35.6 weeks (0.7, 3.1, 5.7, and 35.6 weeks, respectively); and thawed by immersion in a 40°C waterbath (3–4 minutes). The DMSO concentration was reduced to trace amounts by means of a four-step dilution procedure using nutrient medium. The allografts were then immediately fixed for histologic study by immersion using 4% formaldehyde/1% glutaraldehyde in 0.1 *M* phosphate buffer pH 7.4. In addition to the cryopreserved pulmonary valves ($n = 4$), freshly excised ($n = 7$) and antibiotic-treated ($n = 5$) pulmonary valve cusps were fixed for morphologic studies. The morphologic studies included gross examination; nondestructive evaluation of intact cusps using polarized light microscopy; histologic examination of frozen sections stained with oil red O and of sections of glycol methacrylate- and paraffin-embedded tissues stained with hematoxylin-eosin, von Kossa, toluidine blue, Congo red, Masson trichrome, and alcian blue-PAS methods; scanning electron microscopy; and transmission electron microscopy.

The delicate morphologic features of the pulmonary valve were seen following gross and polarized light microscopic examination of intact wet cusps (e.g., immersion fixation). In contrast to the findings in clinical PAV xenografts, the extent and magnitude of collagen bundle waviness or crimp within the fibrosa and collagen cords of the pulmonary cusp were striking (Figs. 5.21–5.24). The degree of collagen waviness was not altered by antibiotic sterilization, cryopreservation, or freezing and thawing.

Histologic and ultrastructural examination demonstrated the presence of a heterogeneous or patchy distribution of endothelial cells on the cuspal surfaces of unprocessed (i.e., warm time less than 9 hours) pulmonary valves (Figs. 5.25–5.27). Progressive loss of endothelial cells was noted following antibiotic treatment, cryopres-

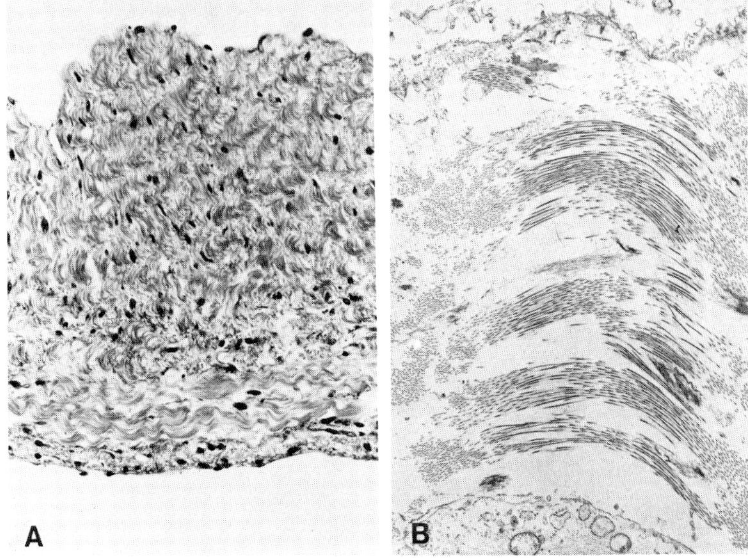

FIGURE 5.22. Histologic (**A**) and ultrathin (**B**) sections demonstrating retention of collagen crimp in an antibiotic-treated, cryopreserved human pulmonary allograft. **A:** 1 μm thick section of glycol methacrylate-embedded tissue; hematoxylin/eosin stain. ×150. **B:** uranyl acetate/lead citrate stain. ×2850.

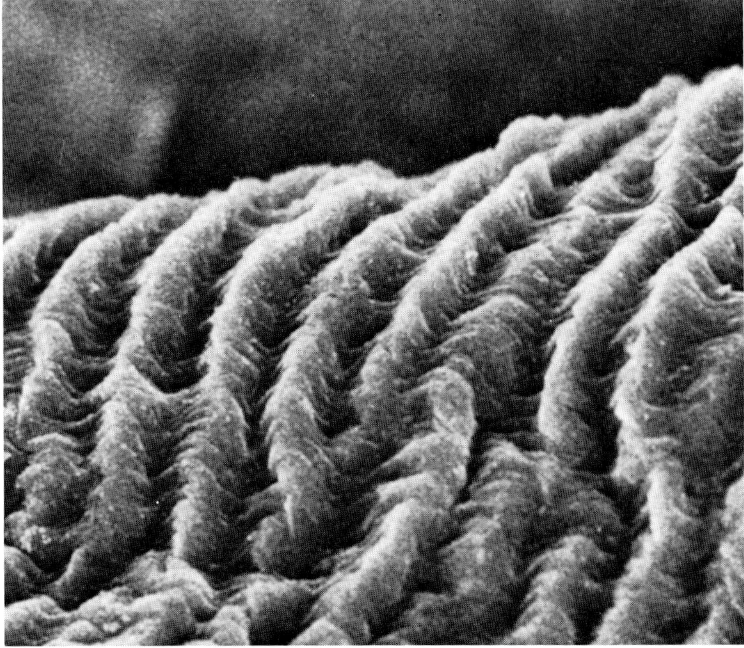

FIGURE 5.23. Representative scanning electron micrograph of the free edge of an antibiotic-treated, cryopreserved, and thawed pulmonary allograft demonstrating marked retention of collagen crimp. ×750.

ervation, freezing, and thawing (Fig. 5.28). Scanning electron microscopy was particularly useful for evaluating these changes (Fig. 5.26). The endothelial cells that remained had prominent round nuclei and few microvilli, and they were randomly distributed on the cuspal surface as either single cells or in clusters. Exposed basement membrane and collagen bundles were seen in regions of denuded endothelial cells.

Proteoglycans, evaluated by staining with alcian blue–PAS, were present throughout the unprocessed allograft cusps, with the largest amount seen within the spongiosa. A progressive loss of proteoglycans occurred during allograft

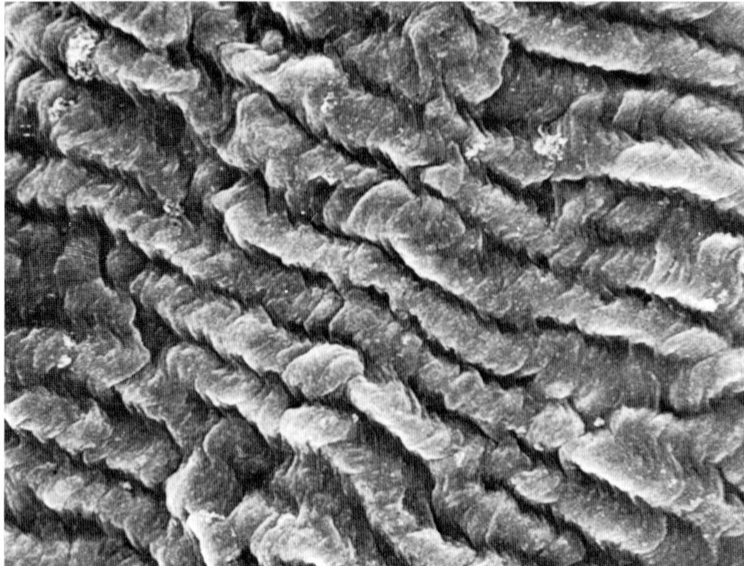

FIGURE 5.24. Representative scanning electron micrograph of the outflow surface of a cryopreserved pulmonary valve allograft illustrating the retention of collagen crimp. ×750.

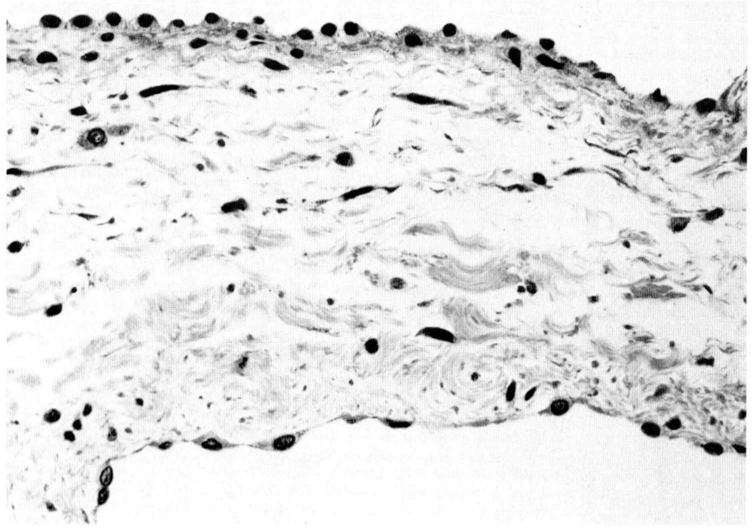

FIGURE 5.25. Histologic section of a human pulmonary valve fixed 5 hours after death demonstrates early morphologic changes in endothelial cells (e.g., nuclear pykosis and loss of their characteristic squamous shape). The outflow surface in on the top. Glycol methacrylate-embedded tissue; hematoxylin/eosin stain. ×240.

collection and preimplantation processing. Proteoglycans remained primarily within the spongiosa following antibiotic treatment, cryopreservation, freezing, and thawing. Although the proteoglycan content was not quantitatively measured, histologic comparisons demonstrated a greater retention of proteoglycans within the spongiosa in antibiotic-treated and cryopreserved pulmonary allografts than in PAV xenografts.

Cholesterol crystals and deposits of calcium, lipid, and amyloid were not observed within the cusps. Occasionally, small focal areas of increased eosinophilia were seen by light microscopy within the fibrosa of unprocessed, antibiotic-sterilized, and cryopreserved cusps. These regions of increased eosinophilia may have resulted from autolytic deterioration of collagen; however, the role played by further processing is unknown.

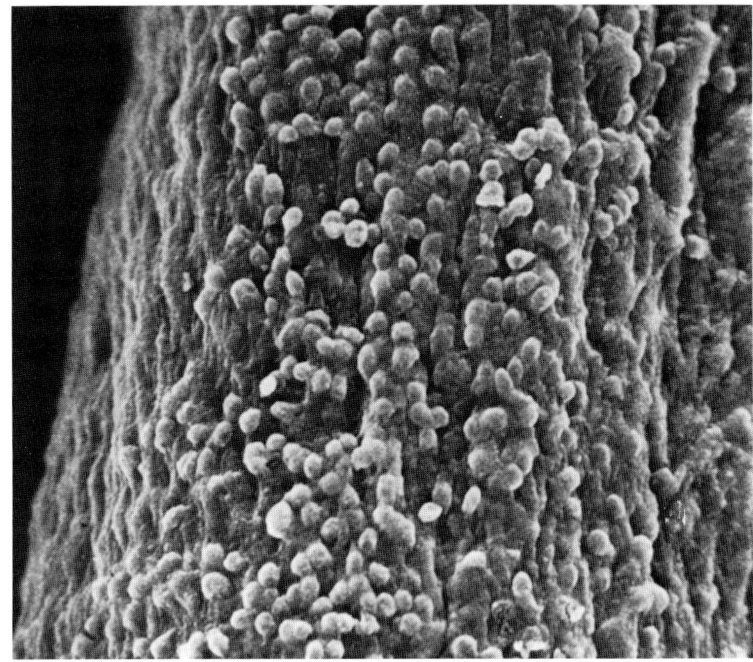

FIGURE 5.26. Scanning electron micrograph illustrating the patchy distribution of clusters of endothelial cells on the free edge of a human pulmonary valve fixed 5 hours after death. The endothelial cells no longer form a continuous monolayer. They have lost their characteristic squamous shape and appear rounded. Compare with Figure 5.25. ×450.

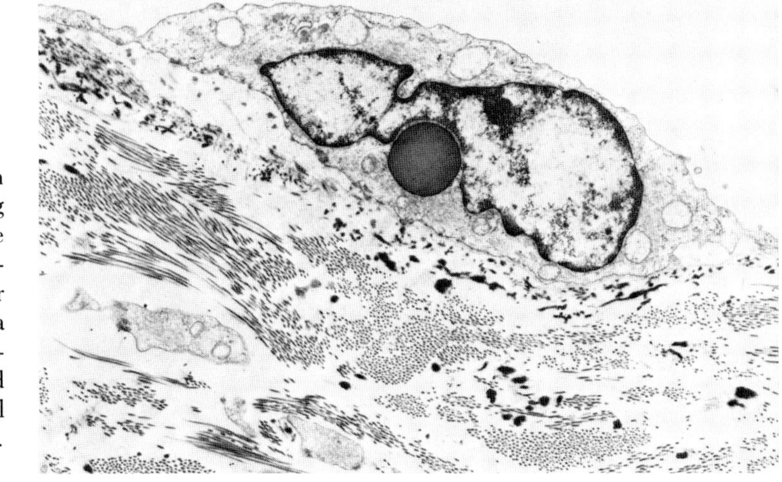

FIGURE 5.27. Transmission electron micrograph showing an intact endothelial cell on the outflow surface of a human pulmonary valve fixed 5 hours after death. Note the presence of a lipid droplet within the cytoplasm of the cell and dilated endoplasmic reticulum. Uranyl acetate/lead citrate stain. ×5400.

The ultrastructural morphology of collagen fibrils and elastic fibers was unremarkable, although prominent collagen bundle waviness was seen within the fibrosa (Fig. 5.22B). The following cell types were observed ultrastructurally: endothelial cells, fibroblasts, myofibroblasts, undifferentiated mesenchymal cells, macrophages, and cardiac myocytes. With additional processing, the overall cellularity (i.e., predominantly fibroblasts) progressively decreased, whereas the number of cells with pyknotic nuclei increased. It could not be determined whether this observed reduction in cellularity and altered nuclear morphology is indicative of cellular injury induced by antibiotic treatment, DMSO treatment, freezing and thawing, or hypoxia.

Fibroblasts and myofibroblasts were the principal cell types seen within the cusp (Fig. 5.29).

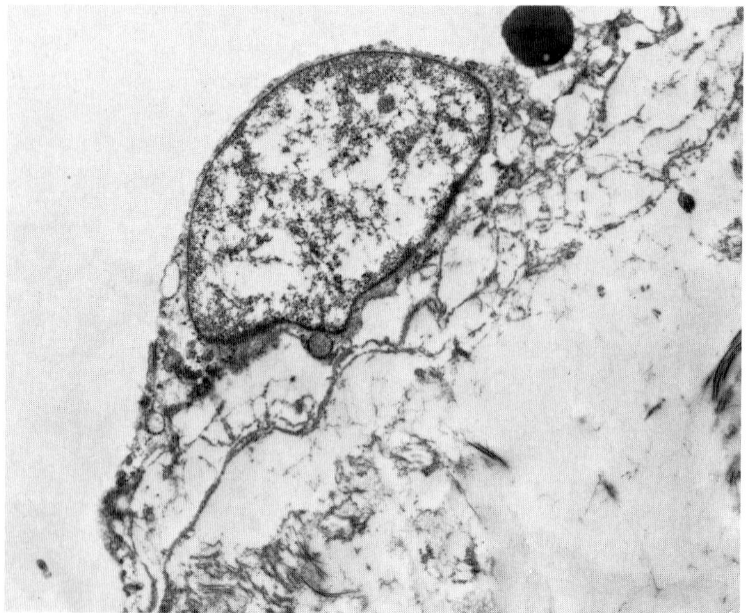

Figure 5.29. Transmission electron micrograph showing an injured endothelial cell on the outflow surface of an antibiotic-treated, cryopreserved human pulmonary valve allograft. Few endothelial cells remained on the valvular surface following cryopreservation; those that were present demonstrated markedly altered morphology. Uranyl acetate/lead citrate stain. ×7200.

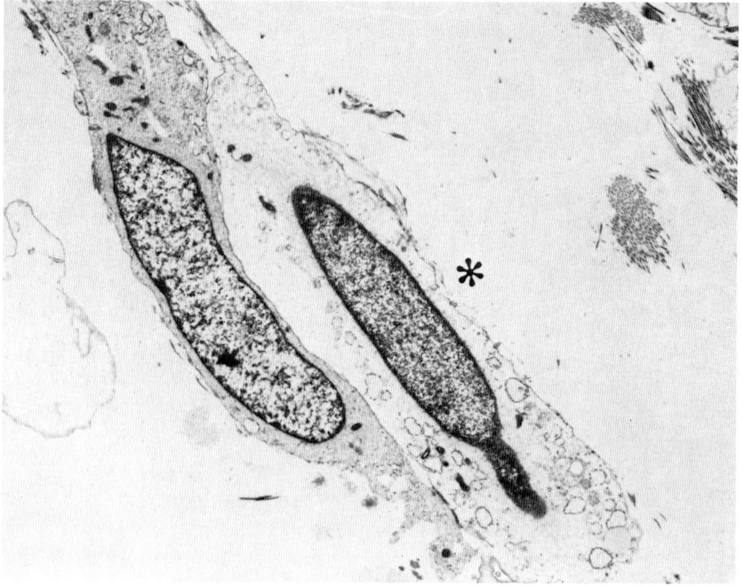

Figure 5.29. Transmission electron micrograph showing two fibroblasts in the fibrosa of a cryopreserved pulmonary valve allograft. One of the cells (asterisk) has been injured, resulting in dilation of endoplasmic reticulum, condensation of nuclear chromatin, and disruption of the plasma membrane; the other fibroblast is intact. Uranyl acetate/lead citrate stain. ×4350.

These cells develop a spectrum of cellular alterations as a result of allograft collection and processing, including cellular and mitochondrial swelling; dilation of endoplasmic reticulum; degranulation of rough endoplasmic reticulum; mitochondrial flocculent densities; autophagic and hydropic vacuoles; nuclear pyknosis, karyorrhexis, and karyolysis; lipid accumulation; membrane blebs; and disruption of organelle and plasma membranes. The longer the time elapsed before preimplantation processing is initiated, the greater the extent of cellular injury observed in the allograft tissue (Fig. 5.30).

Studies investigating the mechanisms of cellu-

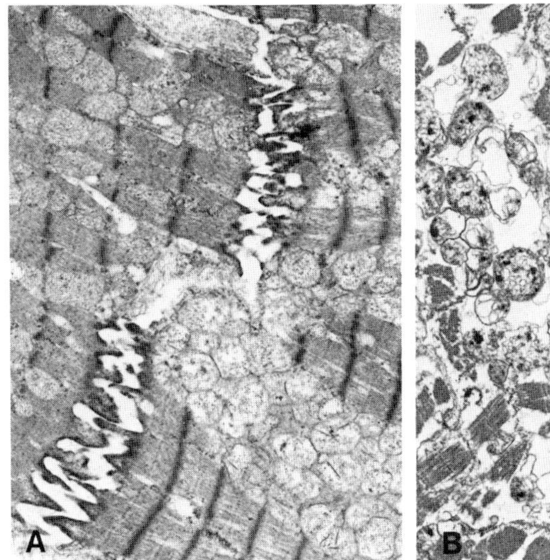

FIGURE 5.30. Transmission electron micrographs showing the morphologic appearance of human cardiac myocytes present in the basal region of the cusp of a cryopreserved pulmonary allograft. Dissociation of intercalated disks (**A**), mitochondrial swelling, and intramitochondrial flocculent densities (**B**) are seen. A: warm time 18 minutes; cold time 18 hours. B: warm time 5 hours 15 minutes; cold time 13 hours 45 minutes. Uranyl acetate/lead citrate stain. ×5400.

lar injury indicate that morphologic alterations such as cellular and mitochondrial swelling, dilation of the endoplasmic reticulum, hydropic vacuoles, and lipid accumulatiion are reversible changes, whereas the appearance of organelle and plasma membrane rupture, karyorrhexis, and karyolysis are hallmarks of irreversible damage. Factors such as cell type, the degree of differentiation, and the level of metabolic activity have been reported to predispose cells to cellular injury.[180] The morphologic findings of our preliminary study of cryopreserved, unimplanted human pulmonary valves suggest that metabolically active cells (e.g., endothelial cells and cardiac myocytes) are more sensitive to irreversible cellular injury resulting from allograft harvesting and preimplantation processing than are fibroblasts, myofibroblasts, mesenchymal cells, and macrophages. Although the total cuspal cellularity is markedly reduced, some cells may survive and remain viable following the implantation of allografts as cardiac valve substitutes. Studies[148,149] involving explanted, cryopreserved allografts have concluded that viability is retained after implantation in allografts prepared using contemporary techniques of cryopreservation (i.e., prompt harvesting, exposure to less toxic antibiotics, reduced storage time in nutrient media). Similarly, studies of cryopreserved human pulmonary valves and cryopreserved canine pulmonary and aortic valves showed good preservation of ultrastructure; fine structural alterations correlated with the total interval of autolysis rather than with the cause of death or other variables and were not uniform in any of the specimens.[181] These findings are in contrast to the results of previous investigations,[143,151] which concluded that allograft viability was lost under various conditions of harvesting and storage (including exposure to high concentrations of antibiotics and prolonged storage in media). Detailed morphologic assessment of the extent of cellular injury and distribution of viable cells within explanted allografts that have undergone preimplantation processing by cryopreservation has not been reported.

Many questions remain to be investigated, such as the length of time the cells that have survived preimplantation processing by cryopreservation technology remain viable, quantitative studies of the distribution of viable cells, the cells' capability of division and protein synthesis, and their contribution to the metabolic turnover of connective tissue. Lastly, it is not known whether the denuded surfaces of cyropreserved, implanted allografts are relined by surviving allograft endothelial cells or by endothelial cells of host origin, as are xenografts. These issues must be addressed in order to validate the preimplantation processing methods and to determine if the retention of cell viability is a crucial determinant of the long-term durability of valvular allografts.

Note. The opinions or assertions about specific products identified by brand name contained herein are the private views of the authors and are not to be construed as conveying either an official endorsement or criticism by the U.S. Department of Health and Human Services, the Food and Drug Administration, or the National Institutes of Health.

References

1. Sebening F, Klovekorn WP, Meisner H, Struck E (eds): *Bioprosthetic Cardiac Valves.* Munich: Deutsches Herzzentrum, München, 1979.
2. Lefrak EA, Starr A (eds): *Cardiac Valve Prostheses.* New York: Appleton-Century-Crofts, 1979.
3. Ionescu MI (ed): *Tissue Heart Valves.* London: Butterworth, 1979.
4. DeBakey ME: *Advances in Cardiac Valves: Clinical Perspectives.* New York: Yorke, 1983.
5. Cohn LH, Gallucci V (eds): *Cardiac Bioprostheses.* New York: Yorke, 1982.
6. Morse D, Steiner RM, Fernandez J (eds): *Guide to Prosthetic Cardiac Valves.* New York: Springer-Verlag, 1985.
7. Bodnar E, Yacoub M (eds): *Biologic and Bioprosthetic Valves.* New York: Yorke, 1986.
8. Bjork VO, Cullhed I, Lodin H: Aortic valve prosthesis (Teflon): two year follow-up. *J Thorac Cardiovasc Surg* 45:635–644, 1963.
9. Braunwald NS, Morrow AG: A late evaluation of flexible Teflon prostheses utilized for total aortic valve replacement: postoperative clinical, hemodynamic and pathologic assessments. *J Thorac Cardiovasc Surg* 49:485–496, 1965.
10. Wisman CB, Pierce WS, Donachy JH, et al: A polyurethane trileaflet cardiac valve prosthesis: in vitro and in vivo studies. *Trans Am Soc Artif Intern Organs* 28:164–168, 1982.
11. Hilbert SL, Ferrans VJ, Tomita Y, et al: Evaluation of explanted polyurethane trileaflet cardiac valve prostheses. *J Thorac Cardiovasc Surg* 94:419–429, 1987.
12. Gabbay S, Frater RWM: The unileaflet heart valve bioprosthesis: new concept. In Cohn LH, Gallucci V (eds): *Cardiac Bioprostheses.* New York: Yorke, 1982, pp. 411–424.
13. Bodnar E, Bowden NL, Drury PJ, et al: Bicuspid mitral bioprosthesis. *Thorax* 36:45–51, 1981.
14. Black MM, Drury PJ, Tindale WB, Lawford PV: The Sheffield bicuspid valve: concept, design and in vitro and in vivo assessment. In Bodnar E, Yacoub M (eds): *Biologic and Bioprosthetic Valves.* New York: Yorke, 1986, pp. 709–717.
15. Zerbini EJ, Puig LB: Experience with dura-mater allograft: long term results. In Sebening F, Klovekorn WP, Meisner H, Struck E (eds): *Bioprosthetic Cardiac Valves.* Munich: Deutsches Herzzentrum München, 1979, pp. 179–197.
16. Senning A: Fascia lata replacement of aortic valves. *J Thorac Cardiovasc Surg* 54:465–470, 1967.
17. Rodewald G, Akrami R, Bantea C, et al: Long-term follow-up of aortic valve replacement using fascia-lata-graft according to Ionescu. In Sebening F, Klovekorn WP, Meisner H, Struck E (eds): *Bioprosthetic Cardiac Valves.* Munich: Deutsches Herzzentrum München, 1979, pp. 161–177.
18. Petch M, Somerville J, Ross DN, et al: Replacement of the mitral valve with autologous fascia lata. *Br Heart J* 36:177–181, 1974.
19. Bodnar E, Ross DN: Mode of failure in 226 explanted biologic and bioprosthetic valves. In Cohn LH, Gallucci V (eds): *Cardiac Bioprostheses.* New York: Yorke, 1982, pp. 401–407.
20. Silver MD, Hudson REB, Trimble AS: Morphologic observations on heart valve prostheses made of fascia lata. *J Thorac Cardiovasc Surg* 70:360–366, 1975.
21. Woodroof EA: The chemistry and biology of aldehyde treated tissue heart valve xenografts. In Ionescu MI (ed): *Tissue Heart Valves.* London: Butterworth, 1979, pp. 347–362.
22. Cheung DT, Perelman N, Ko EC, Nimni ME: Mechanism of crosslinking of proteins by glutaraldehyde. III. Reaction with collagen in tissues. *Connect Tissue Res* 13:109–115, 1985.
23. Cheung DT, Nimni ME: Mechanism of crosslinking of proteins by glutaraldehyde. II. Reaction with monomeric and polymeric collagen. *Connect Tissue Res* 10:201–216, 1982.
24. Broom ND: Simultaneous morphologic and stress-strain studies of fibrous components in wet heart valve leaflet tissue. *Connect Tissue Res* 6:37–50, 1978.
25. Broom N, Christie GW: The structure/function relationship of fresh and glutaraldehyde-fixed aortic valve leaflets. In Cohn LH, Gallucci V (eds): *Cardiac Bioprostheses.* New York: Yorke, 1982, pp. 476–491.

26. Gavilanes JG, Gonzalez de Buitrago G, Lizarbe MA, et al: Stabilization of pericardial tissue by glutaraldehyde. *Connect Tissue Res* 13:37–44, 1984.
27. Sade RM, Greene WB, Kurtz SM: Structural changes in a procine xenograft after implantation for 105 months. *Am J Cardiol* 44:761–766, 1979.
28. O'Brien MF, Clarebrough JK: Heterograft aortic valve transplantatioin for human valve disease. *Med J Aust* 2:228–230, 1966.
29. O'Brien MF: Heterologous replacement of the aortic valve. In Ionescu MI, Ross DN, Woller GH (eds): *Biological Tissue and Heart Valve Replacement*. London: Butterworth, 1972, pp. 445–466.
30. Buch WS, Kosek JC, Angell WW, Shumway SE: Deterioration of formalin-treated aortic valve heterografts. *J Thorac Cardiovasc Surg* 60:673–682, 1970.
31. Dubiel WT, Johansson L, Willen R: Late changes in formalin-treated porchine aortic heterografts replacing human mitral valves. *Scand J Thorac Cardiovasc Surg* 9:16–26, 1975.
32. Bortolotti V, Milano A, Mazzucco A, et al: Longevity of the formaldehyde-preserved hancock porcine heterograft. *J Thorac Cardiovasc Surg* 84:451–453, 1982.
33. Ferrans VJ, Spray TL, Billingham ME, Roberts WC: Structural changes in glutaraldehyde-treated porcine heterografts used as substitute cardiac valves: transmission and scanning electron microscopic observation in 12 patients. *Am J Cardiol* 41:1159–1184, 1978.
34. Yarbrough JW, Roberts WC, Reis RL: Structural alterations in tissue cardiac valves implanted in patients and in calves. *J Thorac Cardiovasc Surg* 65:364–375, 1973.
35. Broom ND, Thomson FJ: Influence of fixation conditions on the performance of glutaraldehyde-treated porcine aortic valves: towards a more scientific basis. *Thorax* 34:166–176, 1979.
36. Swanson WM, Clark RE: Dimensions and geometic relationships of the human aortic valve as a function of pressure. *Circ Res* 35:871–882, 1974.
37. Brewer RJ, Mentzer RM, Deck JD, et al: An in vivo study of the dimensional changes of the aortic valve leaflets during the cardiac cycle. *J Thorac Cardiovasc Surg* 74:645–650, 1977.
38. Deck JD, Thubrikar MJ, Schneider PJ, Nolan SP: Structure, stress and tissue repair in aortic valve leaflets. *Cardiovasc Res* 22:7–16, 1988.
39. Broom ND: An in vitro study of mechanical fatigue in glutaraldehyde-treated procine aortic valve tissues. *Biomaterials* 1:3–8, 1980.
40. Hilbert SL, Ferrans VJ, Swanson WM: Optical methods for the nondestructive evaluation of collagen morphology in bioprosthetic heart valves. *J Biomed Mater Res* 20:1411–1421, 1986.
41. Zerbini EJ, Puig LB: The dura mater allograft valve. In Ionescu MI (ed): *Tissue Heart Valves*. London: Butterworth, 1979, pp. 253–301.
42. Puig LB, Verginelli G, Iryia K, et al: Homologous dura mater cardiac valves: study of 533 surgical cases. *J Thorac Cardiovasc Surg* 69:722–728, 1975.
43. Centers for Disease Control: Rapidly progressive dementia in a patient who received a cadaveric dura mater graft. *MMWR* 36:49–50, 55, 1987.
44. Barnhart GR, Jones M, Ishihara T, et al: Degeneration and calcification of bioprosthetic cardiac valves: bioprosthetic tricuspid valve implantation in sheep. *Am J Pathol* 106:136–139, 1982.
45. Arbustini E, Jones M, Moses RD, et al: Modification by the Hancock T6 process of calcification of bioprosthetic cardiac valves implanted in sheep. *Am J Cardiol* 53:1388–1396, 1984.
46. Jones M, Eidbo EE, Walters SM, et al: Effects of two types of preimplantation processes on calcification of bioprosthetic valves. In Bodnar E, Yacoub M (eds): *Biologic and Bioprosthetic Valves*. New York: Yorke, 1986, pp. 451–459.
47. Fishbein MC, Levy RJ, Ferrans VJ, et al: Calcification of cardiac valve bioprostheses: biochemical, histologic and ultrastructural observations in a subcutaneous implantation model system. *J Thorac Cardiovasc Surg* 83:602–609, 1982.
48. Schoen FJ, Levy RJ, Nelson AC, et al: Onset and progression of experimental bioprosthetic heart valve calcification. *Lab Invest* 52:523–532, 1985.
49. Schoen FJ, Tsao JW, Levy RJ: Calcification of bovine pericardium used in cardiac valve bioprostheses: implication for the mechanism of bioprosthetic tissue mineralization. *Am J Pathol* 123:134–145, 1986.
50. Thiene G, Arbustini E, Bortolotti V, et al: Pathologic substrates of porcine valve dysfunction. In Cohn LH, Gallucci V (eds): *Cardiac Bioprostheses*. New York: Yorke, 1982, pp. 378–400.
51. Schoen FJ, Hobson CE: Anatomic analysis of removed prosthetic heart valves: causes of failure in 33 mechanical valves and 58 bioprostheses, 1980 to 1983. *Hum Pathol* 16:549–559, 1985.
52. Schoen FJ, Kujovich JL, Levy RJ, St John Sutton M: Bioprosthetic valve failure. *Cardiovasc Clin* 18:289–317, 1987.
53. Gallucci V, Bortolotti U, Milano A, et al: The

Hancock porcine valve 15 years later: an analysis of 575 patients. In Bodnar E, Yacoub M (eds): *Biologic and Bioprosthetic Valves*. New York: Yorke, 1986, pp. 91–97.
54. Milano A, Bortolotti V, Talenti E, et al: Calcific degeneration as the main course of porcine bioprosthetic valve failure. *Am J Cardio* 53:1066–1070, 1984.
55. Ferrans VJ, Boyce SW, Billingham ME, et al: Calcific deposits in porcine bioprostheses: structure and pathogenesis. *Am J Cardiol* 46:721–734, 1980.
56. Valente M, Bortolotti U, Thiene G: Ultrastructural substrates of dystrophic calcification in porcine bioprosthetic valve failure. *Am J Pathol* 119:12–21, 1985.
57. Carpentier A, Lemaigre G, Robert L, et al: Biological factors affecting long-term results of valvular heterografts. *J Thorac Cardiovasc Surg* 58:467–483, 1969.
58. Dunn JM, Marmon L: Mechanisms of calcification of tissue valves. *Cardiol Clin* 3:385–396, 1985.
59. Sanders SP, Levy RJ, Freed MD, et al: Use of Hancock porcine xenografts in children and adolescents. *Am J Cardiol* 46:429–438, 1980.
60. Silver MS, Pollock J, Silver MD, et al: Calcification in porcine xenograft valves in children. *Am J Cardiol* 45:685–689, 1980.
61. Gallucci V, Bortolotti U, Milano A, et al: Isolated mitral valve replacement with the Hancock bioprosthesis: a 13-year appraisal. *Ann Thorac Surg* 38:571–577, 1984.
62. Oyer PE, Miller DC, Stinson EB, et al: The performance of the Hancock bioprosthetic valve over an 11½ year follow-up period: a perliminary report. In Duran C, Angell WW, Johnson AD, Oury JH (eds): *Recent Progress in Mitral Heart Valve Disease*. London: Butterworth, 1984, pp. 244–251.
63. Magilligan DJ Jr, Lewis JW Jr, Tilley B, Peterson E: The porcine bioprosthetic valve: twelve years later. *J Thorac Cardiovasc Surg* 89:499–507, 1985.
64. Gallo I, Nistal F, Artinano E: Six- to ten-year follow-up of patients with the Hancock cardiac bioprosthesis: incidence of primary tissue failure. *J Thorac Cardiovasc Surg* 92:14–20, 1986.
65. Foster AH, Greenberg GJ, Underhill DJ, et al: Intrinsic failure of Hancock mitral bioprostheses: 10- to 15-year experience. *Ann Thorac Surg* 44:568–577, 1987.
66. Brofman PR, Carvalho RG, Ribeiro EJ, et al: Dura mater bioprostheses in young patients. In Cohn LH, Gallucci V (eds): *Cardiac Bioprostheses*. New York: Yorke, 1982, pp. 265–272.
67. Ferrans VJ, Boyce SW, Billingham ME, et al: Infection of glutaraldehyde-preserved porcine valve heterografts. *Am J Cardiol* 43:1123–1136, 1979.
68. Ferrans VJ, Ishihara T, Jones M, et al: Pathogenesis and stages of bioprosthetic infection. In Cohn LH, Gallucci V (eds): *Cardiac Bioprostheses*. New York: Yorke, 1982, pp. 346–361.
69. Levy RJ, Schoen FJ, Sherman FS, et al: Calcification of subcutaneously implanted type I collagen sponges. *Am J Pathol* 122:71–82, 1986.
70. Golomb G, Schoen FJ, Smith MS, et al: The role of glutaraldehyde-induced cross-links in calcification of bovine pericardium used in cardiac valve bioprostheses. *Am J Pathol* 127:122–130, 1987.
71. Harasake H, Nose Y, McMahon JT, et al: Calcification in blood pumps. In: *Devices and Technology Branch Contractors Meeting 1987, Program*. Bethesda: Division of Heart and Vascular Diseases, National Heart, Lung and Blood Institute, National Institutes of Health, U.S. Department of Health and Human Services, 1987.
72. Van Buskirk JJ, Kirsch WM, Kleyer DL, et al: Aminomalonic acid: identification in E. coli and atherosclerotic plaque. *Proc Natl Acad Sci USA* 81:722–725, 1984.
73. Koch TH, Bohemier D, Wheelan P, et al: Aminomalonic acid and the calcification of protein. In: *Devices and Technology Branch Contractors Meeting 1987, Program*. Bethesda: Division of Heart and Vascular Diseases, National Heart, Lung and Blood Institute, National Institutes of Health, U.S. Department of Health and Human Services, 1987.
74. Lian JB, Skinner M, Glimcher MJ, Gallop P: The presence of γ-carboxyglutamic acid in the proteins associated with ectopic calcification. *Biochem Biophys Res Commun* 73:349–355, 1976.
75. Levy RJ, Schoen FJ, Levy JT, et al: Biologic determinants of dystrophic calcification and osteocalcin deposition in glutaraldehyde-preserved porcine aortic valve leaflets implanted subcutaneously in rats. *Am J Pathol* 113:143–155, 1983.
76. Levy RJ, Zenker JA, Lian JB: Vitamin K-dependent calcium binding poteins in aortic valve calcification. *J Clin Invest* 65:563–566, 1980.
77. Levy RJ, Zenker JA, Bernhard WF: Porcine bioprosthetic valve calcification in bovine left ventricle-aorta shunts: studies of the deposition

of vitamin K-dependent proteins. *Ann Thorac Surg* 36:187–192, 1983.
78. Bick RL: Anticoagulant and antiplatelet therapy. In Murano G, Bick RL (eds): *Basic Concepts of Hemostasis and Thrombosis*. Boca Raton: CRC Press, 1980, pp. 245–258.
79. Stein PD, Riddle JM, Kemp SR, et al: Effect of warfarin on calcification of spontaneously degenerated porcine bioprosthetic valves. *J Thorac Cardiovasc Surg* 90:119–125, 1985.
80. Carpentier A, Nashef A, Carpentier S, et al: Techniques for prevention of calcification of valvular bioprostheses. *Circulation* 70(suppl I):I165–I168, 1984.
81. Lentz DJ, Pollock EM, Olsen DB, et al: Inhibition of mineralization of glutaraldehyde-fixed Hancock bioprosthetic heart valves. In Cohn LH, Gallucci V (eds): *Cardiac Bioprostheses*. New York: Yorke, 1982, pp. 306–319.
82. Jones M, Eidbo EE, Hilbert SL, et al: Anticalcification treatments of bioprosthetic heart valves: in vivo, in situ studies in the sheep model. *Ann Thorac Surg* (in press).
83. Dmitrovsky E, Boskey AL: Calcium-acidic phospholipid-phosphate complexes in human atherosclerotic aortas. *Calcif Tissue Int* 37:121–125, 1985.
84. Gasser AB, Morgan DB, Fleisch HA, Richelle LJ: The influence of two diphosphonates on calcium metabolism in rats. *Clin Sci* 43:31–45, 1972.
85. Meyer JL, Nancollas GH: The influence of multidentate organic diphosphonates on crystal growth of hydroxyapatite. *Calcif Tissue Res* 13:265–303, 1973.
86. Lamson ML, Fox JL, Higuchi WJ: Calcium and 1-hydroxyethylidene-1, 1-diphosphonic acid: polynuclear complex formation in physiological range of pH. *Int J Pharm* 21:143–154, 1966.
87. Levy RJ, Hawley MA, Schoen FJ, et al: Inhibition by diphosphonate compounds of calcification of porcine bioprosthetic heart valve cusps implanted subcutaneously in rats. *Circulation* 71:349–356, 1985.
88. Schoen FJ, Levy RJ: Pathophysiology of bioprosthetic heart valve calcification. In: Bodnar E, Yacoub M (eds): *Biologic and Bioprosthetic Valves*. New York: Yorke, 1986, pp. 418–441.
89. Levy RJ, Schoen FJ, Lund SA, Smith MS: Prevention of leaflet calcification of bioprosthetic heart valves with diphosphonate injection therapy: experimental studies of optimal dosages and therapeutic durations. *J Thorac Cardiovasc Surg* 94:551–557, 1987.
90. Levy RJ, Wolfrum J, Schoen FJ, et al: Inhibition of calcification of bioprosthetic heart valves by local controlled release diphosphonate. *Science* 228:190–192, 1985.
91. Golomb G, Langer R, Schoen FJ, et al: Controlled release diphosphonate to inhibit bioprosthetic heart valve calcification: dose response and mechanistic studies. *J Contr Rel* 4:181–194, 1986.
92. Levy RJ, Amidon G, Johnston T, Schoen FJ: Cardiovascular calcification: pathophysiology and treatment. In: *Devices and Technology Branch Contractors Meeting, 1987. Program.* Bethesda: Division of Heart and Vascular Diseases, National Heart, Lung and Blood Institutes, National Institutes of Health, Department of Health and Human Services, 1987, p. 142.
93. Urist MR, Adams JM: Effects of various blocking agents upon local mechanisms of calcification. *Arch Pathol* 81:325–342, 1966.
94. Carpentier A, Nashef A, Carpentier S, et al: Prevention of tissue valve calcification by chemical techniques. In: Cohn LH, Gallucci V (eds): *Cardiac Bioprostheses*. New York: Yorke, 1982, pp. 320–327.
95. Menasche P, Hue A, Lavergne A, et al: Selective blockade of collagen-calcium binding sites: new process to decrease bioprosthetic valvular calcification. In Bodnar E, Yacoub M (eds): *Biologic and Bioprosthetic Valves*. New York: Yorke, 1986, pp. 478–483.
96. Golomb G, Levy RJ: Prevention of calcification of glutaraldehyde-treated biomaterials by charge modification. *Transactions of the Society for Biomaterials*, 1987, p. 108.
97. Tsao JW, Schoen FJ, Shanker R, et al: Retardation of bovine pericardial bioprosthetic tissue calcification by a physiologic mineralization inhibitor, phosphocitrate, administered locally. *Transactions of the Society for Biomaterials*, 1987, p. 144.
98. Schryer PJ, Tomasek FR, Starr JA, Wright JTM: Anticalcification effect of glutaraldehyde-preserved valve tissue stored for increasing time in glutaraldehyde. In Bodnar E, Yacoub M (eds): *Biologic and Bioprosthetic Valves*. New York: Yorke, 1986, pp. 471–477.
99. Koorajian S, Frugard G, Stegwell MJ: Sterilization of tissue valves. In Sebening F, Klovekorn WP, Meisner H, Struck E (eds): *Bioprosthetic Cardiac Valves*. Munich: Duetsches Herzzentrum München, 1979, pp. 373–378.
100. Centers for Disease Control: Isolation of mycobacteria species from porcine heart valve prostheses. *MMWR* 26:42–43, 1977.
101. Laskowski LF, Marr JJ, Spernoga JF, et al: Fas-

tidious mycobacteria grown from porcine prosthetic-heart-valve cultures. *N Engl J Med* 297:101–102, 1977.

102. Thubrikar MJ, Skinner JR, Eppink RT, Nolan SP: Stress analysis of porcine bioprosthetic heart valves in vivo. *J Biomed Mater Res* 16:811–826, 1982.
103. Thubrikar M, Piegrass WC, Deck JD, Nolan SP: Stresses of natural versus prosthetic aortic valve leaflets in vivo. *Ann Thorac Surg* 30:230–239, 1980.
104. Thubrikar M, Carabello BA, Aouad A, Nolan SP: Interpretation of aortic root angiography in dogs and humans. *Cardiovasc Res* 16:16–21, 1982.
105. Thubrikar M, Piegrass, Bosher LP, Nolan SP: The elastic modulus of canine aortic valve leaflets in vivo and in vitro. *Circ Res* 47:792–800, 1980.
106. Van Steehoven AA, Veenstra PC, Reneman RS: The effect of some hemodynamic factors on the behavior of the aortic valve. *J Biomech* 15:941–950, 1982.
107. Van Steehoven AA, van Dongen MEH: The role of the trapped sinus vortex in aortic valve closure. In Schneck DJ (ed): *Biofluid Mechanics* 2. New York: Plenum, 1980, pp. 317–325.
108. Chong M, Eng M, Missirlis YF: Aortic valve mechanics. II. A stress analysis of porcine aortic valve leaflets in diastole. *Biomater Med Devices Artif Organs* 6:225–244, 1978.
109. Reis RL, Hancock WD, Yarbrough JW, et al: The flexible stent: a new concept in the fabrication of tissue heart valve prostheses. *J Thorac Cardiovasc* 62:683–689, 1971.
110. Thomson FJ, Barratt-Boyes BG: The glutaraldehyde-treated heterograft valve. *J Thorac Cardiovasc Surg* 74:317–321, 1977.
111. Wright JTM, Eberhart CE, Gibbs ML, et al: Hancock II—an improved bioprosthesis. In Cohn LH, Gallucci V (eds): *Cardiac Bioprostheses*. New York: Yorke, 1982, pp. 425–444.
112. Carpentier AF, Lane E: Supported bioprosthetic heart valve with compliant orifice ring. US Patent 4,106,129, 1978.
113. Borkon AM, McIntosh CL, Jones M, et al: Inward stent-post bending of a porcine bioprosthesis in the mitral position: cause of bioprosthetic dysfunction. *J Thorac Cardiovasc Surg* 83:105–107, 1982.
114. Salomon NW, Copeland JG, Goldman S, Larson DF: Unusual complication of the Hancock porcine heterograft: strut compression in the aortic root. *J Thorac Cardiovasc Surg* 77:294–296, 1979.
115. Magilligan DJ, Fisher E, Alam M: Hemolytic anemia with porcine xenograft aortic and mitral valves. *J Thorac Cardiovasc Surg* 79:628–631, 1980.
116. Schoen FJ, Schulman LJ, Cohn LH: Quantitative anatomic analysis of "stent creep" of explanted Hancock standard porcine bioprostheses used for cardiac valve replacement. *Am J Cardiol* 56:110–114, 1985.
117. Levine FH, Buckley MJ, Austen WG: Hemodynamic evaluation of the Hancock modified orifice bioprosthesis in the aortic position. *Circulation* 58(suppl I):33–35, 1978.
118. Carpentier A, Dubost C, Lane E, et al: Continuing improvements in valvular bioprostheses. *J Thorac Cardiovasc Surg* 83:27–42, 1982.
119. Wright JTM: Porcine or pericardial valves? Now and the future: design and engineering considerations. In Bodnar E, Yacoub M (eds): *Biologic and Bioprosthetic Valves*. New York: Yorke, 1986, pp. 567–579.
120. Schoen FJ, Fernandez J, Gonzalez-Lavin L, Cernaianu A: Causes of failure and pathologic findings in surgically removed Ionescu-Shiley standard bovine pericardial heart valve bioprostheses: emphasis on progressive structural deterioration. *Circulation* 76:618–627, 1987.
121. Wheatley DJ, Fisher J, Reece IJ, et al: Primary tissue failure in pericardial heart valves. *J Thorac Cardiovasc Surg* 94:367–374, 1987.
122. Walley VM, Keon WJ: Patterns of failure in Ionescu-Shiley bovine pericardial bioprosthetic valves. *J Thorac Cardiovasc Surg* 93:925–933, 1987.
123. Gabbay S, Bortolotti U, Wasserman F, et al: Long-term follow-up of the Ionescu-Shiley mitral pericardial xenograft. *J Thorac Caradiovasc Surg* 88:758–763, 1984.
124. Brais MP, Bedard JP, Goldstein W, et al: Ionescu-Shiley pericardial xenografts: follow-up to 6 years. *Ann Thorac Surg* 39:105–111, 1985.
125. Reul GJ, Cooley DA, Duncan JM, et al: Valve failure with the Ionescu-Shiley bovine pericardial bioprosthesis: analysis of 2680 patients. *J Vasc Surg* 2:192–203, 1985.
126. Nistal F, Garcia-Satue E, Artinano E, et al: Comparative study of primary tissue valve failure between Ionescu-Shiley pericardial and Hancock porcine valves in the aortic position. *Am J Cardiol* 57:161–164, 1986.
127. Cooley DA, Ott DA, Reul GJ, et al: Ionescu-Shiley bovine pericardial bioprostheses: clinical results in 2701 patients. In Bodnar E, Yacoub M (eds): *Biologic and Bioprosthetic Valves*. New York: Yorke, 1986, pp. 177–198.

128. Bortolotti U, Milano A, Thiene G, et al: Early mechanical failures of the Hancock pericardial xenograft. *J Thorac Cardiovasc Surg* 94:200–207, 1987.
129. Yoganathan AP, Woo YR, Sung HW, et al: In vitro hemodynamic characteristics of tissue bioprostheses in the aortic position. *J Thorac Cardiovasc Surg* 92:198–209, 1986.
130. Jones M, Eidbo EE, Rodriguez R, et al: Ventricular aneurysms produced by the struts of bioprosthetic valves implanted in sheep. *J Thorac Cardiovasc Surg* (in press).
131. Heng MK, Baratt-Boyes BG, Agnew TM, et al: Isolated mitral replacement with stent-mounted antibiotic-treated aortic allograft valves. *J Thorac Cardiovasc Surg* 74:230–235, 1977.
132. Christie GW, Gavin JB, Barratt-Boyes BG: Graft detachment, a cause of incompetence in stent-mounted aortic valve allografts. *J Thorac Cardiovasc Surg* 90:901–906, 1985.
133. Murray G: Homologous aortic-valve-segment transplants as a surgical treatment for aortic and mitral insufficiency. Angiology 7:466–471, 1956.
134. Barratt-Boyes BG: Homograft aortic valve replacement in aortic incompetence and stenosis. *Thorax* 19:131–150, 1964.
135. Ross DN: Homograft replacement of the aortic valve. *Lancet* 2:487, 1962.
136. Ross DN, Somerville J: Correction of pulmonary atresia with a homograft aortic valve. *Lancet* 2:1446–1447, 1966.
137. Foster JH, Collins AH, Jacobs JK, Scott HW Jr: Long term follow-up of homografts used in the treatment of coarctation of the aorta. *J Cardiovasc Surg* 6:111–120, 1965.
138. Ross D, Yacoub M: Homograft replacement of the aortic valve: a critical review. *Prog Cardiovasc Dis* 11:926–929, 1965.
139. Davies H, Lessof MH, Robert CI, Ross DN: Homograft replacement of the aortic valve. *Lancet* 1:926–929, 1965.
140. Barratt-Boyes BG, Roche HG, Brandt PWT, et al: Aortic homograft valve replacement: a long-term follow-up of an initial series of 101 patients. *Circulation* 40:763–775, 1969.
141. Barratt-Boyes BG, Roche AHG, Whitlock RML: Six year review of the results of freehand aortic replacement using an antibiotic sterilized homograft valve. *Circulation* 55:353–361, 1977.
142. Angell WW, Shumway NE, Kosek JC: A five year study of viable aortic valve homografts. *J Thorac Cardiovasc Surg* 64:329–338, 1972.
143. Virdi IS, Monro JL, Ross JK: Eleven year experience of aortic valve replacement with antibiotic sterilized homograft valves in Southhamptom. *J Cardiovasc Surg* (in press).
144. Yacoub M, Kittle CF: Sterilization of valve homografts by antibiotic solution. *Circulation* 41(suppl II):II29–II31, 1970.
145. Wain WH, Pearce HM, Riddell RW, Ross DN: A re-evaluation of antibiotic sterilization of heart valve allografts. *Thorax* 32:740–742, 1977.
146. Malm JP, Bowman FO Jr, Harris PD, Kovalik ATW: An evaluation of aortic homografts sterilized by electron geam energy. *J Thorac Cardiovasc Surg* 54:471–477, 1967.
147. Aparicio SR, Donnelly RJ, Dexter F, Watson DA: Light and electron microscopic studies on homograft and heterograft heart valves. *J Pathol* 115:147–162, 1975.
148. Angell WW, Angell JD, Oury JH, et al: Long-term follow-up of viable frozen aortic homografts: a viable homograft valve bank. *J Thorac Cardiovasc Surg* 93:815–822, 1987.
149. O'Brien MF, Strafford EG, Gardner MAH, et al: A comparison of aortic valve replacement with viable cryopreserved and fresh allograft valves, with a note on chromosomal studies. *J Thorac Cardiovasc Surg* 94:812–823, 1987.
150. Bodnar E, Wain WH, Martelli V, Ross DN: Long term performance of 580 homograft and autograft valves used for aortic valve replacement. *Thorac Cardiovasc Surg* 27:31–38, 1979.
151. Barratt-Boyes BG, Roche AHG, Subramanyan R, et al: Long-term follow-up of patients with the antibiotic-sterilized aortic homograft valve inserted free-hand in the aortic position. *Circulation* 75:768–777, 1987.
152. Wain WH, Greco R, Ingegneri A, et al: 15 Years' experience with 615 homograft and autograft aortic valve replacements. *Int J Artif Organs* 3:169–172, 1980.
153. Harris PD, Kovalik AJW, Marks JA, Malm JP: Factors modifying aortic homograft structure and function. *Surgery* 63:45–59, 1968.
154. Hudson REB: Pathology of human aortic valve homografts. *Br Heart J* 28:291–301, 1966.
155. Smith JC: The pathology of human aortic valve homografts. *Thorax* 22:114–138, 1967.
156. Roe FJC, Glendenning OM: The carcinogenicity of beta-propiolactone for mouse skin. *Br J Cancer* 10:357–362, 1956.
157. Kolman A, Naslund M, Calleman CJ: Genotoxic effects of ethylene oxide and the relevance to human cancer. *Carcinogenesis* 7:1245–1250, 1986.
158. Davies H, Missen GAK, Blandford G, et al: Homograft replacement of the aortic valve: a

clinical and pathologic study. *Am J Cardiol* 22:195–217, 1968.

159. Barratt-Boyes BG: Long-term follow-up of aortic valve grafts. *Br Heart J* 33(suppl):60–65, 1971.
160. Ingegneri A, Wain WH, Martelli V, et al: An 11 year assessment of 93 flash frozen homograft valves in the aortic position. *Thorac Cardiovasc Surg* 27:304–397, 1979.
161. Livi U, Abdel-Kadir A, Parker R, et al: Viability and morphology of aortic and pulmonary homografts: a comparative study. *J Thorac Cardiovasc Surg* 93:755–760, 1987.
162. Pate JW, Sawyer PN: Freeze dried aortic grafts: a preliminary report of experimental evaluation. *Am J Surg* 86:3–13, 1953.
163. Reichenbach DD, Mohri H, Merendino KA: Pathological changes in human aortic valve homografts. *Circulation* 39(suppl I):I47–I56, 1969.
164. Brock RC: Long-term degenerative changes in aortic segment homografts with particular reference to calcification. *Thorax* 23:249–255, 1968.
165. Knaghani A, Dhalla N, Penta A, et al: Patient status 10 years or more after aortic valve replacement using antibiotic sterilized homografts. In Bodnar E, Yacoub M (eds): *Biologic and Bioprosthetic Valves.* New York: Yorke, 1986, pp. 38–46.
166. Ferrans VJ, Hilbert SL, Tomita Y, et al: Morphology of collagen in bioprosthetic heart valves. In Nimni M (ed): *Collagen, Vol. 3: Biotechnology.* Boca Raton: CRC Press, 1988, pp. 145–189.
167. *Polystan Bioprostheses Information Bulletins BPA, BPC, BPD, BPE, BPF,* and *BP1.* Copenhagen: Polystan A/S, 1980.
168. Ishihara T, Ferrans VJ, Jones M, et al: Structure of bovine parietal pericardium and of unimplanted Ionescu-Shiley pericardial valvular bioprostheses. *J Thorac Cardiovasc Surg* 81:747–757, 1981.
169. Ferrans VJ, Thiedemann KU: Ultrastructure of the normal heart. In Silver MD (ed): *Cardiovascular Pathology.* New York: Churchill Livingstone, 1983, pp. 31–86.
170. Gross L, Kugel MA: Topographic anatomy and histology of the valves in the human heart. *Am J Pathol* 7:445–473, 1931.
171. Sell S, Scully RE: Aging changes in the aortic and mitral valves: histologic and histochemical studies, with observations on the pathogenesis of calcific aortic stenosis and calcification of the mitral annulus. *Am J Pathol* 46:345–365, 1965.
172. Khanna SK, Ross JK, Monro JL: Homograft aortic valve replacement: seven years' experience with antibiotic-treated valves. *Thorax* 36:330–337, 1981.
173. Ross DN, Martelli V, Wain WH: Allograft and antograft valves used for aortic valve replacement. In Ionescu MJ (ed): *Tissue Heart Valves.* London: Butterworth, 1979, pp. 127–172.
174. Kay PH, Ross DN: Fifteen years' experience with the aortic homograft: the conduit of choice for right ventricular outflow tract reconstruction. *Ann Thorac Surg* 40:360–363, 1985.
175. Shabbo FP, Wain WH, Ross DN: Right ventricular outflow reconstruction with aortic homograft conduit: analysis of long-term results. *Thorac Cadiovasc Surg* 28:21–25, 1980.
176. Fontan F, Choussat A, Peville C, et al: Aortic valve homografts in the surgical treatment of complex cardiac malformations. *J Thorac Cardiovasc Surg* 87:649–657, 1984.
177. Jonas RA, Freed MD, Mayer JF, Castaneda AR: Long-term follow-up of patients with synthetic right heart conduits. *Circulation* 72(suppl II):II77–II83, 1985.
178. Miller DC, Stinson ES, Oyer PE, et al: Durability of porcine xenograft valves and conduits in children. *Circulation* 66(suppl I):172–185, 1982.
179. Ferrans VJ, Arbustini E, Eido EE, Jones M: Anatomic changes in right ventricular-pulmonary artery conduits implanted in baboons. In Bodnar E, Yacoub M (eds): *Biologic and Bioprosthetic Valves.* New York: Yorke, 1986, pp. 316–339.
180. Robbins SL: Cell injury and cell death. In: *Pathologic Basis of Disease.* Philadelphia: Saunders, 1974, pp. 21–54.
181. Armiger LC, Thomson RW, Strickett MG, Barratt-Boyes BG: Morphology of heart valves preserved by liquid nitrogen freezing. *Thorax* 40:778–786, 1985.

Section II—Surgical Techniques

6—Left Ventricular Outflow Tract Reconstructions

RICHARD A. HOPKINS

The developing role for allograft transplants is reviewed in chapters 1 and 2. The major controversy resides in the issue of durability. The hemodynamic performance of a properly placed allograft is clearly superior to stented xenograft or mechanical valve and the advantages concerning resistance to infection and the avoidance of anticoagulation are becoming more evident and attractive. Good long-term performance is dependent on an excellent technical surgical result. The surgeon must view the use of allograft tissue as a tool for the reconstruction of the left ventricular outflow tract rather than as an implant of a device. This requires mastering both the analysis of the outflow tract as well as multiple methods for its reconstruction.

"Freehand" Aortic Valve Replacement with Aortic Allograft Valve Transplant

The early allograft aortic valve replacements were referred to as "freehand" in the sense that the valve was sewn directly into the aortic root without stents. This "freehand" approach encompasses a range of techniques which must account for variations in annulus, aortic root, and coronary anatomy as well as ensuring the continued perfect function of the allograft semilunar aortic valve mechanism.

Indications and Contraindications

Although some authors have recommended that the allograft valve is the prosthesis of choice for all aortic valve replacements, limitation of availability and the requisite increase in aortic cross-clamp time requires selection.[1] In addition, there are anatomic situations that may increase the difficulty of inserting an allograft valve. In general, allograft valve transplant is considered for the following indications: (1) all aortic valve replacements and left ventricular outflow tract reconstructions in patients with more than a 10-year life expectancy in whom anticoagulation is undesirable (e.g., children, young women of childbearing age, and young active adults); (2) aortic root replacement; (3) aortoventriculoplasty; (4) small aortic annulus; (5) bacterial endocarditis;[2] (6) reoperation for failure of an aortic valve prosthesis, particularly in patients with accelerated degeneration of a porcine bioprosthesis.

Relative contraindications to insertion of an allograft valve include the following: (1) severe assymetric annular calcification precluding uniform, smooth "seating" or extensive calcification extending into the septum, mitral valve, and fibrous trigones; (2) lack of availability; (3) unfavorable coronary anatomy that precludes adjustment of the geometry; (4) aortic root ectasia exceeding a diameter of 30 mm;[3] (5) aortic valve replacement being a small component of the total amount of cardiac surgery necessary in which cross-clamp times would be expected to exceed 120 minutes; (6) severe left ventricular dysfunction; and (7) connective tissue disorders such as Marfan's syndrome or cystic medial necrosis.

Sizing of Aortic Root for Allograft Insertion

Careful matching of allograft size to aortic annulus is important for optimal performance. It requires a slightly different set of assumptions for the surgeon accustomed to using rigid stented prostheses, as the measured diameter of the allograft is the internal diameter (in contrast to the external diameter for standard prostheses) and thus allowance must be made for wall thickness. In addition, the hemodynamic performance of the smaller allograft aortic valves is markedly superior to mechanical or bioprostheses such that a 19- to 20-mm (internal diameter, ID) allograft valve is usually adequate for most adults and hemodynamically analogous to a much larger prosthesis (see Appendix: Valve Diameters). A 16- to 17-mm or larger valve can usually be placed in patients who weigh more than 20 kg.

Preoperative estimation of the allograft size required for a given patient has been approached angiographically and echocardiographically. Yankah, from Germany, recommended angiographic measurement of the aortic "annulus" for preoperative determination of size. This technique involves an angiogram obtained in the lateral position during both systole and diastole, with the measurements being performed 1 mm above the sinuses.[4] However, others have thought that aortography gives unreliable estimates of aortic annulus size and, to be useful, the left ventriculography requires precise methodology.[5]

We have found a simple echocardiographic technique most helpful. A parasternal long axis view is obtained of the left ventricular outflow tract. The internal diameter of the outflow tract is measured at the point of the continuity of the anterior leaflet of the mitral valve and the aortic annulus just beneath the valve leaflet attachment and across to the septum (Fig. 6.1). Multiple measurements are made, but the most important is during early systolic ejection, as a useful correlation within 1–2 mm is possible with this measurement (Fig. 6.2). The ultimate inter-

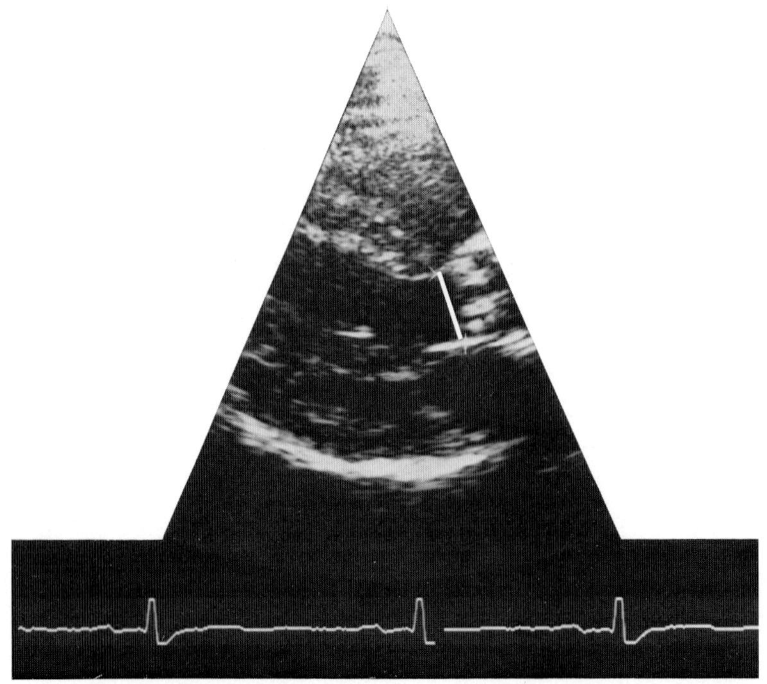

Figure 6.1. Parasternal, long axis two-dimensional echocardiographic view for allograft sizing. The white bar shows the plane in which the left ventricular outflow tract diameter is measured during the initial portion of systole for sizing for freehand aortic valve replacement.

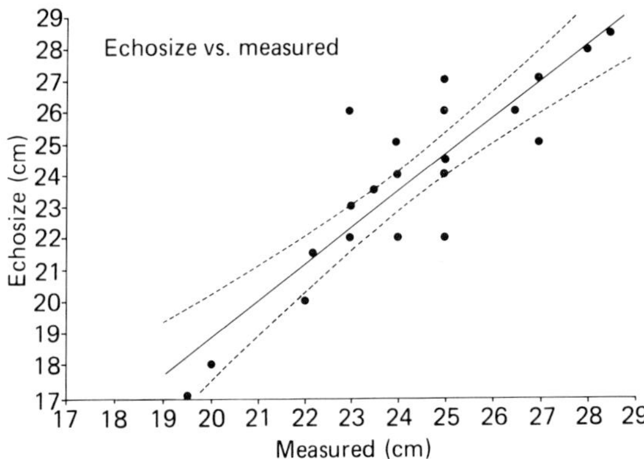

FIGURE 6.2. Correlation between internal diameter measurement of aortic "annulus" at surgery with the echocardiographic preoperative measurement. Dotted line represents ± 1 SD. $n = 21$. Best fit: $y = 1.15x + (-4.12)$. Analysis of variance: $r^2 = 0.7769$.

nal diameter measurement is made during surgery. The measured estimated diameter of the base of the aortic outflow minus 3–4 mm provides a "target size" so that a span of allograft sizes can be readily available.

Some authors have recommended external aortic root diameter measurement at the time of surgery as a guide to the internal diameter. The formula is approximately 8 mm less than the external diameter measurement as measured by forceps at the base of the aortic root. This technique has been unreliable in our hands.

Direct internal measurements are made at operation after opening the aorta and excising the native valve. After adequate débridement, the size of the aortic outflow is measured with Hegar dilators. Hegar dilators are preferred, as commercial prosthesis sizers vary significantly from their nominal measurements owing to purposely introduced manufacturers' "fudge factors."[6] This measurement can be made prior to the final meticulous débridement of the annulus but at such time that the actual size of the outflow is readily apparent. This measurement is then used to calculate the size of the aortic valve allograft selected. Because the wall thickness of an allograft is approximately 2 mm, it is necessary to subtract 4 mm from the measured internal diameter to obtain the size of the allograft to implant. If there is not a large amount of calcium, in general one can increase the size of the allograft by 1–2 mm such that only 2–3 mm are subtracted from the internal diameter size. For example, if the internal measurement is 24 mm, we would use a 21-mm aortic allograft; but if there is much calcium, a 20-mm allograft would be selected. If the measurement is 21.5 mm, we would select an 18- or 19-mm allograft. The more calcium in the annulus, the more one avoids a large allograft.

Preparation of Allograft for Insertion

The allograft is thawed as described in Chapter 4. On obtaining the allograft, the surgeon inspects the aorta for cracks and the valve itself for fenestrations or congenital abnormalities. The aortic allograft is then filled with saline to test for aortic valve insufficiency, and the muscle at the base of the valve on the septal side is trimmed meticulously. As much of this tissue as can be removed safely is débrided. This step is easily accomplished by gently placing the wet gloved finger through the valve and using the curved portion of the scissors to gently pare away the muscle (Fig. 6.3). Sufficient muscle must be removed that the fibrous skeleton can be visualized for accurate placement of the sutures. In addition, reducing the muscle bulk allows placement of a slightly larger prosthesis and reduces the need to rotate the valve. When the muscle has been meticulously removed, the aortic valve can be placed orthotopically without rotation in virtually all aortic roots. For the standard freehand aortic valve insertion, the anterior leaflet of the mitral valve is excised, leaving a 2-mm remnant.

Cannulation

Cannulate the ascending aorta as high as possible, close to the innominate artery. If the proximal aortic root is short, we recommend cannulating the femoral artery or the aortic arch.

Cardiopulmonary Bypass Management

A single atrial return cannula and left ventricular venting via the right superior pulmonary vein

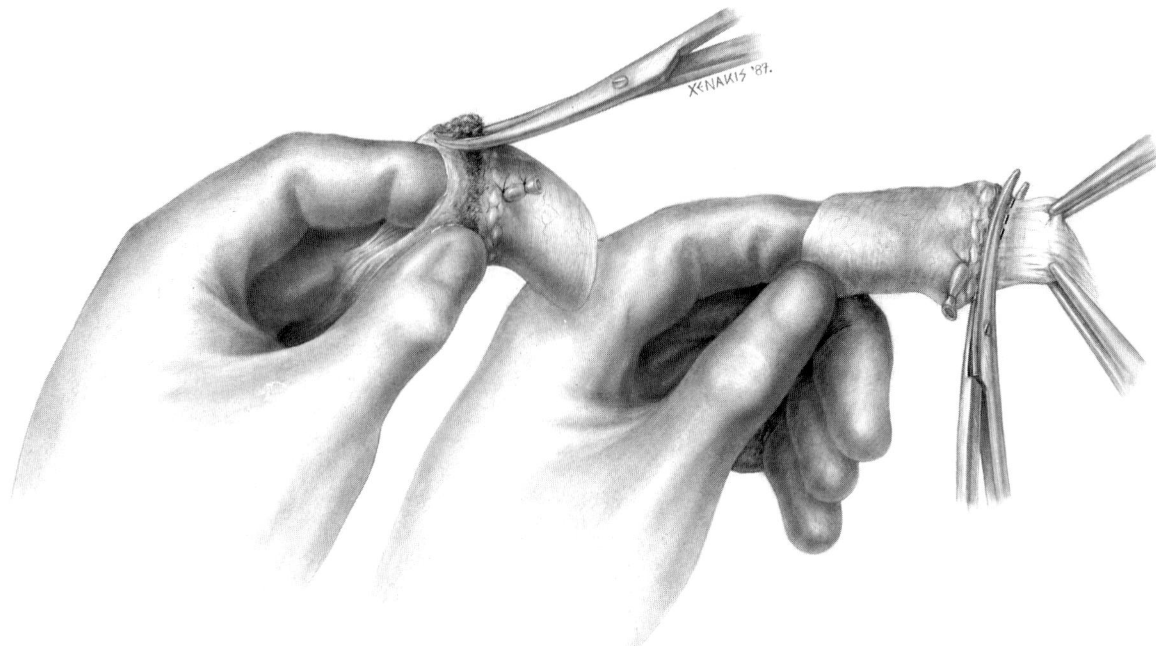

Figure 6.3. Trimming of the thawed allograft is begun by removing muscle at the base of the fibrous skeleton. The allograft is kept moist with saline during all manipulations.

are used for aortic valve replacement, as is moderate total body hypothermia with cardioplegic arrest supplemented by topical cooling. Multiple doses of cardioplegia are delivered via direct coronary cannulas at 20-minute intervals.

Aortotomy

The aortotomy for aortic valve replacement should be different when using an allograft from that used when implanting other prostheses. A reverse "lazy S" incision is begun 4–5 cm vertically above the right coronary artery and is brought down to a level that is well above a point at which the allograft commissural pillars are estimated to reach; it is then deviated virtually transversely until reaching the midpoint above the noncoronary cusp—thus leaving space for the suspended commissural pillar between the right and noncoronary cusp (Fig. 6.4). The incision is then completed by aiming down toward the anterior leaflet of the mitral valve; unless an extensive aortoplasty or annuloplasty is definitely planned, however, the incision is stopped well above the annulus, approximately at or just below the level of the aortic sinus ridge, to the right of the pillar between the left and noncoronary cusps. The exposure of this aortotomy is greatly facilitated by placement of three stay sutures, two on the left "flap" and one on the surgeon's side of the aortotomy (Fig. 6.5). This incision gives good exposure, leaves adequate native aortic wall for placement of the commissural posts, provides the option of extending the incision for annuloplastic maneuvers, and allows aortoplastic augmentation or reduction. Other incisions have been suggested, including oblique standard incisions and transverse incisions. The transverse incision, although adequate if nothing needs to be done to the aortic root, is limiting if enlargement procedures or alterations in aortic root geometry are necessary. A standard oblique incision, as is usually performed for mechanical prostheses, can make placement of the allograft commissural pillar between the right and noncoronary sinuses more difficult because it is usually lower and would encroach on this region.

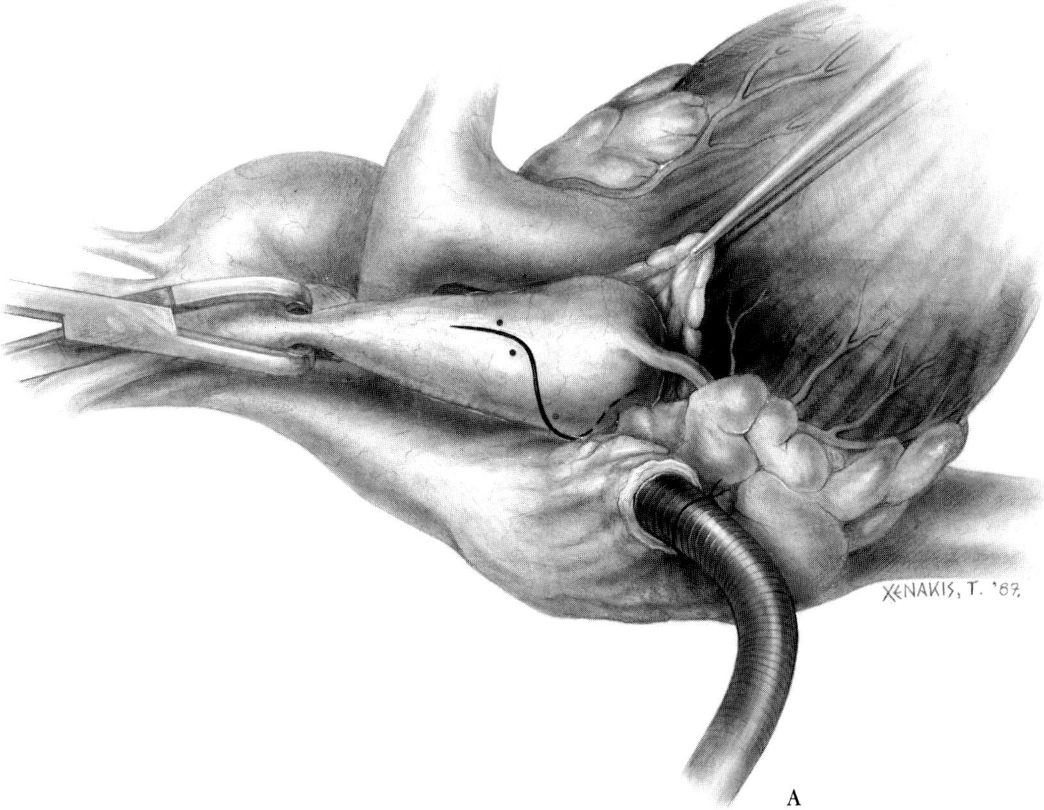

A

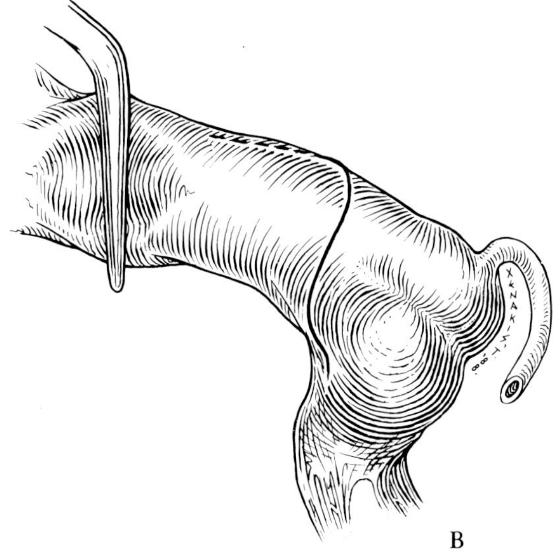

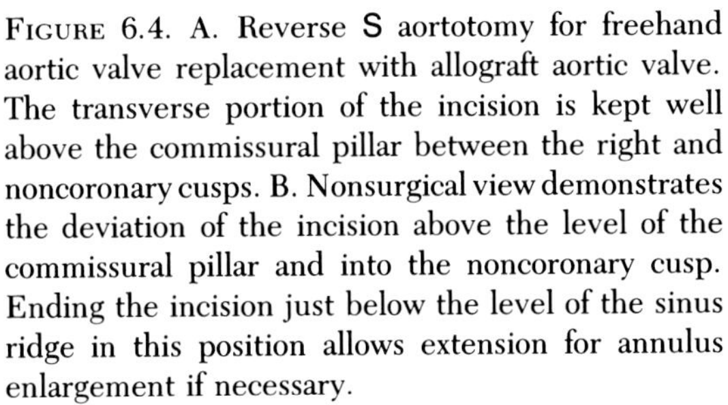

FIGURE 6.4. A. Reverse S aortotomy for freehand aortic valve replacement with allograft aortic valve. The transverse portion of the incision is kept well above the commissural pillar between the right and noncoronary cusps. B. Nonsurgical view demonstrates the deviation of the incision above the level of the commissural pillar and into the noncoronary cusp. Ending the incision just below the level of the sinus ridge in this position allows extension for annulus enlargement if necessary.

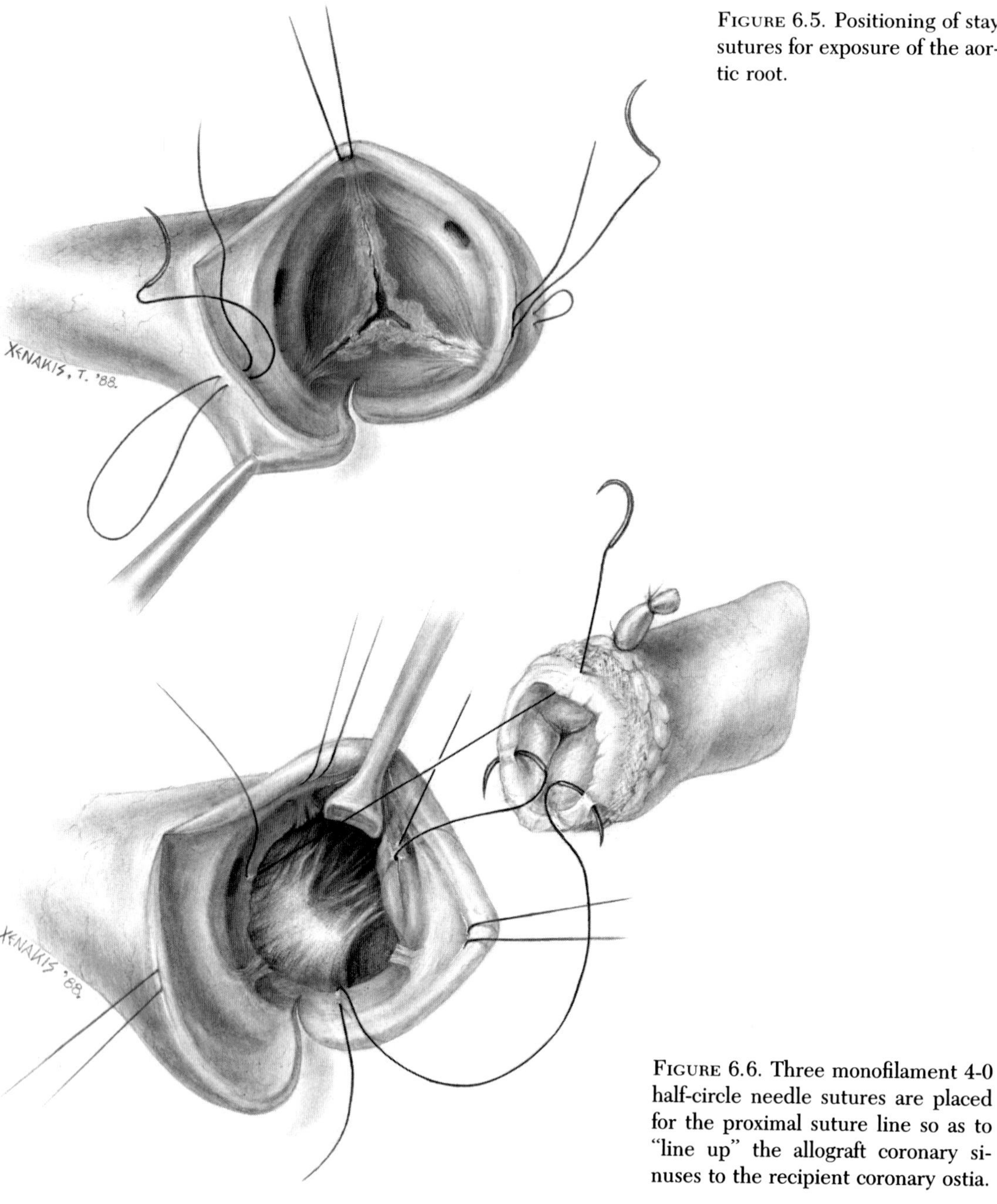

Figure 6.5. Positioning of stay sutures for exposure of the aortic root.

Figure 6.6. Three monofilament 4-0 half-circle needle sutures are placed for the proximal suture line so as to "line up" the allograft coronary sinuses to the recipient coronary ostia.

Surgical Technique for Standard Aortic Valve Replacement with Freehand Insertion of an Allograft Aortic Valve

Proximal Suture Line

After preparation of the allograft and resection of the native valve, three sutures of 4-0 monofilament polypropylene on a taper-point half-circle needle are placed as simple sutures, relating the middle of each recipient sinus to the donor coronary ostia (Fig. 6.6). They are placed as simple sutures beginning with the base of the left sinus of the allograft lined up to a position directly underneath the left coronary of the recipient (Fig. 6.7). Similarly, a simple suture is

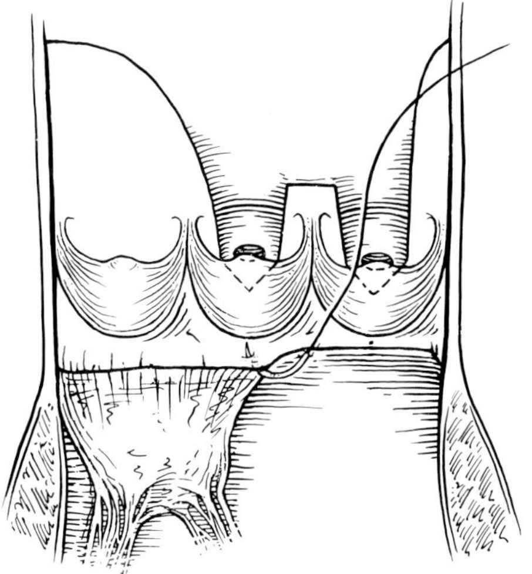

FIGURE 6.7. The first suture is placed at a point underneath the left coronary ostia of the recipient and lined up to the midpoint of the coronary sinus of the allograft. When the sinus geometry between recipient and transplant are symmetric, the second suture relates the midpoint of the recipient right sinus below the right coronary ostia of the donor mid-sinus point.

placed between the midportion of the right coronary sinus of the transplant and a point just underneath the right coronary ostia (presuming both coronary ostia are in the middle of their respective sinuses). The valve is thus placed orthotopically without rotation.

When the second suture is placed, an "adjustment" may be necessary. If either of the native coronary ostia are off center from their coronary sinuses (which they often are), the allograft left coronary sinus is centered to the left coronary ostia. A rotational adjustment is then needed for positioning the midportion of the right coronary sinus to a point relevant to the recipient right coronary ostia (see the section on minirotation, below). This adjustment makes placement of the distal suture line possible without deviating the line of the commissural post to avoid the right coronary ostium, which would cause semilunar dysfunction. The third suture starts in the midportion of the noncoronary sinus through the fibrous skeleton of the base of the transplant valve and is then placed at a point equidistant from each of the other two sutures (midway on both recipient and transplant). These three sutures fix the rotation of the valve.

The valve is inverted into the left ventricular cavity (Fig. 6.8). Beginning with the left suture, a running suture line is constructed with four or five simple sutures being taken with each limb such that the sutures meet at a midpoint between the starting points (usually underneath

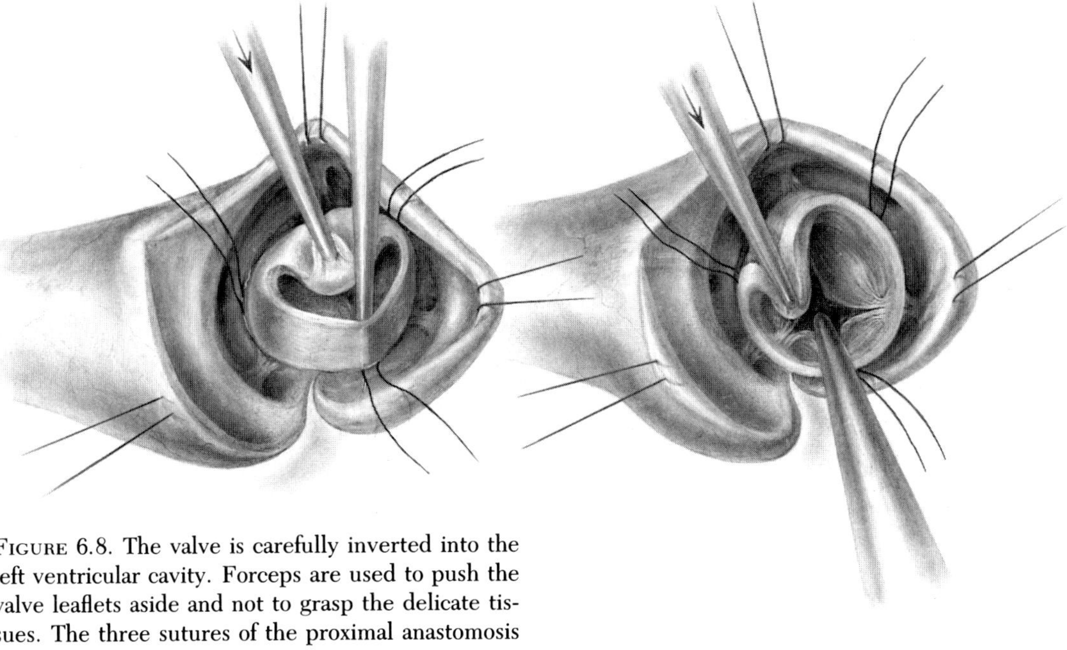

FIGURE 6.8. The valve is carefully inverted into the left ventricular cavity. Forceps are used to push the valve leaflets aside and not to grasp the delicate tissues. The three sutures of the proximal anastomosis are kept on light tension with rubber-shod clamps.

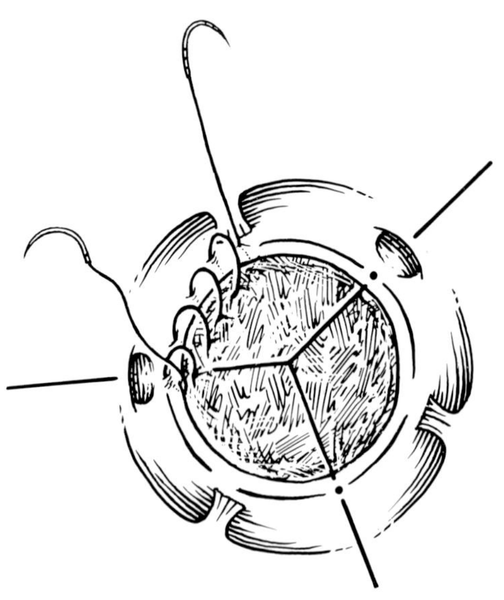

Figure 6.9. The three sutures are begun at the points indicated by the dots, and the six hemisutures are each run to a midpoint between their starting places, taking approximately four bites apiece.

the commissures) (Fig. 6.9). This measure allows a continuous suture line but on which tension needs to be placed for only four or five suture "bites" to allow tightening without drag or cutting into the delicate allograft tissue; once all six hemisutures have been run to the midportions, they are snugged and tied (Fig. 6.10). This point is a good time to repeat the cardioplegia with direct coronary cannulae (Spencer's). The valve is reverted (Fig. 6.11).

Distal Suture Line

Guide traction sutures of 4-0 monofilament are placed at the apex of each commissural post (Fig. 6.12) and the allograft coronary sinuses excised with scissors to provide an opening sufficient to suture around the native coronary ostia (Fig. 6.13). We defer this step until now because it is at this time that the position of the coronary ostia relative to the transplanted coronary sinus can be best ascertained, thereby avoiding unnec-

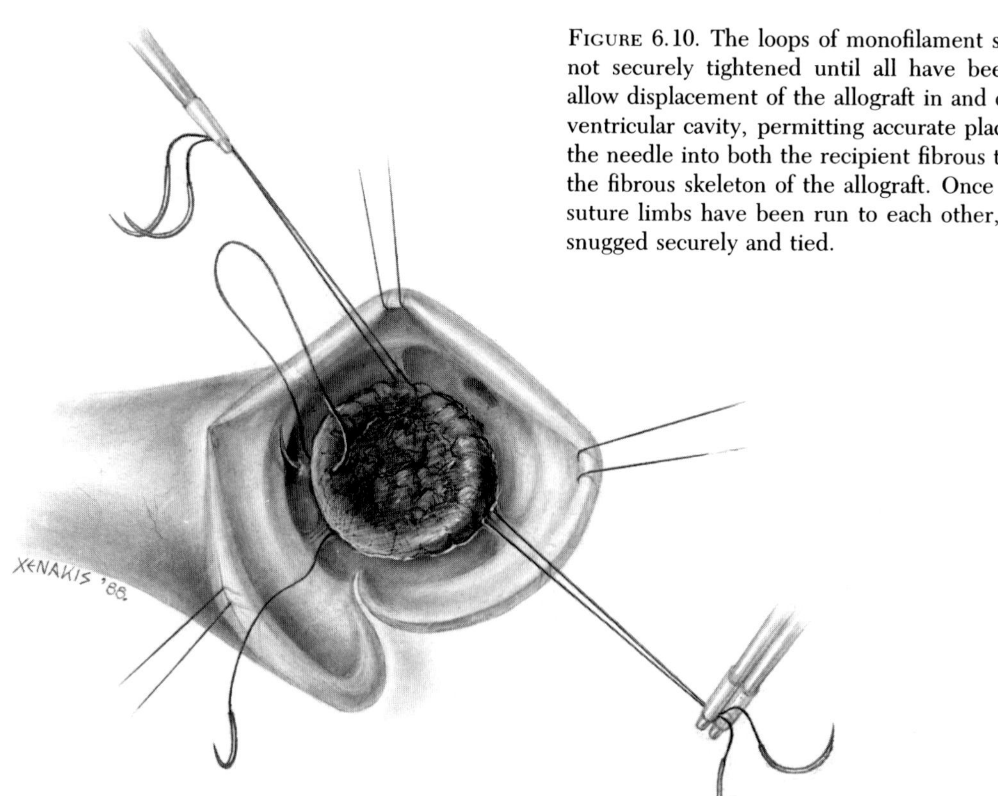

Figure 6.10. The loops of monofilament suture are not securely tightened until all have been run to allow displacement of the allograft in and out of the ventricular cavity, permitting accurate placement of the needle into both the recipient fibrous tissue and the fibrous skeleton of the allograft. Once all of the suture limbs have been run to each other, they are snugged securely and tied.

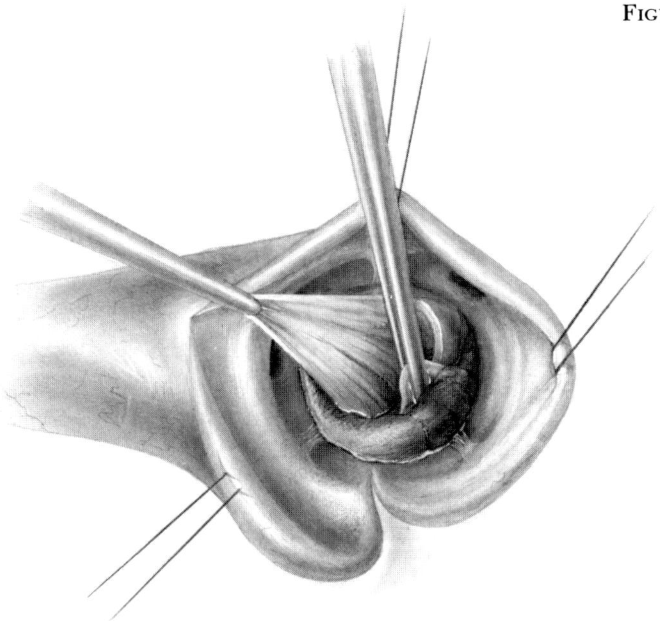

FIGURE 6.11. The valve is carefully reverted.

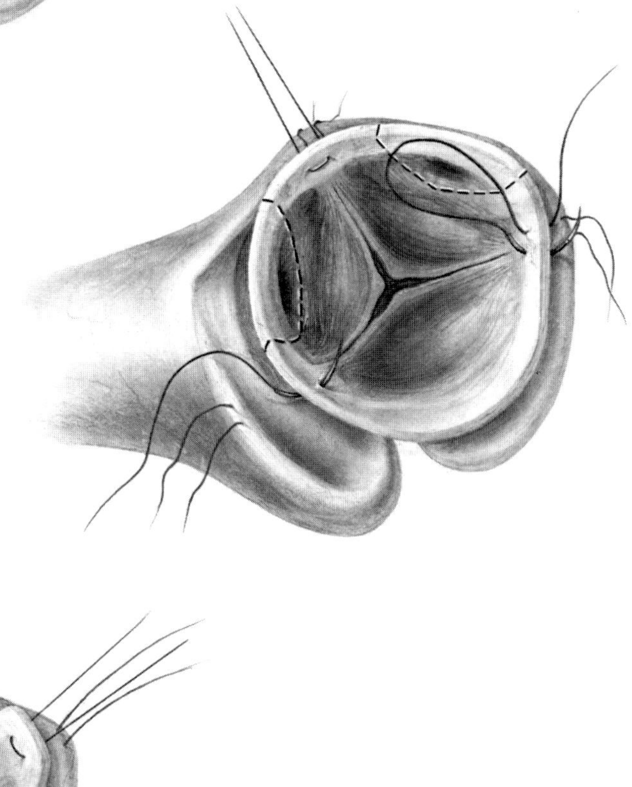

FIGURE 6.12. Monofilament guide sutures are placed at the apex of each allograft commissural pillar. They are then controlled by the assistant, which gives exposure of the sinuses and allows some stretch to be placed on the pillars during excision of sinus walls and the creation of the distal suture line.

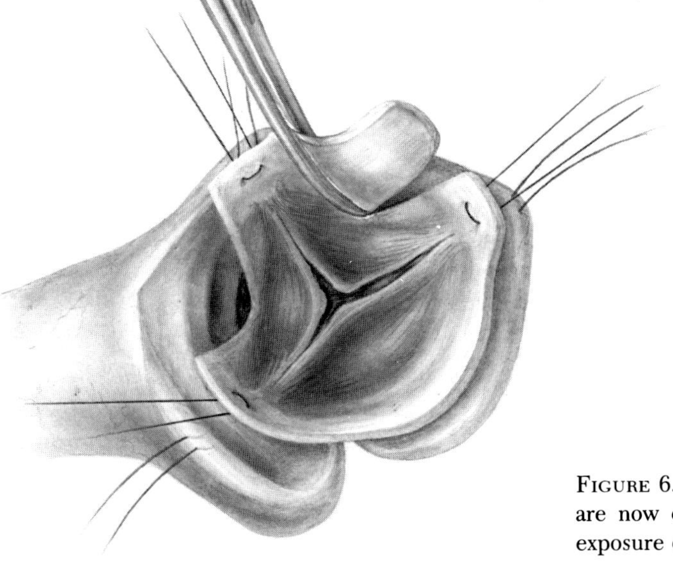

FIGURE 6.13. The coronary sinuses of the allograft are now excised as deeply as necessary to allow exposure of the native coronary ostia.

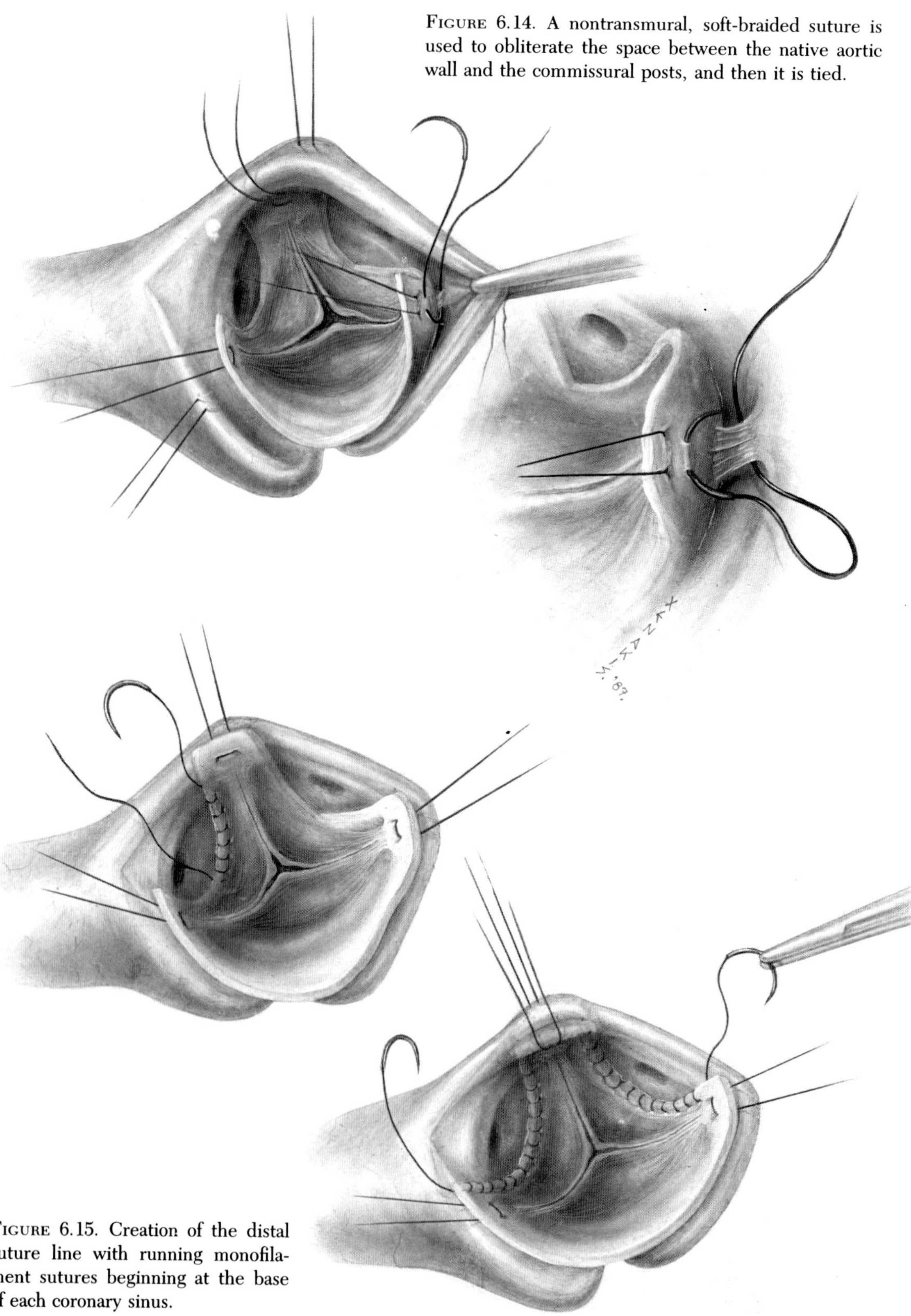

Figure 6.14. A nontransmural, soft-braided suture is used to obliterate the space between the native aortic wall and the commissural posts, and then it is tied.

Figure 6.15. Creation of the distal suture line with running monofilament sutures beginning at the base of each coronary sinus.

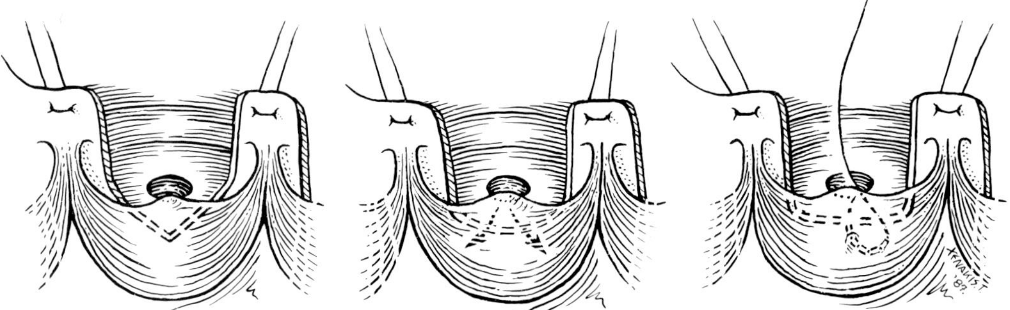

FIGURE 6.16. The base of the suture line underneath the coronary ostia is kept "flat" to avoid encroachment.

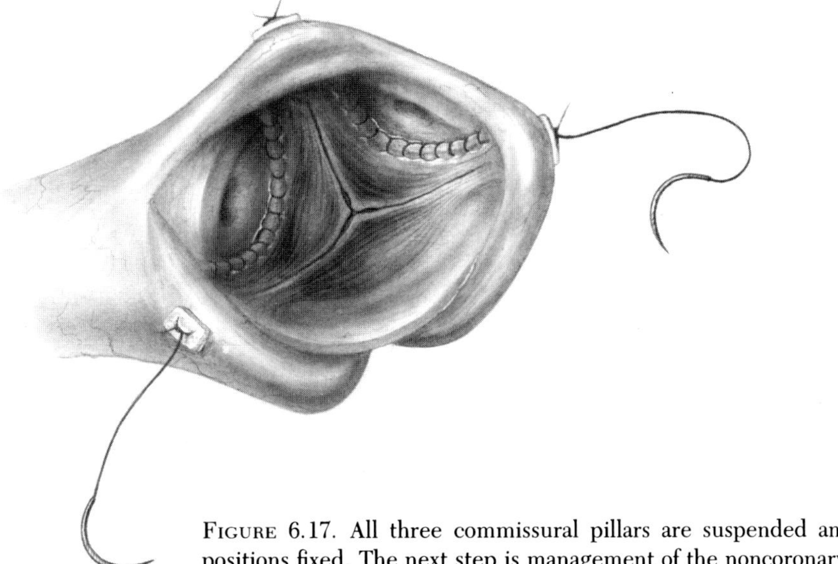

FIGURE 6.17. All three commissural pillars are suspended and their positions fixed. The next step is management of the noncoronary sinus.

essary dissection. 4-0 Soft braided sutures (e.g., Tycron) are then placed behind the commissural posts to the native aortic wall as nontransmural simple sutures to accomplish obliteration of that space (Fig. 6.14) (analogous to the vertical mattress through-and-through suture of Barratt-Boyes and Roche[7]). Then, with modest tension on the commissural posts by the assistant, 4-0 monofilament sutures on half-circle needles are started at the bottom of each coronary sinus (usually starting with the left) and the suture line run to the tops of each commissural post where the suture is brought outside the native aorta (Fig. 6.15). Sutures are used to run from the bottom of each sinus, taking care to keep the lower portion of the distal suture line "flat" and to maintain commissural suspension for enhancement of semilunar function (Fig. 6.16). These sutures are tied over pledgets outside the aorta (Fig. 6.17).

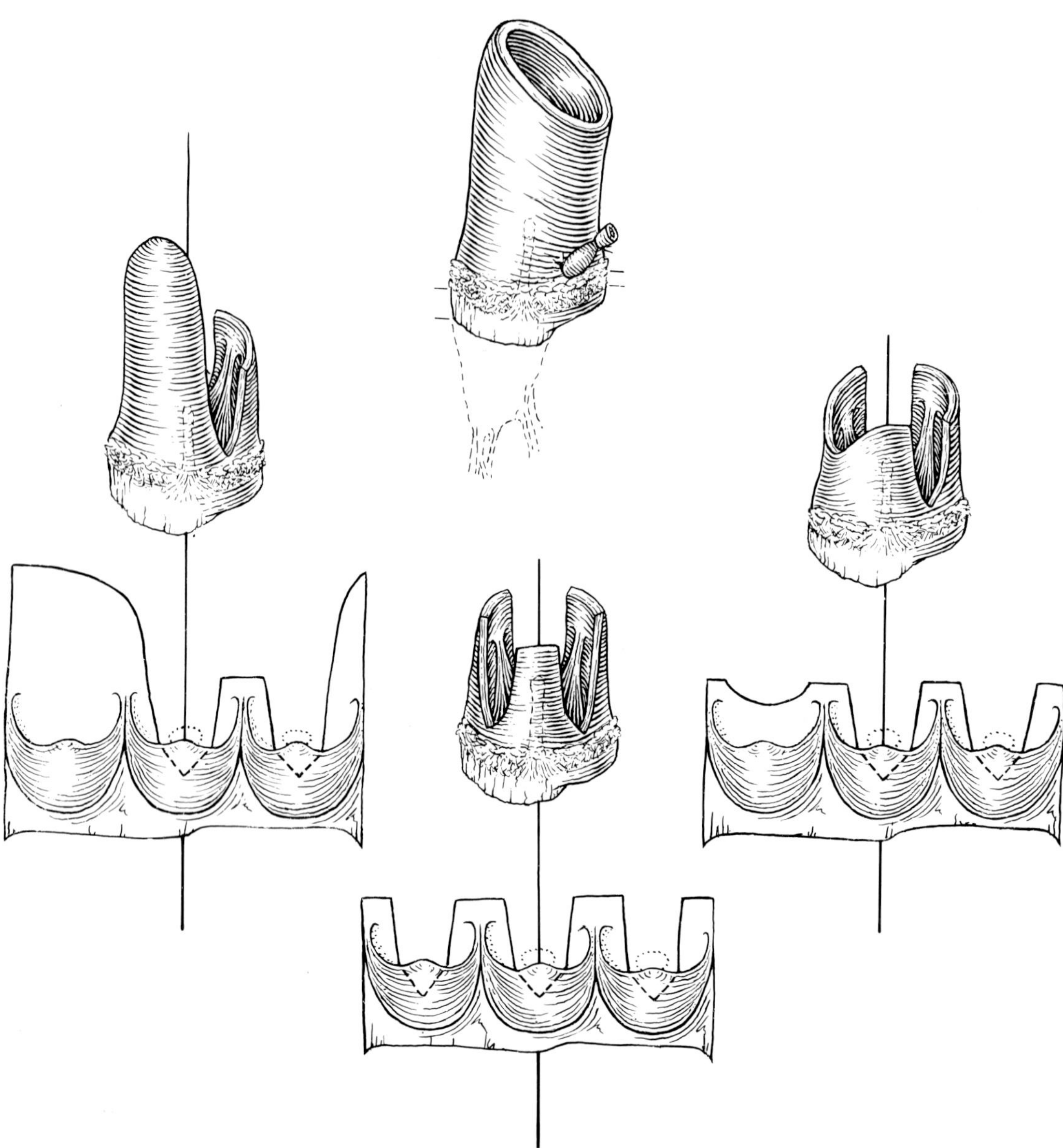

FIGURE 6.18. Representation of the three basic techniques for managing the noncoronary sinus, particularly the distal suture line. *Flange technique* (on the left) allows allograft augmentation of the noncoronary sinus, which when accomplished with annulus enlargement can enlarge the entire aortic root for placement of a larger valve. In the *classic technique* (middle) the sinuses of the allograft are excised and the suture lines run around each pillar, taking care to suspend the pillars for semilunar valvular function. It is the best technique when "rotation" of the allograft is planned within the recipient aortic root (i.e., aligning the allograft left sinus to the recipient right sinus). In the *scallop technique* (on the right) only a shallow scallop is removed from the noncoronary sinus. This maneuver allows primary closure of the aortotomy with deviation of the suture line of that sinus below the aortotomy site, but it does not remove much allograft tissue in that sinus, which helps preserve the alignment of the pillars.

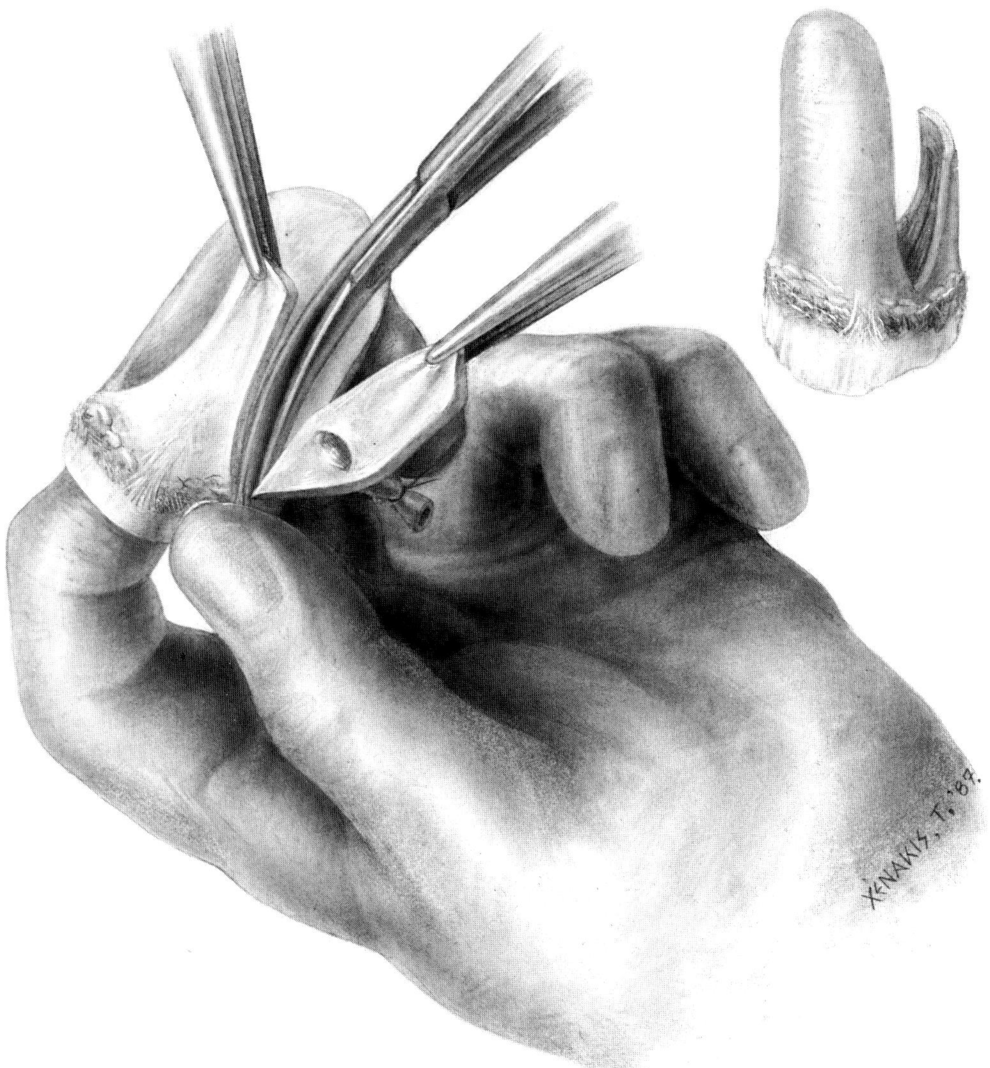

FIGURE 6.19. Trimming of the allograft for the flange technique of handling the distal suture line. It can be accomplished prior to the proximal suture line construction when aortic augmentation aortoplasty is definitely required or after reversion, if preferred.

There are basically three methods for handling the noncoronary sinus (Fig. 6.18).

1. *Flange technique*. In our practice, the "flange" technique of preparing the allograft is the most routine, as it leaves ample allograft tissue for sculpturing of the aortic root to ensure uniform commissural post architecture.

The allograft is trimmed as demonstrated (Fig. 6.19). Care is taken to leave the length of the aorta in the region of the noncoronary sinus long—longer than one would think necessary. The three bottom sutures are placed as previously described and the proximal suture line accomplished in the usual fashion (Fig. 6.20). The valve is reverted, and the right and left coronary ostia are excised, leaving the commissural pillar between the right and left sinuses isolated but the noncoronary sinus and its flange of aorta intact (Fig. 6.21). Stay sutures are placed at the top of each pillar. The distal suture line

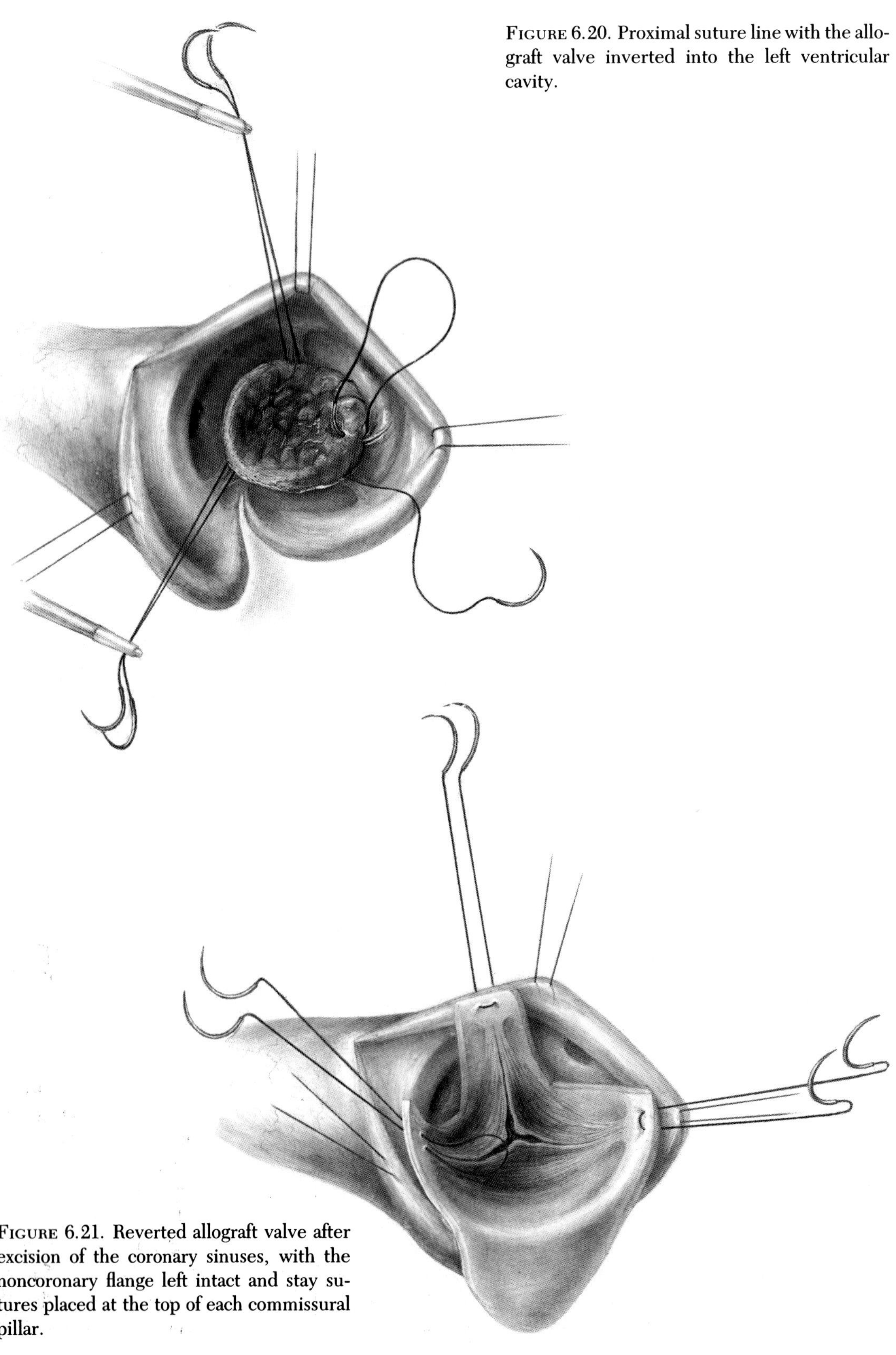

Figure 6.20. Proximal suture line with the allograft valve inverted into the left ventricular cavity.

Figure 6.21. Reverted allograft valve after excision of the coronary sinuses, with the noncoronary flange left intact and stay sutures placed at the top of each commissural pillar.

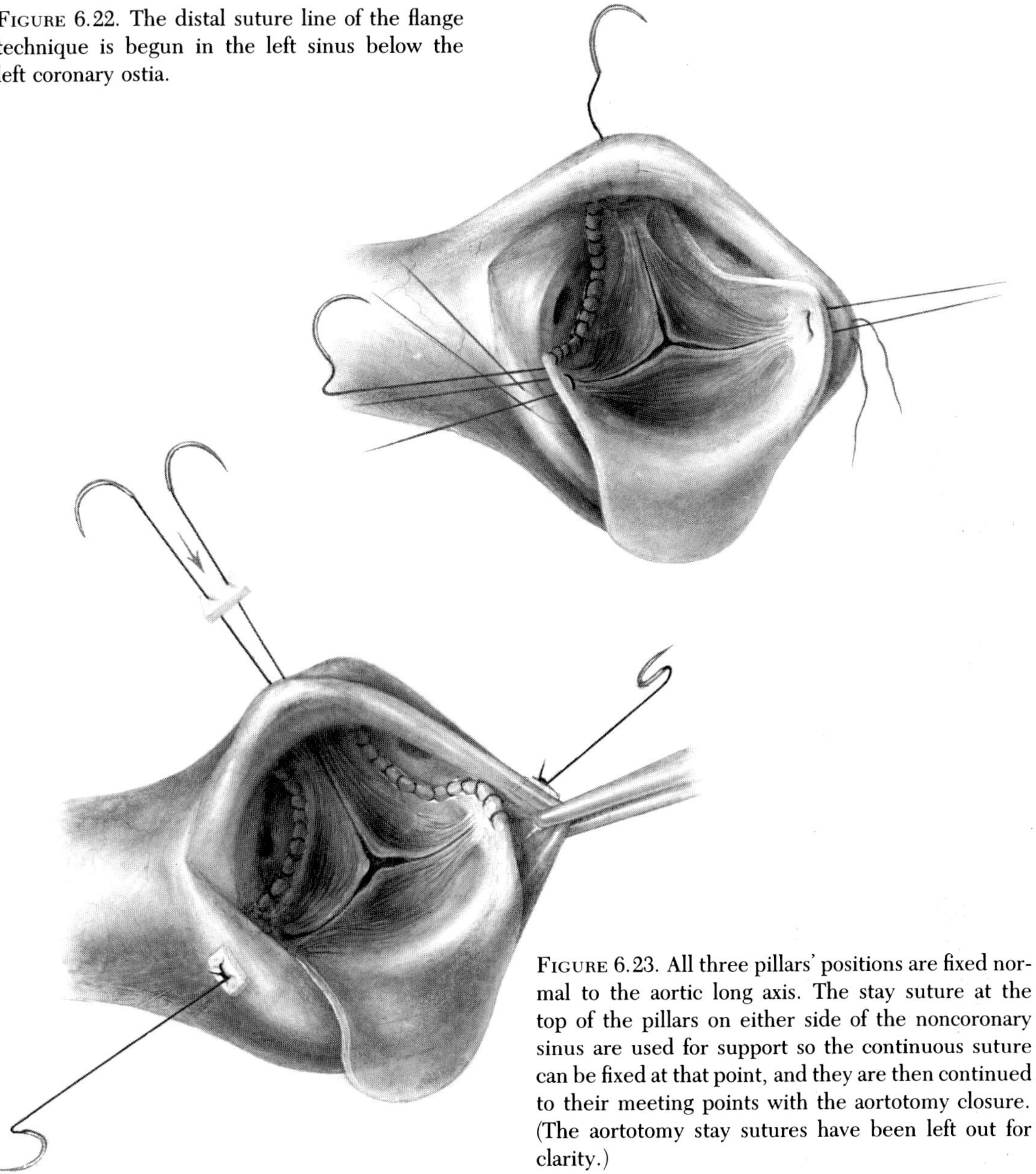

FIGURE 6.22. The distal suture line of the flange technique is begun in the left sinus below the left coronary ostia.

FIGURE 6.23. All three pillars' positions are fixed normal to the aortic long axis. The stay suture at the top of the pillars on either side of the noncoronary sinus are used for support so the continuous suture can be fixed at that point, and they are then continued to their meeting points with the aortotomy closure. (The aortotomy stay sutures have been left out for clarity.)

is then begun with a running 4-0 polypropylene suture on a half-circle taper-point needle. The suturing is begun at the base of the left coronary sinus (Fig. 6.22). Care is taken to keep the suture line flat underneath the left coronary ostia. The suture line is run to the top of the pillar between the left and right coronary ostia, where it is brought outside the aorta. The right coronary sinus is handled similarly. The suture line is brought to the top of the other two pillars and outside the aorta. The stay sutures at the top of these two pillars are brought to the outside of the aorta, through a pledget, and tied (Fig. 6.23). This measure fixes the commissural posts but leaves the aortic wall of the allograft to fill however much is necessary of the noncoronary sinus to maintain the aortic root geometry (Fig. 6.24).

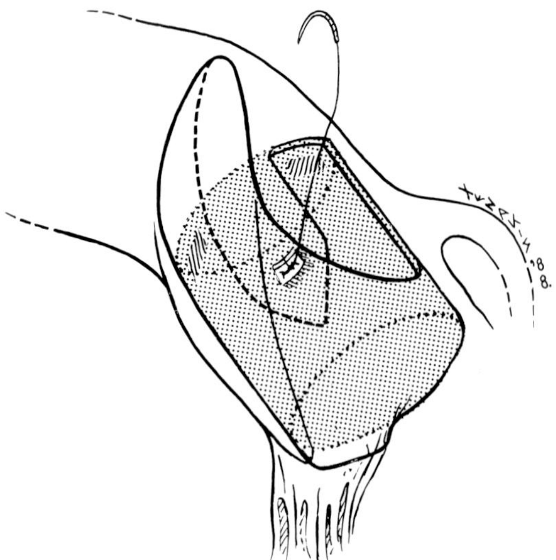

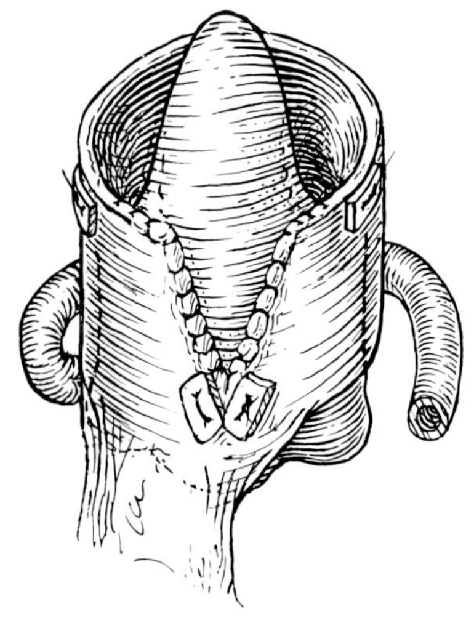

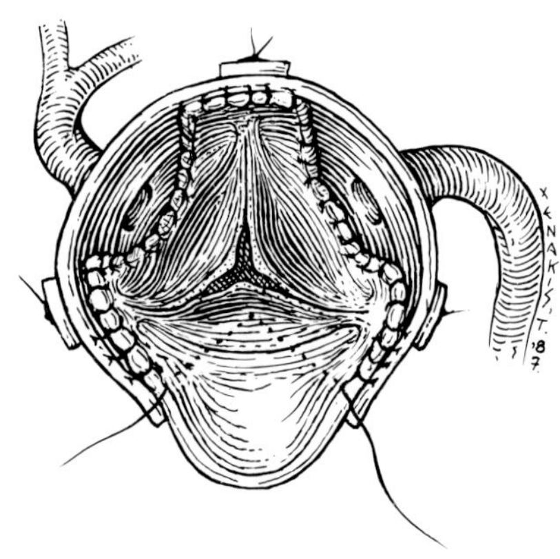

Figure 6.24. The flange of the allograft allows reconstruction of the aortic root to a symmetric cylinder, with the amount of augmentation necessary to maintain alignment of the pillars. If no augmentation is necessary, the flange can be excised or left to reenforce the aortotomy.

Figure 6.25. The distal suture line is continued to the points where the aortotomy closure sutures meet them, and they are then tied together. If no augmentation aortoplasty is necessary, the sutures are run to the top of a truncated flange and tied together outside the native aorta.

The aortotomy closure is begun at the base of the noncoronary sinus with a pledgetted suture (Fig. 6.25). The suture is advanced superiorly along the aortic closure with transmural suturing through the native aorta to the wall of the allograft aortic wall. This suture line is run to the point where the distal line meets the aortotomy, then converted to a running edge-to-edge closure of the allograft aortic wall flange and the native aorta (Fig. 6.26). The flange (trimmed as necessary) fills the aortotomy up into its transverse portion (Fig. 6.27), providing controlled expansion of the noncoronary sinus.

If only a small amount of expansion of the noncoronary sinus is required, the suture line can be deviated away from the native aortic edge. Sutures are transmural through the native aorta and nontransmural through the allograft until the top of the pillar is reached. At this point, the edge of the allograft is sutured to the inside of the aorta until the triangulation point is reached (Fig. 6.28). The operation is completed by simply suturing the remainder of the aortotomy with a pledgetted technique, de-airing, and removing the cross clamp.

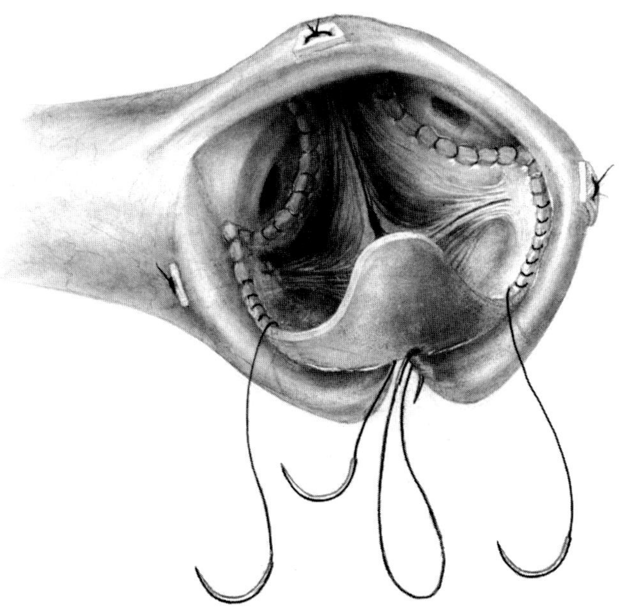

Figure 6.26. The inner distal suture line is continued to the edge of the aortotomy closure.

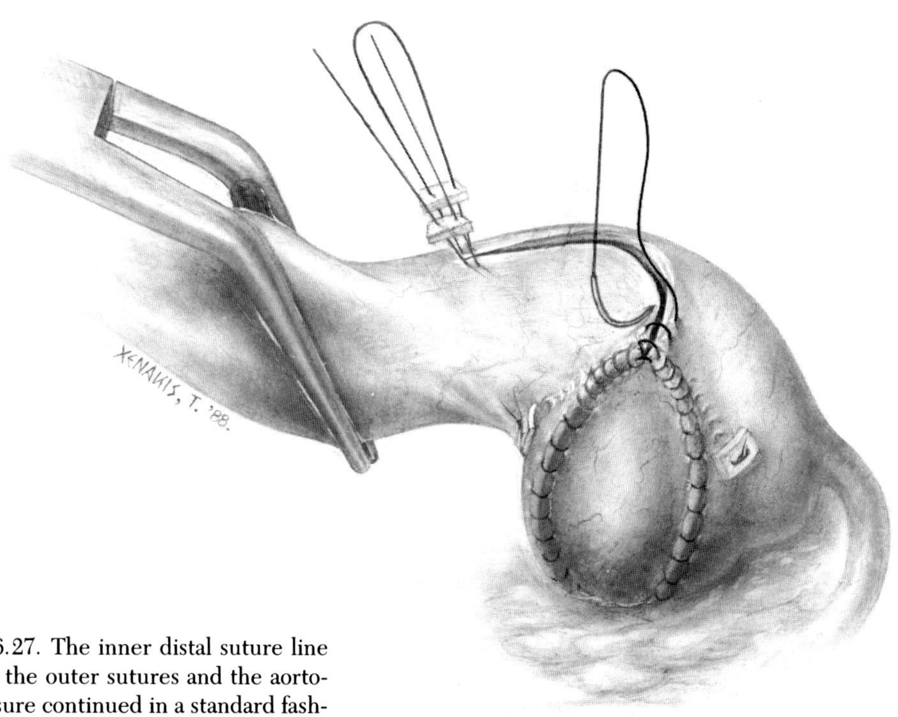

Figure 6.27. The inner distal suture line is tied to the outer sutures and the aortotomy closure continued in a standard fashion.

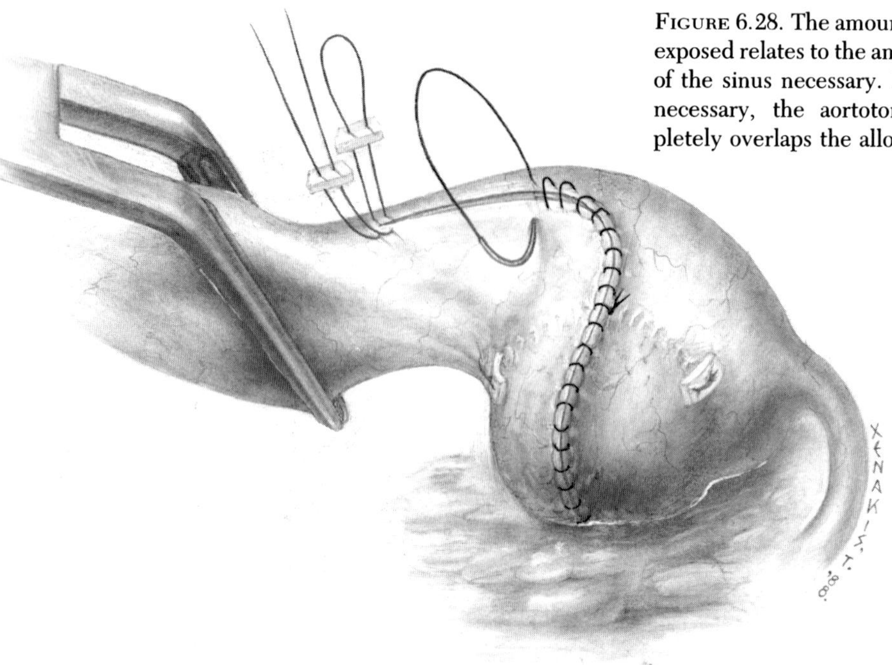

FIGURE 6.28. The amount of allograft aorta exposed relates to the amount of expansion of the sinus necessary. If no expansion is necessary, the aortotomy closure completely overlaps the allograft flange.

2. *Classic technique*. With the classic technique (similar to that originally developed by Barratt-Boyes, Ross, Karp, and others) minimal allograft aorta is retained, and the allograft is dissected prior to beginning the proximal suture line (Fig. 6.29).[8–11] All three sinuses are excised, leaving the commissural pillars as three posts, as in a crown (Fig. 6.18). This technique is selected for an aortic root in which commissural post placement can be accomplished in such a manner that primary closure of the aortotomy incision results in appropriate architecture without splaying or narrowing of the posts or if rotation of the sinuses is desired. The distal suture

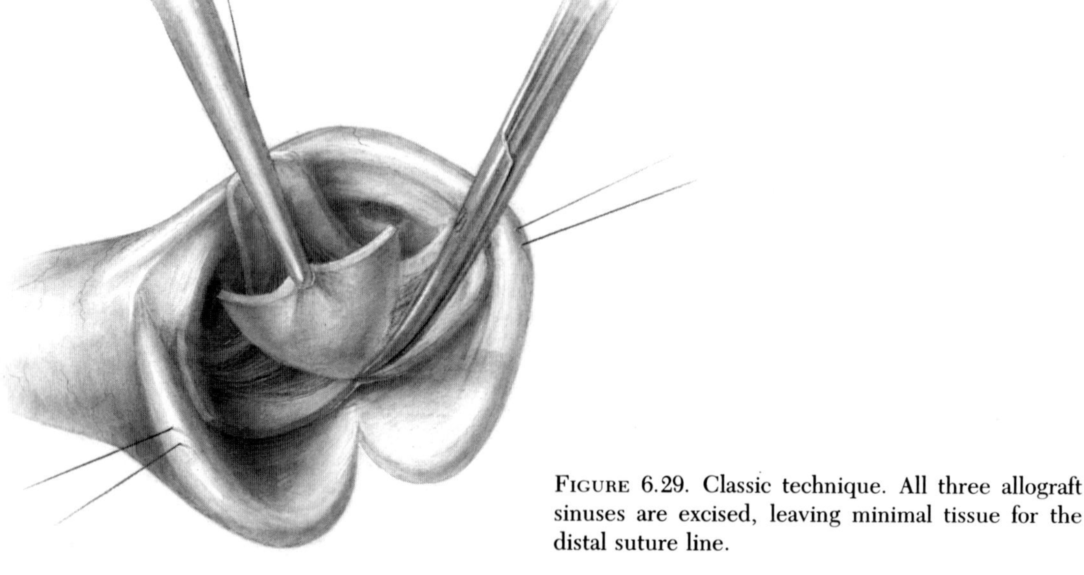

FIGURE 6.29. Classic technique. All three allograft sinuses are excised, leaving minimal tissue for the distal suture line.

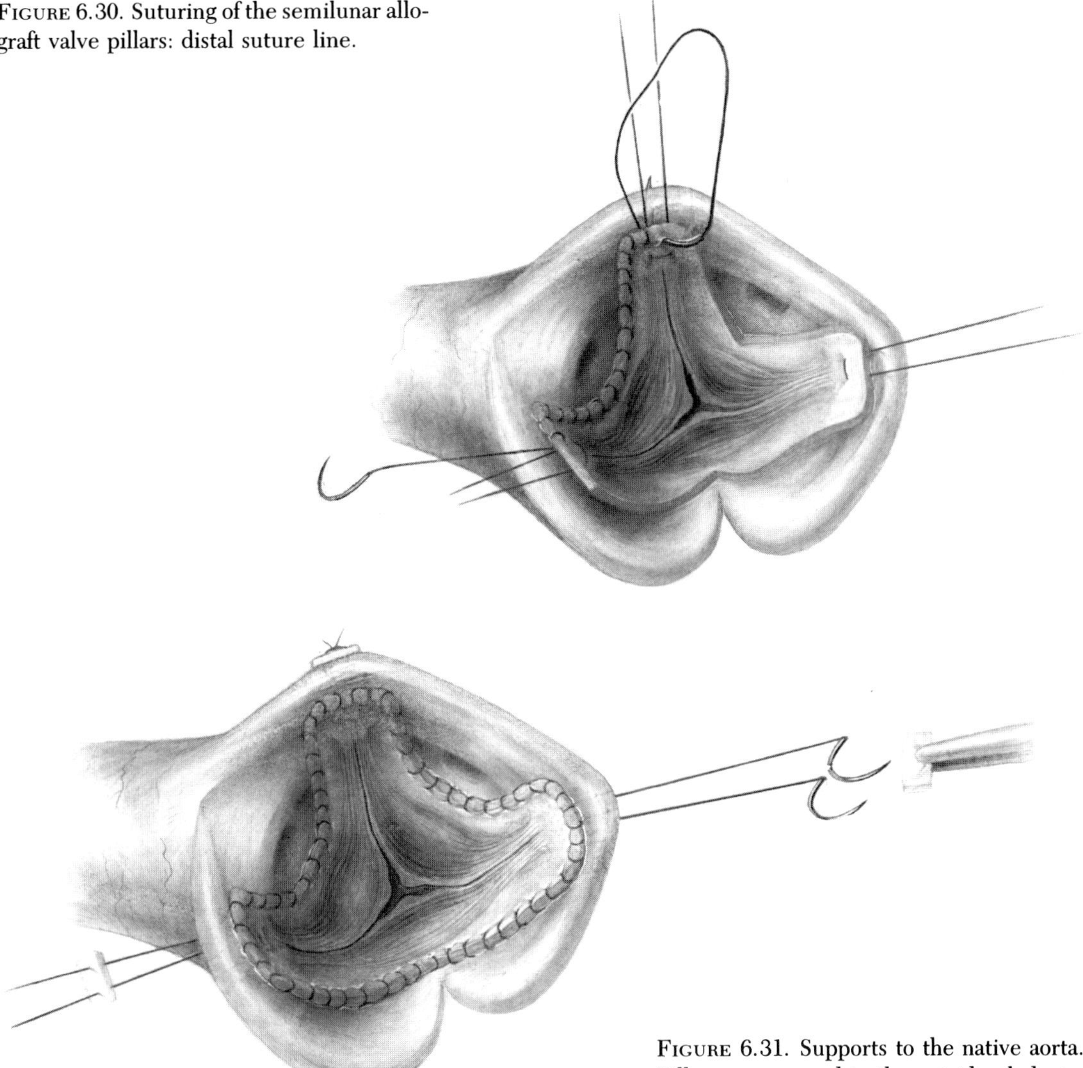

FIGURE 6.30. Suturing of the semilunar allograft valve pillars: distal suture line.

FIGURE 6.31. Supports to the native aorta. Pillars are secured to the outside pledgets.

line is constructed with three 4-0 polypropylene sutures, each begun at the bottom of a sinus and run to meet each other at the top of the pillars (Figs. 6.30 and 6.31).

Although appearing to be the simplest technique conceptually, the classic technique limits later options for sculpturing the aortic root. The spatial geometry of the noncoronary sinus must be reassessed after suturing the allograft commissural posts. If the noncoronary sinus of the native aorta cannot be closed without deforming the commissures on either side, a patch of prosthetic material must be inserted (Fig. 6.32). Air removal maneuvers are performed and the aortotomy closed with a running monofilament suture technique. The "classic" method of aortic valve replacement is best used when there is sufficient dilatation of aortic root to allow "sacrifice" of enough aorta at the aortotomy for adequate closure without distorting the noncoronary sinus and causing inward deflection of the commissural posts at the aortic sinus ridge. If the implant cannot be made in this way, attention to aortic root geometry mandates some minor changes in this method (vida infra).

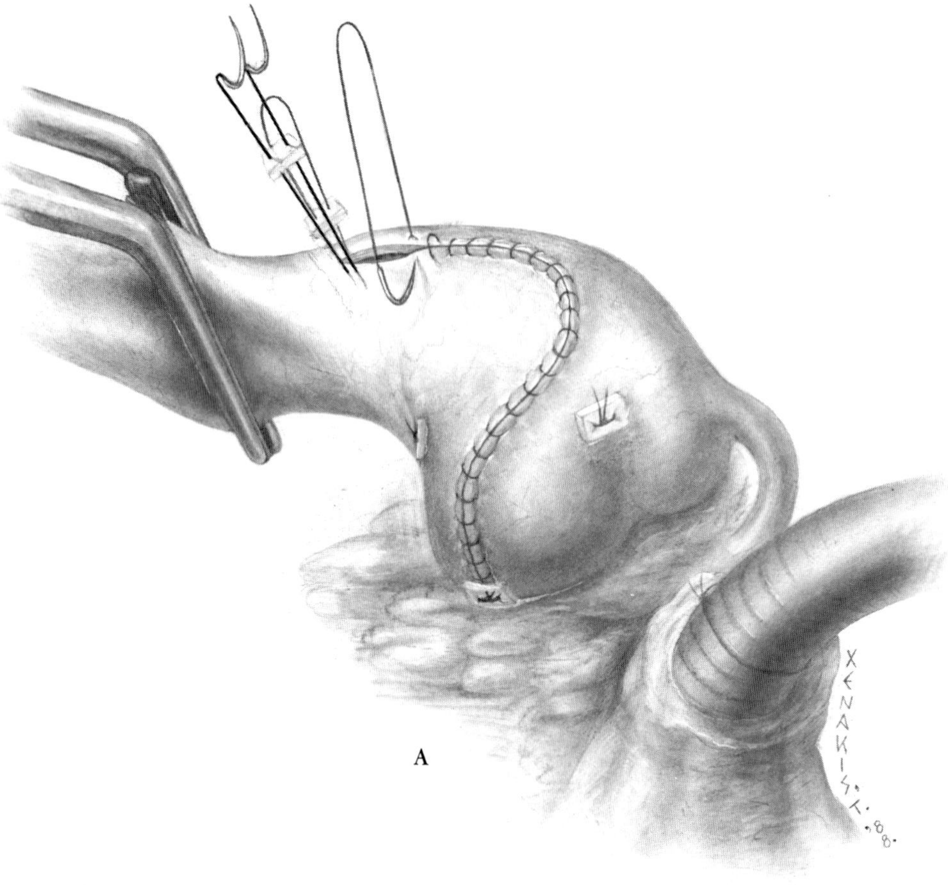

A

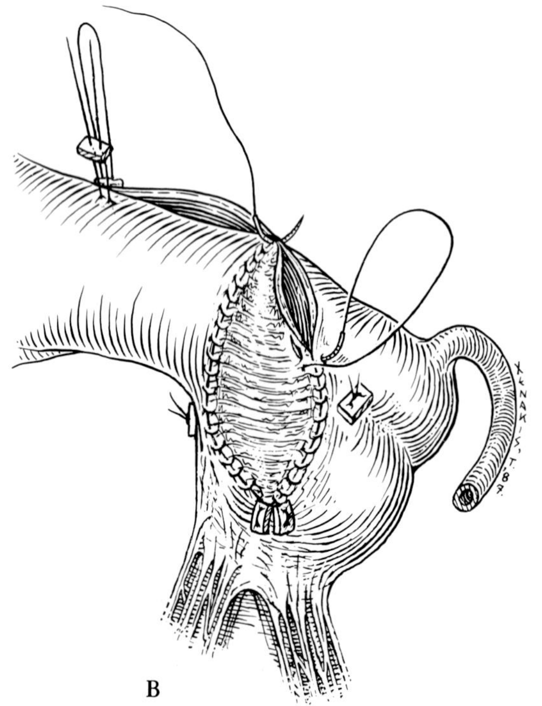

Figure 6.32. Aortotomy closure in the classic "pillars only" technique without (A) and with (B) a prosthetic patch.

3. *Scallop technique*. The scallop technique is similar to the later method of Ross,[12] as it leaves the noncoronary sinus relatively intact to buttress, or fill, the base of the aortotomy incision and allows deferral of the decision on what to do with the aortic root geometry until after the proximal suture line has been completed (Fig. 6.18). To use this technique, the native aortic root must not need annulus enlargement or an augmentation aortoplasty at the level of the sinus ridge. The noncoronary sinus is only minimally "scalloped" (Fig. 6.33). The usual aortotomy incision is performed but can be stopped at the top of the native commissures (the sinus ridge). The proximal suture line is the same as

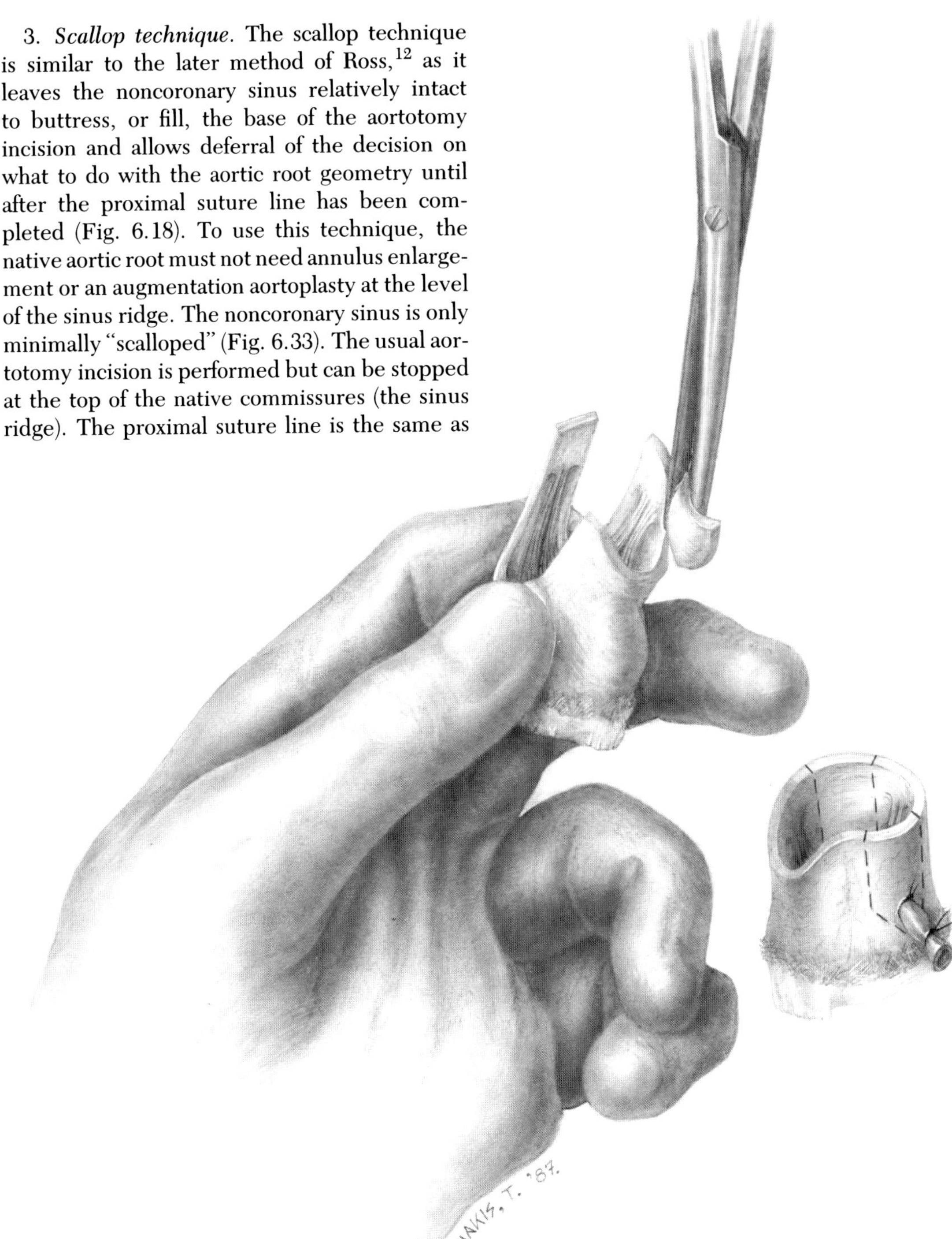

FIGURE 6.33. Sinus excisions for the scallop technique.

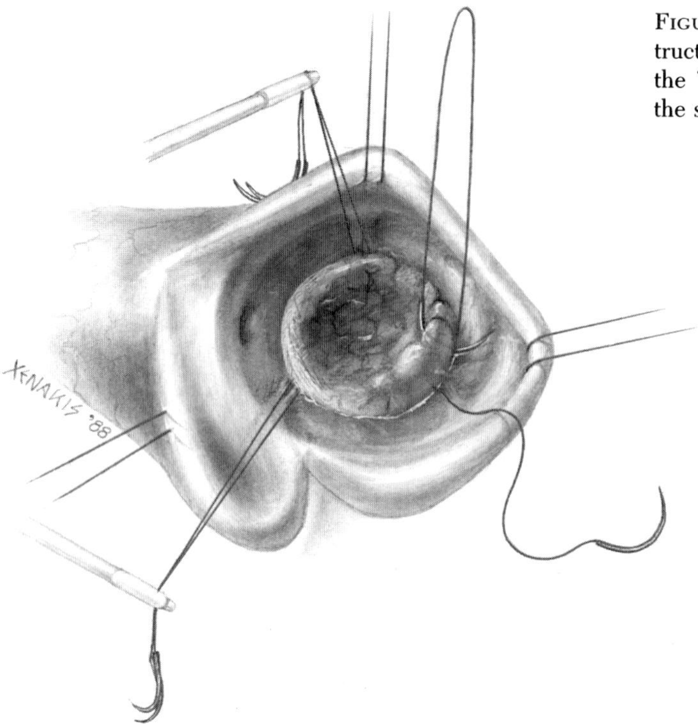

Figure 6.34. Proximal suture line contructed with three continuous sutures. Note the "shallower" aortotomy stopping above the sinus ridge.

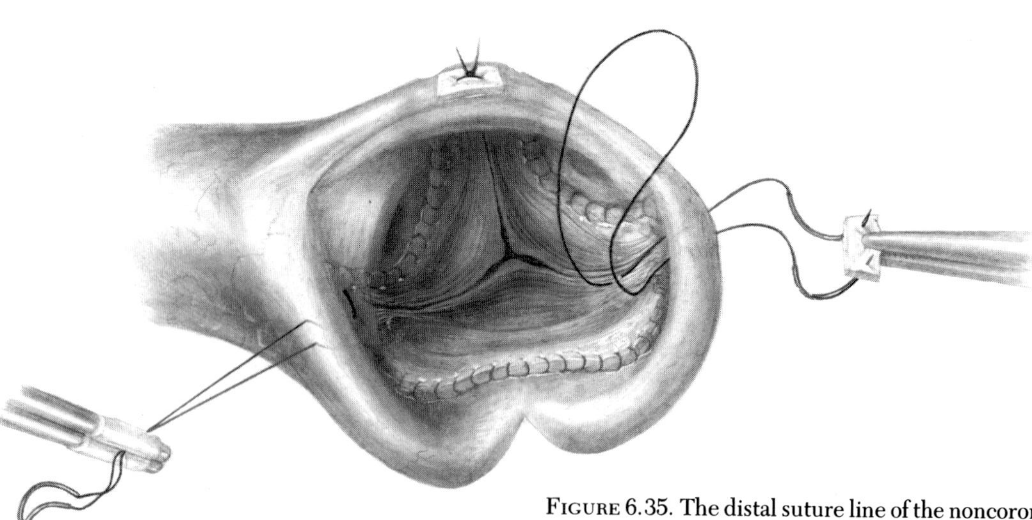

Figure 6.35. The distal suture line of the noncoronary sinus runs just below the aortotomy. The pillars are fixed to pledgets outside the native aorta.

for all the other methods (Fig. 6.34). The distal suture line is constructed in a fashion similar to that for the classic technique except the noncoronary sinus scallop is shallow (Fig. 6.35). A suture is begun at the base of this scallop, run to the top of each commissural post, and tied over a pledget outside the native aorta. The spaces behind the pillars on either side of this noncoronary sinus have been obliterated with nontransmural 4-0 braided suture. The noncoronary sinus is only minimally scalloped so as to place the distal suture line of this portion of the allograft below the level of the aortotomy (Fig. 6.36). Closure is accomplished with a pledgetted simple technique (Fig. 6.37).

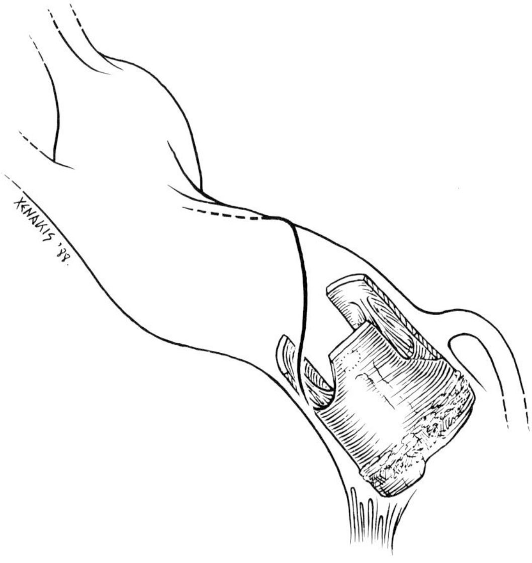

FIGURE 6.36. Position of the allograft within the aortic root, demonstrating retention of the pillar architecture.

Hints

Mistakes to avoid in "freehand" aortic valve replacement include stretching the commissural

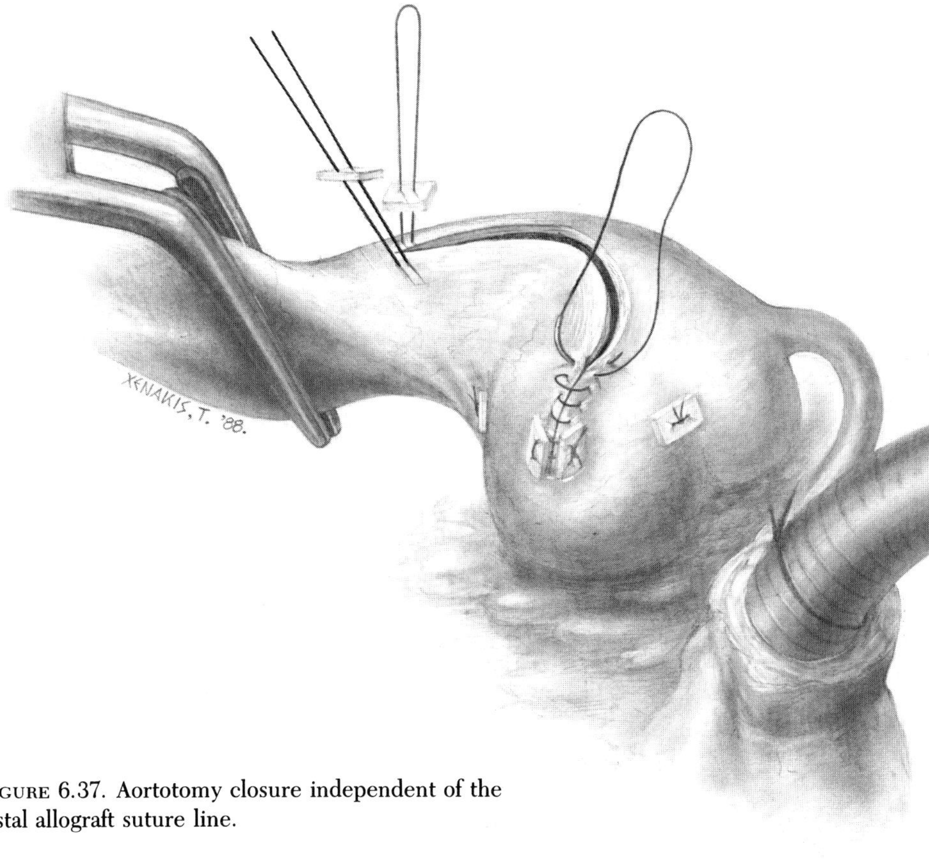

FIGURE 6.37. Aortotomy closure independent of the distal allograft suture line.

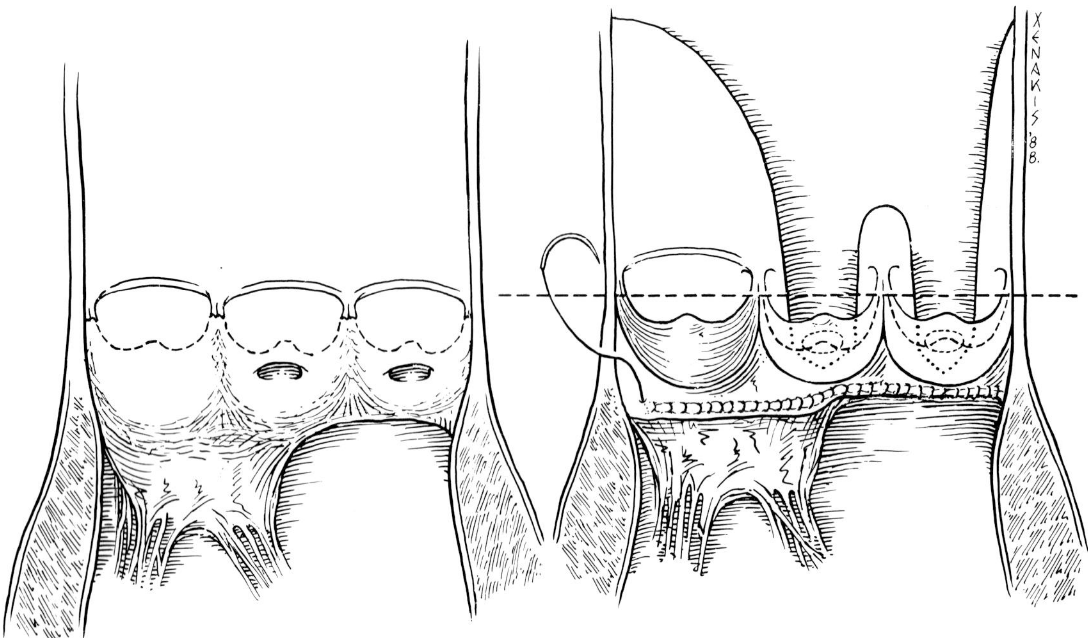

Figure 6.38. The dotted line is at the sinus ridge. Allograft pillars are "hitched" higher than the native pillars.

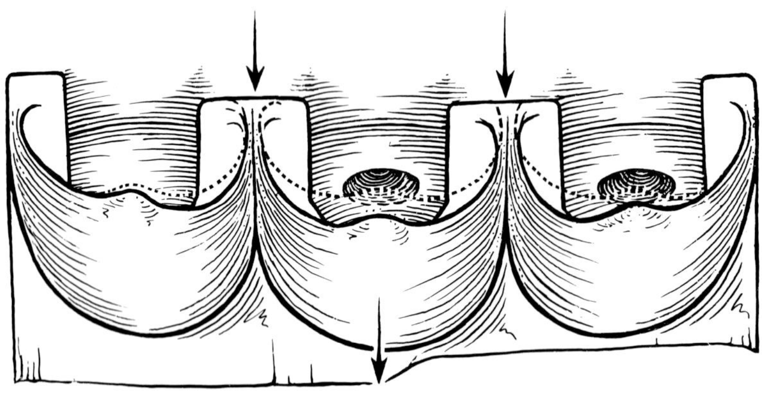

Figure 6.39. Sagging of commissures when the pillar suspension is not maintained. The dotted lines indicate the optimal leaflet edge positions.

posts over dilated aortic sinuses and deviation of commissural post suspensions. The latter can be minimized by sighting the line of the new commissural post relative to the old commissures in native trileaflet valves. In the ideally simple implant, they are orthotopic to the native commissures. Most often, one or two allograft commissural posts are shifted parallel to the native commissural line (while being kept straight axially) so as to account for aortic root geometry and positioning of coronary ostia. If suspension of pillars is not maintained, sagging of semilunar cusps result in regurgitation; thus the tops of the allograft pillars are usually brought to a point superior to the native pillars (Figs. 6.38 and 6.39). Severe calcification that extends heavily into the anterior leaflet of the mitral valve and the trigones causes some risk for "cracking" and bleeding with a continuous proximal suture line. In these cases either an allograft should not be used or consideration is given to a pledgetted interrupted technique.

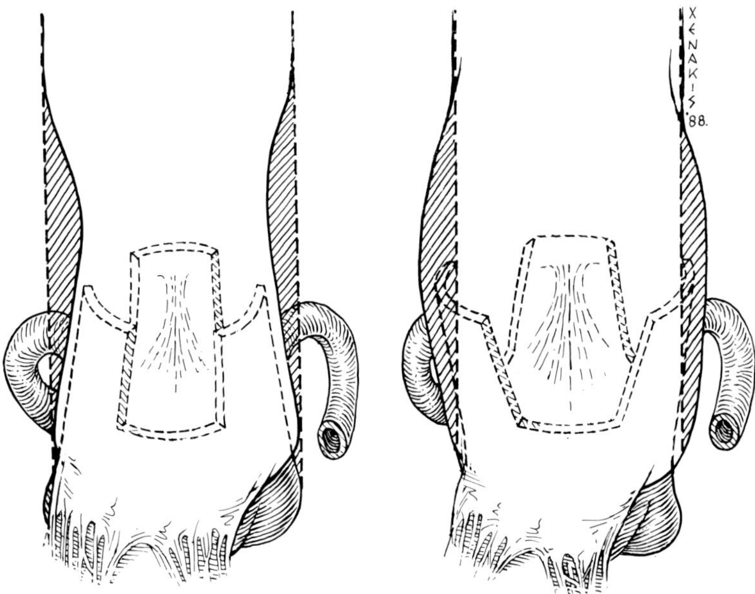

FIGURE 6.40. If the pillars converge, or splay, the distortion can alter semilunar function, resulting in insufficiency. The sinus ridge circumference must approximate the circumference of the base of the normal aortic valve.

Variations in Technique

The preceding techniques are clearly derived from those described by the pioneers of allograft valve transplantation. Variations have been suggested by many authorities.

Placement of the initial three sutures can be underneath the commissural post rather than at the base of each sinus. A 120° counterclockwise rotation can be used as originally described by Barratt-Boyes.[10] We have found it easier to align the native coronary ostia to the analogous portions of the allograft coronary sinuses and allow the commissural posts to assume their necessary positions within the aortic root rather than the reverse. Doty recommended Teflon pledgets at the top of each commissural post on the inside of the aorta, whereas we prefer to place the pledgets outside in order to reduce thrombotic potential.[13,14] Ross did not recommend rotation of the allograft within the aortic root and left the allograft noncoronary sinus intact, forming a backing to the aortotomy.[12] When using this method (Scallop technique), the aortotomy should be stopped above the level of this minimally scalloped sinus unless aortoplasty of the noncoronary aortic sinus is necessary. Similar to Ross, we find it easier not to rotate the allograft except in special situations, e.g., extreme left ventricular hypertrophy with a bulging septum. In this situation, it is advantageous to place the allograft with the least amount of annular bulk (i.e., aortic/mitral continuity) over the septum. Similarly, routine use of the orthotopic position lends itself to variations in annulus enlargement, as described below. Obviously, for applications such as an extended aortic root replacement with Konno, as described by Clarke and associates,[15,16] rotation is mandatory. Barratt-Boyes recommended complete scalloping of all three sinuses and 120° rotation of the allograft (i.e., classic technique).[10] Minor degrees of rotation to account for cusp asymmetry and coronary ostia asymmetry are an essential part of the technique (vida infra).

Barratt-Boyes' aortotomy appears similar to ours with perhaps a slightly less exaggerated transverse component. He also emphasized the subannular suturing of the proximal suture line. Like Ross and Yacoub, we have found this step not to be essential except when the native coronary ostia are very close to the fibrous attachment of the semilunar cusps.[17] In these cases subannular placement of the proximal suture line is critical (vida infra). Also, Barratt-Boyes has emphasized *not* utilizing monofilament suture material as he believes it tends to slice through homograft tissue (personal communication). Others have used an interrupted proximal suture line technique for both aortic root replacements and freehand aortic valve replacements.[18] We recommend the continuous suture technique for the freehand aortic valve replacement because of speed and hemostasis, but we use the interrupted technique for aortic root replacement.

Barratt-Boyes has emphasized reduction aortic root tailoring involving excision of a wedge of aortic root to avoid splaying of the commissural post, which leads to central incompetence when transplanting allografts into dilated aortic roots.[3] Avoidance of splaying or sagging is critically important, being one of the keys to the success of the procedure (Fig. 6.40).[19]

Bailey has recommended a technique to avoid splaying of the sinus ridge region of the allograft by leaving this portion of the graft intact until final sutures are placed.[20] We have not used this technique as it appears cumbersome; our delaying the excision of the allograft sinuses until completion of the proximal suture line (similar to Ross) accomplishes the same important geometric goal.

Surgical Technique for Annulus Enlargement in the Small Aortic Root for Concomitant Use with Allografts

Indications

Usually placement of a mechanical prosthetic valve smaller than 21–23 mm is not recommended because of the risk of inducing prosthetic aortic stenosis.[21,22] Allograft aortic valves have superior hydraulic performance. Hemodynamically, a 17-mm allograft functions better than a 21-mm prosthesis. In the presence of a small aortic annulus, enlargement can be accomplished with techniques similar to that used for prosthetic valves, but the use of allograft tissue simplifies the technique. Aortic annulus enlargement can be used for absolute size increases as well as for altering the rotational geometry of the aortic root (vida infra). This technique can also be used for aortic valve replacement in children so that an adult-sized aortic valve can be positioned into which the child may "grow." The Appendix, which gives aortic valve diameters, is a good guide to the need for aortic annulus enlargements. If a patient of body surface area (BSA) 1.6 m^2 (or one who is expected to grow to that size) has a native annulus of 19 mm or less, he or she should not be left with an allograft smaller than 17 mm or risk the creation of aortic stenosis hemodynamics. As a practical matter, a BSA 2.0 m^2 individual, as a large adult, has a 20- to 24-mm diameter aortic valve. Thus we rarely leave a patient with a valve smaller than 19–20 mm. Conversely, except in small children, it is usually possible to place a 17-mm or larger aortic valve allograft with the techniques described below.

"Manouguian" Technique

The method described by Manouguian and Seybold-Epting for prosthetic valve placement and enlargement utilizing a pericardial patch sutured into the anterior leaflet of the native mitral valve can be adapted to a technique applicable to freehand allograft insertion.[23] The aortotomy is extended somewhat more posteriorly than usual through the region of the native commissure above the midpoint of the anterior leaflet of the mitral valve (Fig. 6.41). The depth of the incision into the left atrium and mitral valve is determined by the amount of enlargement necessary but can extend for a distance of 4–8 mm. The incision into the roof of the left atrium is closed with pledgetted sutures.

The defect in the anterior leaflet of the mitral valve is filled with a shallow piece of residual anterior mitral valve leaflet left on the allograft (Fig. 6.42). When a relatively deep V is created in the anterior leaflet of the mitral valve, these sutures are placed as horizontal interrupted 4-0 monofilaments until the level of the true annulus is reached (Fig. 6.43). At this point, an additional suture is placed on either side, tied, and used as a running suture. A third suture is placed underneath the right coronary ostia of both the allograft and the native valves. The valve is inverted into the ventricular cavity and the proximal suture line constructed by running each suture toward the middle (Fig. 6.44). Unless there is a very bulbous root, the flange technique is usually used for the distal aortic closure (Fig. 6.45).

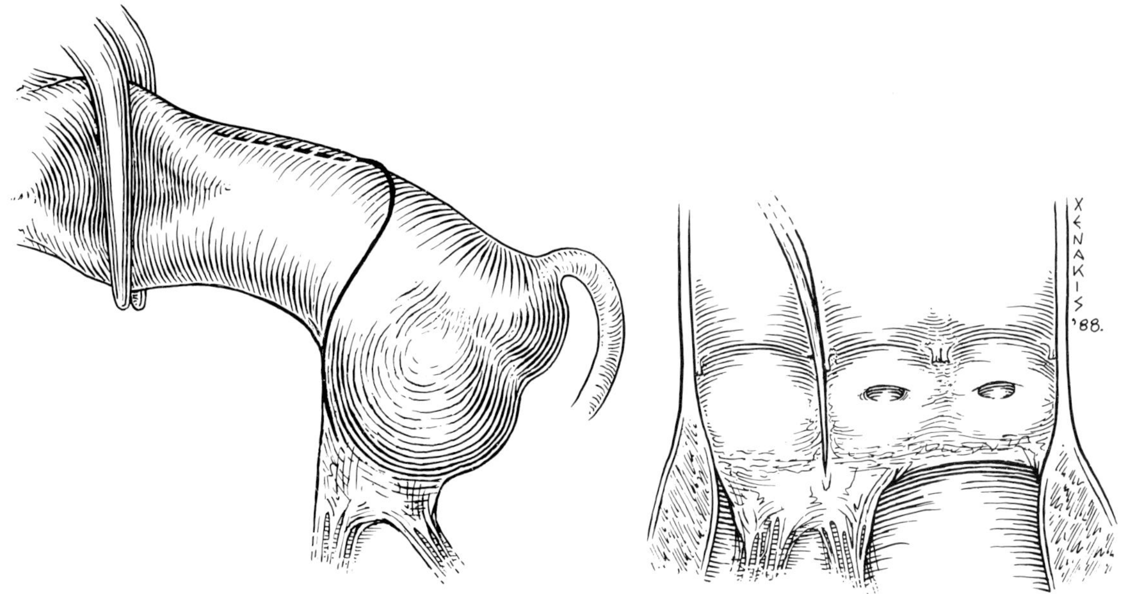

FIGURE 6.41. Aortotomy for enlargement of the annulus when using the Manouguian approach.

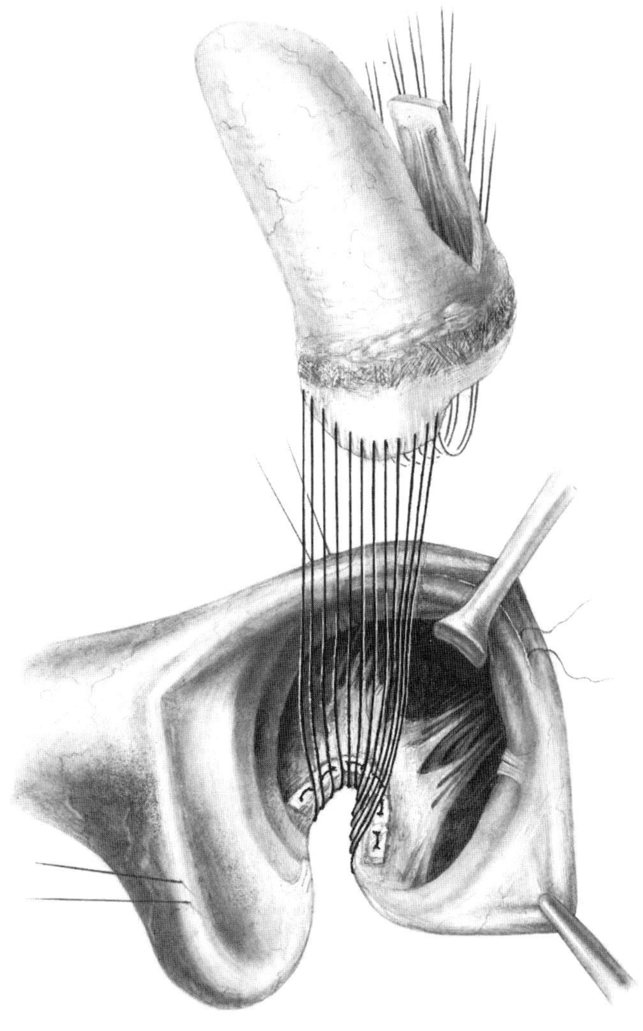

FIGURE 6.42. Enlargement of the annulus by filling the incision into the anterior leaflet of the mitral valve with mitral valve tissue of the allograft.

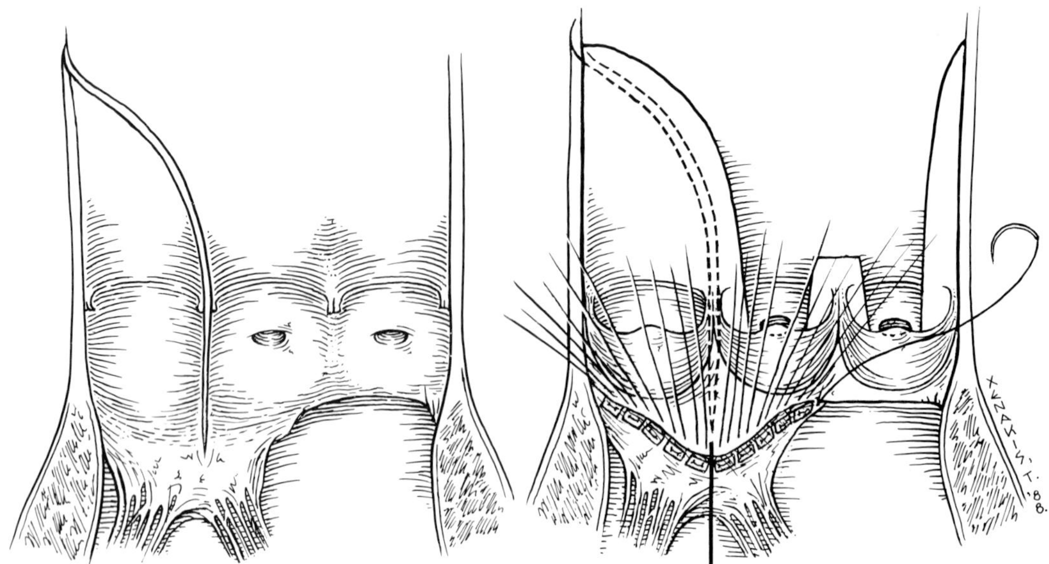

FIGURE 6.43. Pledgetted technique used for mitral to mitral valve tissue closure. Running sutures are used for the remainder of the proximal suture line.

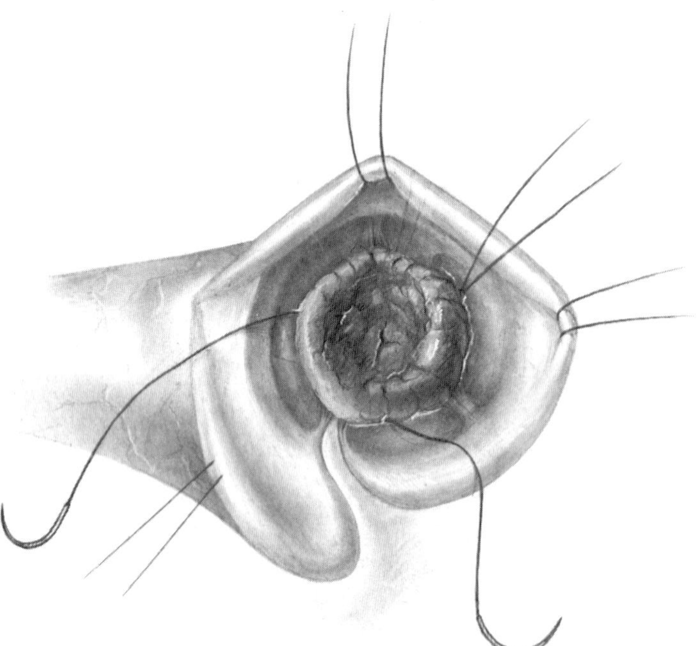

FIGURE 6.44. Proximal suture line with three running sutures. The third suture is begun at a point equidistant from the two begun near the fibrous trigones, where the mitral pledgetted sutures stop.

"Nicks" Technique

The method of Nicks and coworkers can be adapted for use with allografts.[24] It is an incision similar to that originally described by Barratt-Boyes.[10] The incision across the annulus is made to the right of the commissure between the left and noncoronary sinuses of the native aortic root and extended into the anterior leaflet of the mitral valve (Fig. 6.46). It is posterior to the bundle of His. If only a small amount of enlargement

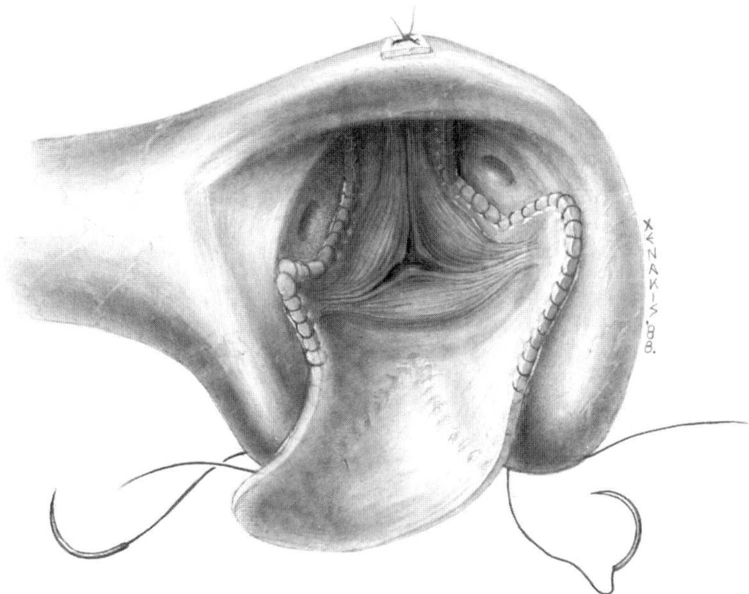

FIGURE 6.45. Closure after annulus enlargement usually requires augmentation aortoplasty.

is necessary, the annulus is simply "nicked," which allows an enlargement of 1–2 mm without actually entering the left atrium. If additional enlargement is necessary, the incision is continued into the anterior leaflet of the mitral valve, and reconstruction is accomplished in a manner similar to the Manouguian technique, utilizing the anterior leaflet of the allograft mitral valve (Fig. 6.47). In this case, interrupted sutures are placed; the remnant of mitral valve tissue is somewhat asymmetric and not in the middle of the leaflet but rather slightly displaced toward the noncoronary sinus (Fig. 6.48). It is usually simplest to use the flange technique for the distal suture line, but the classic method can also be used. Whichever method is chosen, care must be taken to symmetrically reestablish the noncoronary sinus.

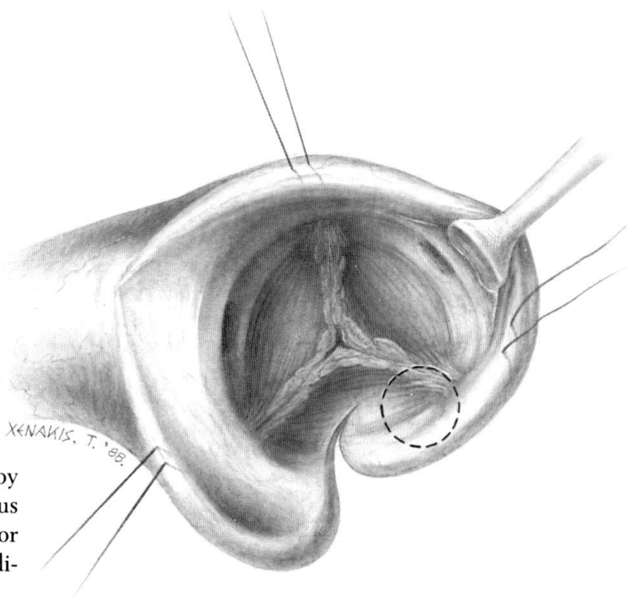

FIGURE 6.46. Enlargement of the annulus by extension of the aortotomy across the annulus anterior to the native commissure and posterior to the membranous septum. Dotted circle indicates the region of the AV node.

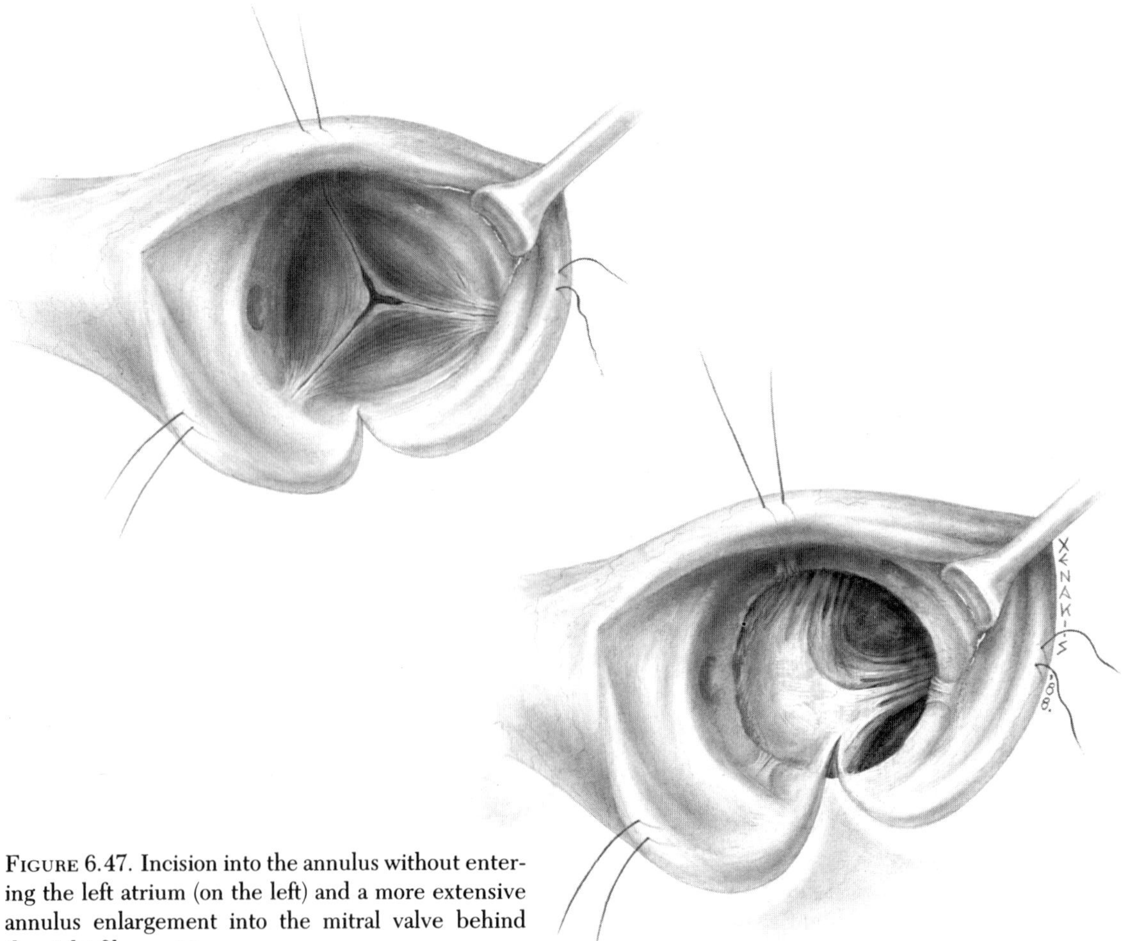

FIGURE 6.47. Incision into the annulus without entering the left atrium (on the left) and a more extensive annulus enlargement into the mitral valve behind the right fibrous trigone.

FIGURE 6.48. Annulus enlargement when a more anterior extension of the incision into the mitral valve is chosen. Care is taken to remain posterior to the AV node.

Aortoplastic Techniques for Problematic Aortic Root Geometry

Indications and Contraindications

One of the major reasons for failure of freehand aortic valve implants is lack of attention to aortic root geometry and its effect on the functional anatomy of the allograft. Barratt-Boyes and associates clearly demonstrated the problem of native aortic root dilatation causing failure.[3] Aortoplastic techniques can be applied to both dilated

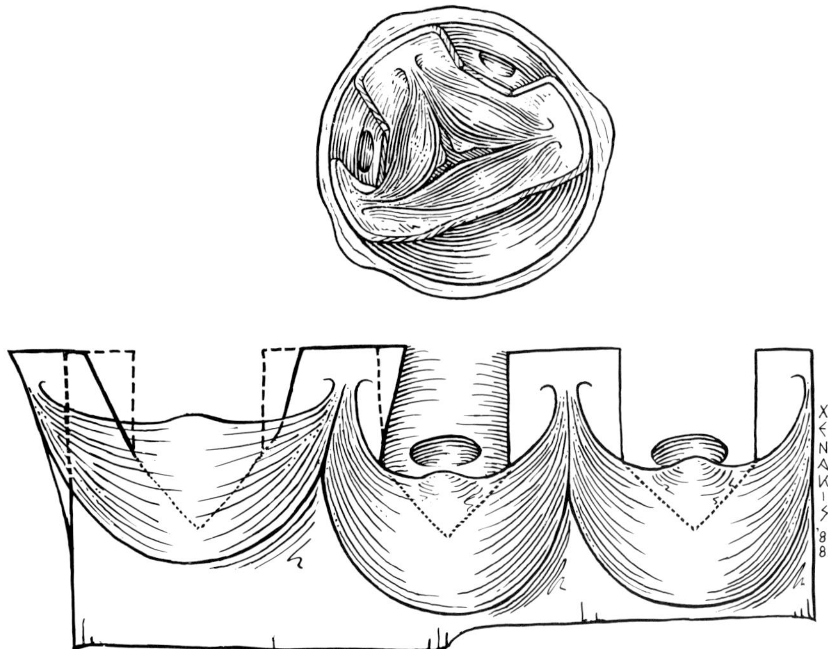

FIGURE 6.49. Effect of splaying and convergence of pillars on semilunar valve function. One of the major technical errors leading to early insufficiency is deviation of the allograft pillars off the long axis of the aortic outflow.

and constricted aortic roots, and they are also applicable to the "normal" aortic root for which closure of the aortotomy would result in narrowing at the sinus ridge level. Contraindications to aortic root tailoring include connective tissue disease and grossly distorted roots with asymmetric sinuses, the latter is best treated with root replacement.

Functional Aortic Valve Anatomy

As has been reviewed by many authors, the aortic valve function depends on semilunar valvular anatomy. This design function depends on leaflet suspension to maintain apposition to the other two leaflets.[25] In an allograft, it depends on adequate suspension of the pillars to maintain the semilunar mechanism and avoidance of splaying, which causes central incompetence or convergence of the pillars, which in turn can result in sagging of the cusps (Figs. 6.38, 6.39, 6.49, and 6.50). As has been pointed out by Frater,[19] the intercommissural distance at the sinus rim level must be maintained and seen to approximate the cylindrical diameter of the fibrous skeleton of the heart forming the base of the aortic root (Fig. 6.51). If these geometric principles are recreated with the freehand technique, the semilunar aortic valve mechanism is preserved and valve competence is maintained. If the suspension of the semilunar valve is lost owing to incorrect placement of the pillars, sagging, or distortion, incompetence results from prolapse of a valve leaflet. Some technical adjustment to aortic root anatomy has been required in 30% of our cases.

Reduction Aortoplasty

Barratt-Boyes[11] and Ross and associates[26] have emphasized the role of aortic root reduction, or "tailoring," to reduce the size of the aortic root. One of the major reasons cited for failure in Barratt-Boyes' 1987 review was dilated aortic root. His group advised against placement of an allograft in a root larger than 30 mm in diameter, although they did recommend placement if the aortic root can be tailored to a diameter of 30 mm or less. We basically use his technique, as published in 1965, for reduction aortoplasty.[11]

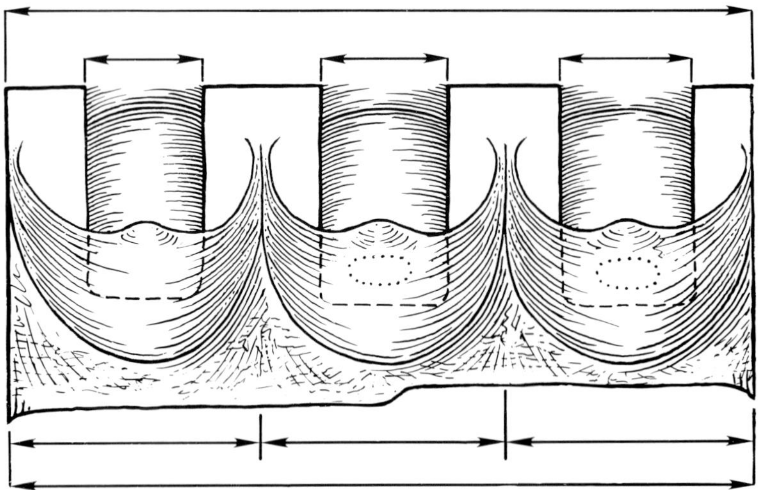

FIGURE 6.50. Relation of aortic base to sinus ridge.

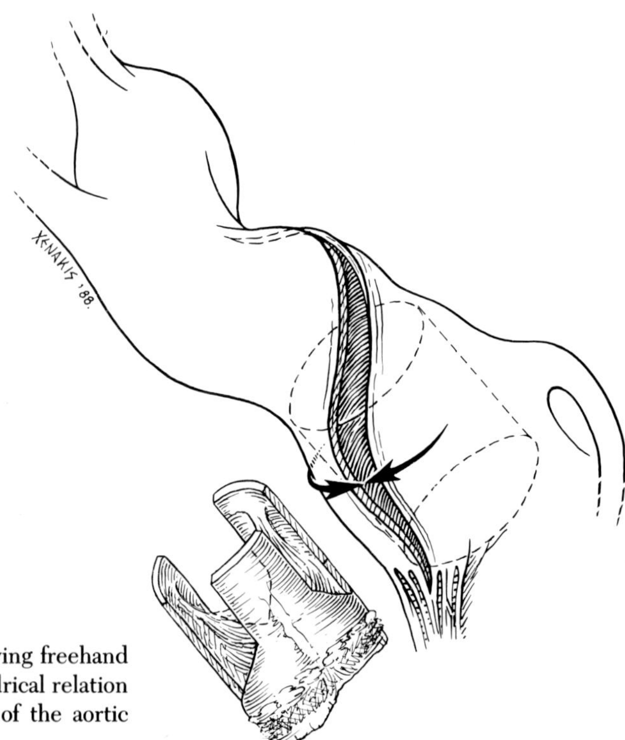

FIGURE 6.51. Closure of the aortic root following freehand aortic valve insertion must maintain the cylindrical relation of the sinus ridge, pillars, and fibrous base of the aortic valve.

The aortotomy is extended just into the mitral leaflet posterior to the right fibrous trigone, which is similar to the incision location of Nicks and associates ("nicked Nicks").[24] Native aorta is excised, and the aortotomy is closed to "reef" the excess aortic root tissue, thereby reducing the diameter of the aortic cylinder between the aortic base and the top of the new sinus ridge (Fig. 6.52). Interrupted sutures are placed at the base of this incision prior to beginning the allograft implant. This measure allows later tying of these sutures after placement of the allograft (Fig. 6.53). Two to three such sutures may be required. It is important when reducing the size

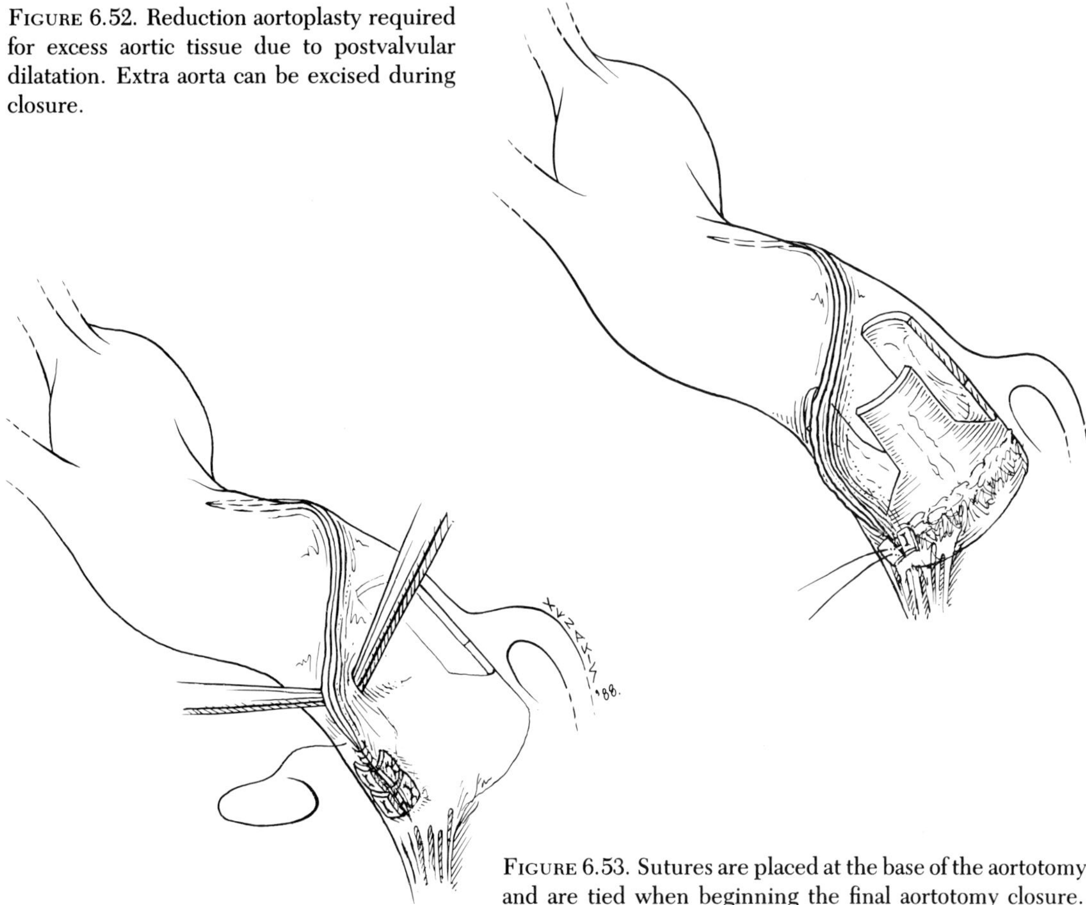

FIGURE 6.52. Reduction aortoplasty required for excess aortic tissue due to postvalvular dilatation. Extra aorta can be excised during closure.

FIGURE 6.53. Sutures are placed at the base of the aortotomy and are tied when beginning the final aortotomy closure.

of the aortic root in the region of the noncoronary sinus that compensation for pillar positioning is performed so as to avoid splaying the allograft pillars toward the reduction aortoplasty. The base of the pillars is relatively orthotopic, but the line of pillar suturing must be deviated away from the reduction aortoplasty rather than being parallel to the native commissural line. If desired, the stay sutures at the top of the pillars can be passed through the native aorta at selected points to test the orientation prior to freehand suturing of the distal suture line.

Augmentation Aortoplasty

When the postvalvular aortic root is small, the aorta can be enlarged to maintain the diameter of the proximal root and new sinus ridge after allograft implantation. With a small or deformed aortic root, it is obvious that this step must be done and can be accomplished either with Dacron material, a separate piece of allograft, or using an aortoplastic technique that utilizes a flange of the allograft left attached (preferred technique). Augmentation is always necessary in the "normal" aortic root when allografts are used for aortic valve replacement, as the aortotomy cannot be closed without displacing orthotopically positioned pillars on either side of the noncoronary sinus, as would occur, for example, during aortic valve replacement for acute bacterial endocarditis in a young patient.

The allograft is sewn with a standard proximal suture line, and the right and left coronary ostia are aligned as usual. The pillars are placed on either side of the noncoronary sinus but deviated toward the aortotomy and not parallel to native commissures. The noncoronary sinus is closed

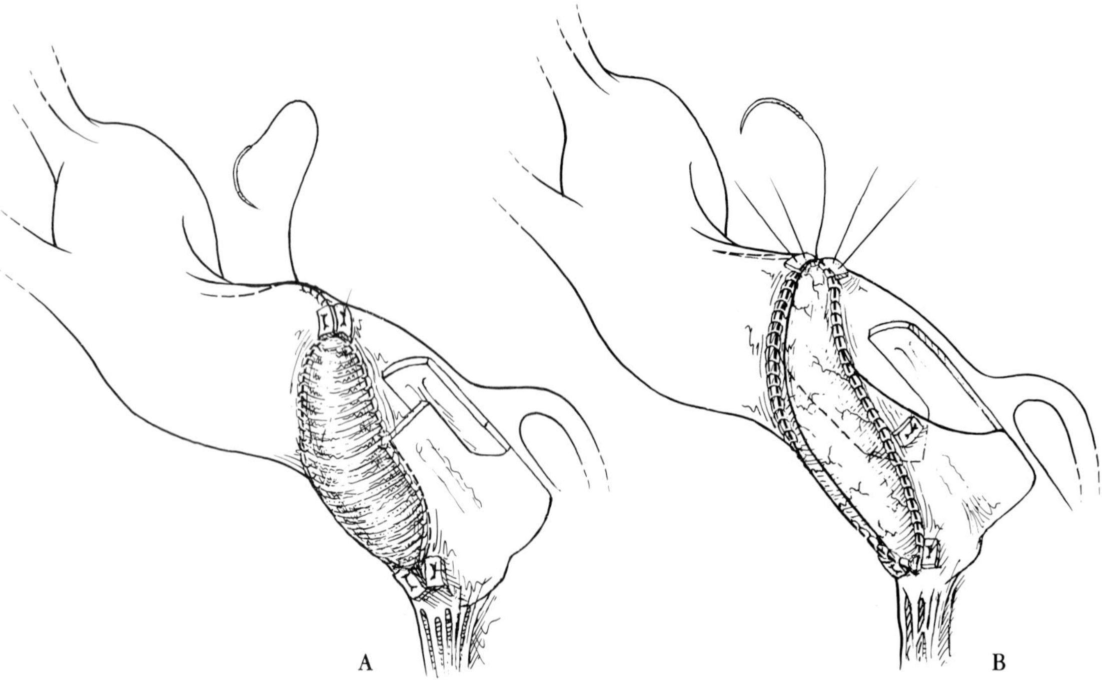

Figure 6.54. Aortic root geometry and the size of the noncoronary sinus are maintained using the classic technique plus augmentation for a small aortic root. Direct closure of the noncoronary sinus would have deformed and converged the pillars toward the aortotomy suture line. Use of a Dacron patch (A) and the flange aortoplasty technique (B).

with an oval patch of Dacron or free patch of allograft aortic wall (Fig. 6.54).

A perhaps easier and more asesthetically pleasing method is the flange technique, which leaves the noncoronary portion of the allograft aorta intact and uses it to enlarge the aortotomy to the point of the transverse component (vida supra). When it is obvious at the time of analysis that this enlargement, or augmentation, of the noncoronary sinus is required, this portion of the allograft is not trimmed. The right and left coronary sinuses are constructed in the usual way, but the top of the pillars on either side of the noncoronary sinus are completed by suturing the running suture from the bottom of the coronary sinus to the stay sutures, which have been brought through the aortic wall and tied over a pledget. The aortotomy is then closed by starting a pledgetted suture at the base of the aortotomy to the outside of the allograft aortic annulus. This suture is tied and each limb run superiorly along the inside of the aortotomy to the allograft flange. The suturing is completed to the point where the transverse aortotomy turns superiorly; the flange fills the proximal aortotomy (Fig. 6.54B). It augments the aortic root and, in addition, maintains the geometry of the allograft aortic root. It should now be clear why the original aortotomy is so important. The lower portion of the incision should cross the sinus ridge and go to the annulus parallel to the long axis, thereby providing the correct orientation for any necessary augmentation.

Augmentation Aortoplasty with Concomitant Annulus Enlargement

Aortic root augmentation aortoplasty can be combined with an annuloplasty to place a larger aortic allograft inside a small aortic root while maintaining accurate aortic root geometry. When annulus enlargement is required, an aug-

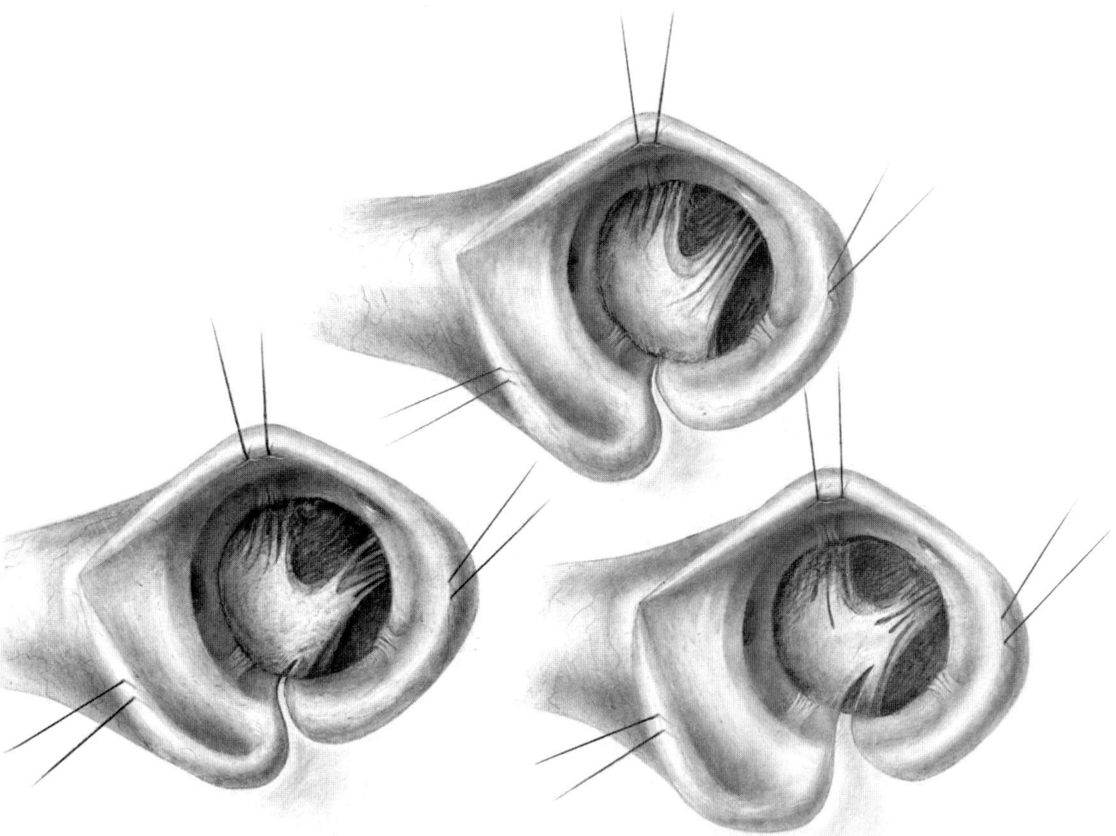

FIGURE 6.55. Extent of the incision across the annulus depends on the amount of annuloplasty required. Demonstrated are incisions into the annulus (top) and through the annulus (bottom left). The bottom right drawing represents a formal extension well into the mitral leaflet.

mentation aortoplasty is usually necessary to maintain aortic root geometry. The original aortotomy is extended across the annulus toward the mitral valve.[27] It can then be extended into the mitral leaflet, as originally suggested by Nicks and Barratt-Boyes, or using the more posterior incision of Manouguian.[10] If only another 2 mm of circumference is required, this incision does not need to enter the left atrium. The left atrial tissue is reflected off the aortic-mitral region external to the aortic root; if additional enlargement is required, the incision can be extended into the anterior leaflet of the mitral valve, as described above for the annuloplasty technique (Fig. 6.55). The defect in the mitral valve leaflet is then filled by leaving a portion of the allograft anterior leaflet attached (Fig. 6.56). The enlargement of the noncoronary sinus is continued by utilizing the flange technique of aortic root augmentation (Fig. 6.57). When using this technique, the alteration in the pillar positions on either side of the right and left coronary sinuses needs to be carefully analyzed when the first three proximal sutures are placed because although the enlargement is obtained within the noncoronary sinus it is partly transferred to the coronary sinuses by parallel shifting of the pillars toward the surgeon.

Management of Complicating Coronary Anatomy

In the idealized aortic valve, the sinuses are of equal size, and the right and left coronary ostia are at 120° angles.[14] Techniques have been described as though one perfectly symmetric valve

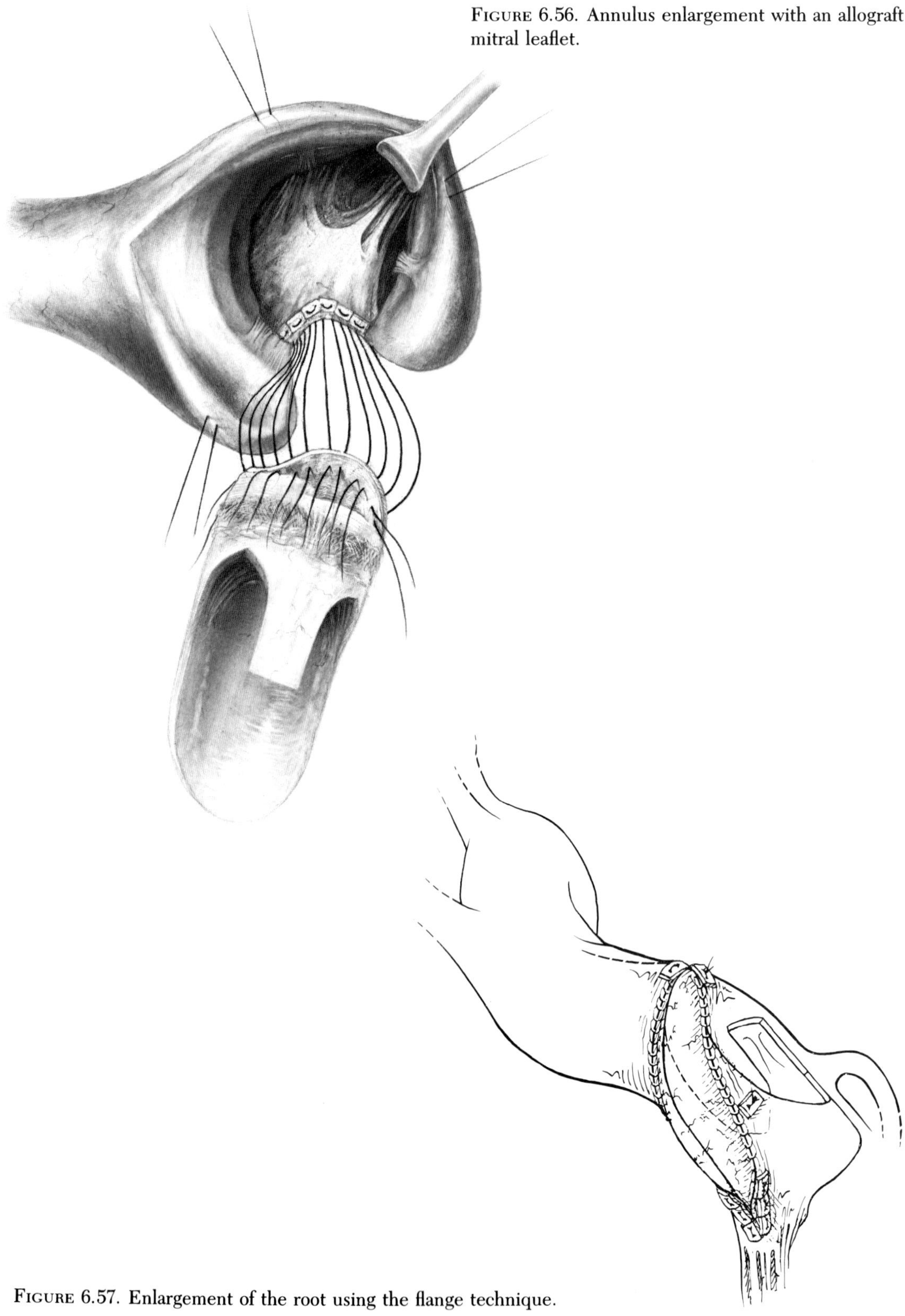

Figure 6.56. Annulus enlargement with an allograft mitral leaflet.

Figure 6.57. Enlargement of the root using the flange technique.

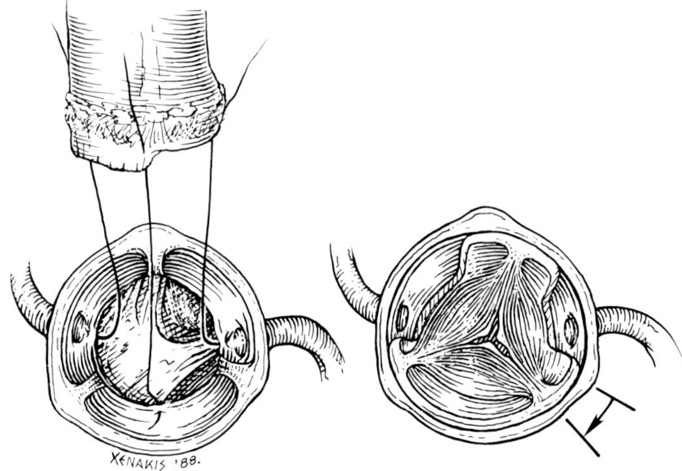

FIGURE 6.58. Placement of sutures to manage coronary ostia approaching 180° orientation. Arrow indicates the "mini-rotation" of the allograft within the root.

is always inserted into another symmetric annulus. However, just as the ancient concept of the idealized human fitting into a perfect circle was wrong, rarely is the human aortic valve so symmetric. The pathology of aortic insufficiency and stenosis further alters the native symmetry. These alterations in coronary ostia and sinus relations must be accounted for in the freehand aortic valve insertion surgical technique.

As was pointed out by McAlpine, the sinuses are variable in size; in general the disparity in annular circumference encompassing the various sinuses can be as great as 20–25% in "normal" valves.[28] The order of size, from large to small, is right, left, and noncoronary. In addition, asymmetric placement of the coronary ostia within the coronary sinuses increases the problem for the surgeon performing the freehand suturing. A methodical approach to placing the first three sutures allows management of these geometric problems in virtually all cases.

Asymmetric Placement of Coronary Ostia Within Native Sinuses: Minirotation

A common geometry involves rotational displacement of the right coronary orifice to the right within its sinus such that the right and left coronary ostia begin to approach 180° (Fig. 6.58). Occasionally, asymmetry of the allograft sinuses allows management by rotating sinuses (e.g., allograft left to recipient right). Usually placement of an allograft inside this geometry requires a slight rotation, placing the left coronary ostia closer to the pillar between the left and noncoronary sinuses such that the pillar between the right and noncoronary sinuses is shifted away from the native coronary ostia and the extremely close native commissure. Placing the allograft in the orthotopic position and utilizing the placement of the first three sutures as the architectural guide assists in this "minirotation." The first suture is placed through the native aortic annulus at a point immediately underneath the left coronary ostia. The suture is then passed as a simple suture through the annulus of the allograft at a point counterclockwise from the bottom of the sinus, which then "sets up" the minirotation. The second suture is then placed below the native right coronary ostia and passed as a simple suture through the annulus of the allograft at a point in the right coronary sinus that allows suturing around the native coronary ostia and effects a similar minirotation of the anterior pillar to the right. The third suture for the proximal suture line is placed at a point equidistant between the first two sutures on both the allograft and the native annulus. The allograft is inverted into the ventricle and the suture lines completed in the usual manner, avoiding tilting of the allograft pillars.

A somewhat similar asymmetry can occur when the right coronary sinus of the native aorta is small even without rightward displacement of the right coronary ostia but with leftward displacement of the pillar. The allograft pillar is

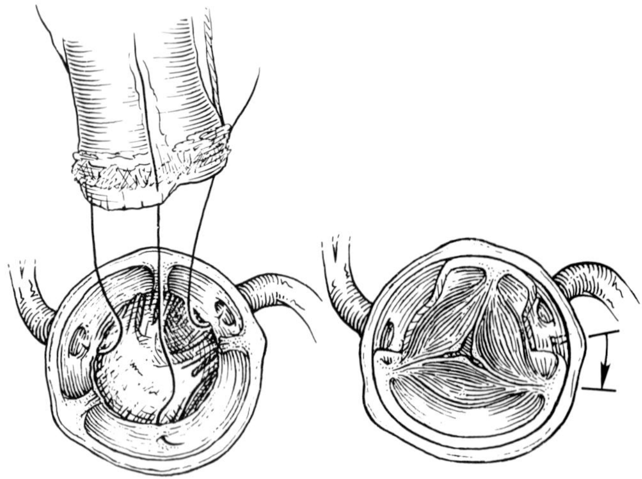

Figure 6.59. A small right recipient sinus requires suturing an allograft pillar to the surgeon's side of the native commissural post. The "rotation" to move the pillar is at the level of the annulus.

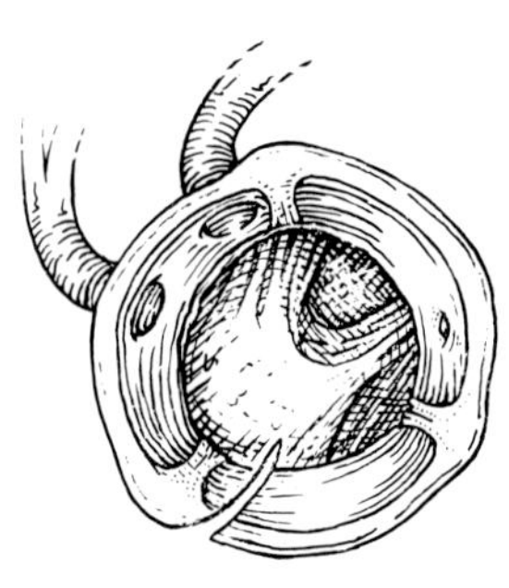

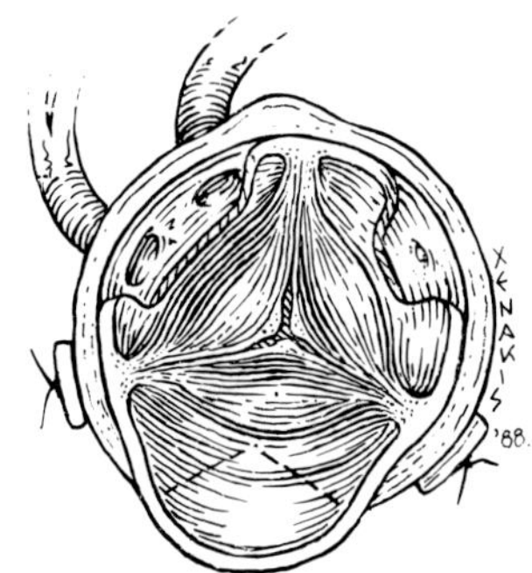

Figure 6.60. Large native left coronary sinus with origins of both coronary ostia. Note the small coronary artery arising from the right sinus. A large allograft is placed to accommodate the large left sinus using the combined technique of annulus enlargement plus augmentation aortoplasty.

sutured to the surgeon's side of the native pillar (Fig. 6.59). The principle of aligning the new pillar parallel to the recipient commissural post is followed.

Both Coronaries Arising from a Single Sinus

A variation on the asymmetry problem occurs when both right and left coronary ostia arise from the left coronary sinus of the recipient aortic root. The native left coronary sinus is usually larger, and the problem is to place a smaller allograft valve inside the native annulus without splaying the pillars on either side of the dual coronary ostia. This problem can be solved by combining the techniques of rotation with augmentation aortoplasty. It is done by enlarging the noncoronary sinus with an augmentation aortoplasty (vida supra), which enlarges the total aortic root and allows a larger allograft to be inserted (Fig. 6.60).

The largest sinus (or the left sinus when they are relatively equal) of the allograft valve is then selected to match the native left coronary sinus, and the three guide sutures are placed. The first suture is placed at the bottom of the native left coronary sinus to the bottom of the allograft sinus. The other two sutures are then placed at 120° angles from the first and the pillars allowed to rotate to their imperative positions. The augmentation aortoplasty can be done with either prosthetic material or an allograft (flange technique).

Bicuspid Aortic Valve with 180° Coronary Ostia

In a situation where the coronary ostia are at 180° angles from each other in the native aortic root, simple orthotopic placement of a trileaflet valve would be defeated. Once again, if the allograft aortic valve is clearly the optimal choice for the patient, it can be managed with enlargement of the noncoronary sinus region of the native aortic root with or without an annulo-

FIGURE 6.61. Management of a bicuspid aortic valve with 180° coronary ostia by combining the techniques of annulus enlargement with aortoplasty to rotate the right coronary ostium to the left while maintaining aortic root geometry.

▷

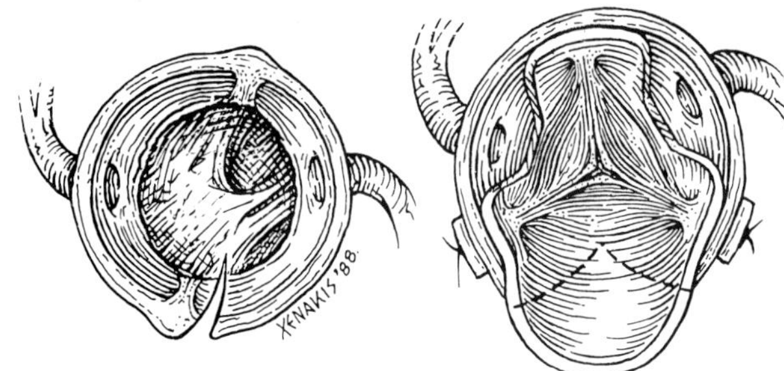

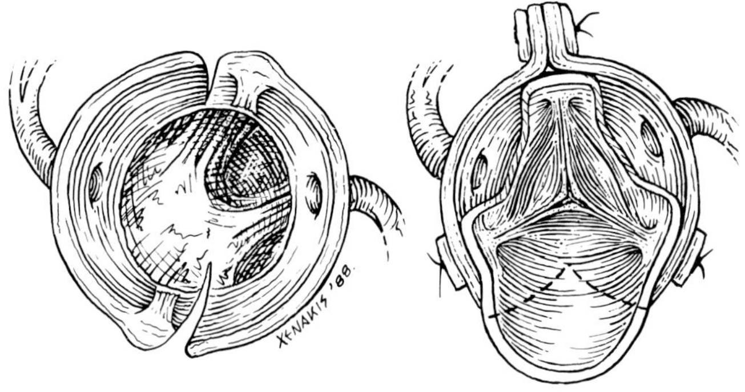

FIGURE 6.62. Counterincision in the aortic root, posterior to the commissural region between the right and left coronaries. This incision does *not* extend to the annulus but takes advantage of poststenotic dilatation of the aortic root to "pull" the coronary ostia toward each other.

plasty. Most often, an annuloplasty is also required that rotates the native coronary ostia toward each other (Fig. 6.61). When the aortic root is significantly dilated, this technique can be combined with an incision between the right and left coronary ostia on the left side of the aorta, which is then sutured with a pledgetted technique (Fig. 6.62). This measure further rotates the coronary ostia toward each other and, with the enlargement of the aortic root on the noncoronary side, allows displacement of the 180° coronary ostia into the right and left coronary sinuses of the allograft. The pillar borders hug the noncoronary side of each ostia. An alternate solution is aortic root replacement with suturing of the coronary buttons to the right and left coronary sinuses.

Coronary Ostia Arising Low in the Sinuses

When the native coronary ostia are low in their sinuses and are close to the leaflet attachment, placement of the proximal suture line must be more in the subleaflet position, as originally described by Barratt-Boyes.[8,10] If the proximal suture line is displaced 2–3 mm below the leaflet attachment, there is ample room for the proximal suture line to "roll" the allograft aortic wall below the coronary ostia of the recipient aorta (Figs. 6.62 and 6.63).

Coronary Ostia Arising High in the Sinuses

In the case of the coronary ostia arising high in the sinuses, the problem for the surgeon is simplified. Resection of the allograft coronary sinus can be minimized, and the proximal suture line placed conveniently at the bottom of the sinus at the level of the native leaflet attachment (Fig. 6.64). The distal suture line is comfortably created around the coronary orifice. Note that the proximal suture line does not follow the semilunar cusp attachment superiorly but, rather, crosses the base of the pyramid of the commissural pillars. The "annulus" of the aortic valve is not a true circular fibrous ring like an atrioventricular (AV) valve annulus.

Aortic Root Replacement with Aortic Allograft Conduit

In certain left ventricular outflow tract reconstructions, one encounters abnormalities extending beyond that of the native valvular leaflets or severe distortion of the aortic root, which

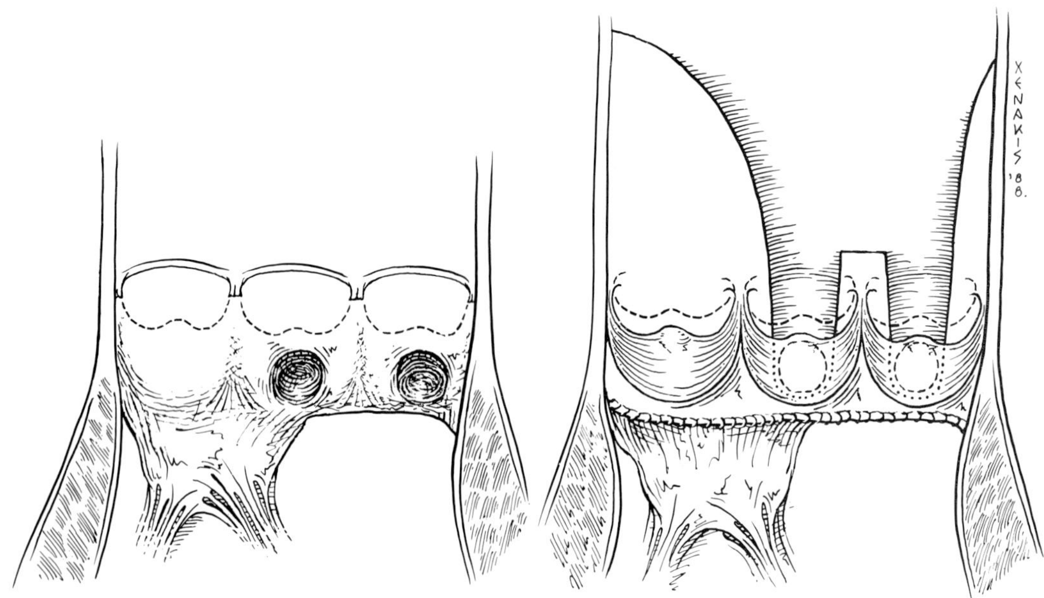

Figure 6.63. The proximal suture line is placed underneath the origin of the native leaflets in a "subannular" position to maintain a subcoronary distal suture line.

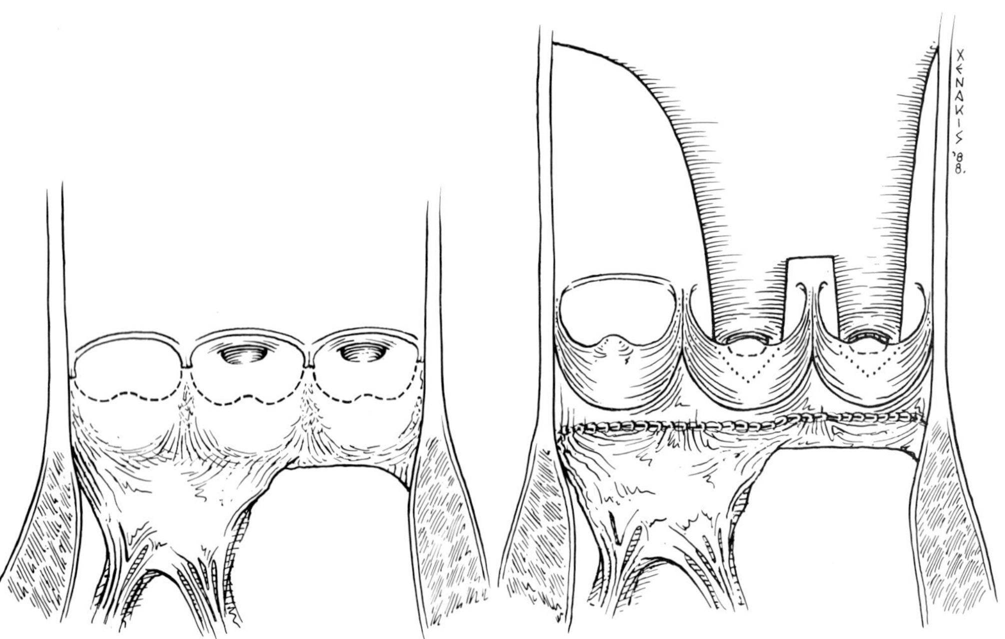

Figure 6.64. The proximal suture line is at the level of the base of the native leaflet attachments when the coronary ostia are relatively high in their sinuses.

are best treated with total aortic root replacement. The solution for this spectrum of difficulties was introduced by Ross, Yacoub, and colleagues.[29–31a] Aortic root replacement is indicated for reconstruction of the left ventricular outflow tract in which diffuse hypoplasia coexists with the valvular abnormality or in children, where it is desirable to place an adult-sized aortic outflow tract into which the child may grow. Aortic root replacements involve moving the coronary ostia on buttons. Complex coronary anatomy can also be managed by aortic root replacement.

In many ways, an aortic root replacement with reimplantation of the coronary ostia is a simpler technique than freehand aortic valve replacement. Nevertheless, we do not recommend it as the routine allograft replacement technique. There are some concerns about later re-replacement in such a setting, although such operations have been reported without difficulty by groups in New Zealand, London, and other centers.[32] Aortic root replacement is indicated for bacterial endocarditis in which loss of aortic continuity with the heart offers a technical challenge. The allograft is a superb prosthetic choice in this setting. Aortic root replacement is also useful in patients with greatly deformed aortic roots in which severe aortic stenosis coexists with asymmetric bulbar dilatations of the aortic sinuses, causing horrendous difficulties in the freehand technique. In the latter anatomic situation, a mechanical prosthesis or xenograft should be placed or an aortic root replacement utilized. We have found that when an aortic root replacement is used for hypoplastic aortic stenosis complex, a myomectomy is almost always required.

Indications

Aortic root replacement may be indicated for: (1) tunnel aortic stenosis (valvular, subvalvular, supravalvular) in which the subvalvular component is moderate or can be relieved with an accompanying myomectomy—there is always a relatively hypoplastic annulus; (2) aortic valvular stenosis with hypoplastic annulus; (3) aortic valve stenosis—the "solution" for severely distorted valvular anatomy for which freehand allograft valve replacement cannot be done but in a patient in whom it is preferred that an allograft be positioned[31]; (4) aortic root replacement in children, allowing an adult-sized valve to be placed into which the child can grow (e.g., tunnel aortic stenosis, subacute bacterial endocarditis); (5) a possible solution for aortic insufficiency with proximal aortic root dilatation in which distortion makes simple reduction aortoplasty accompanying a freehand aortic valve replacement difficult (in the absence of Marfan's syndrome or other connective tissue disorders); (6) possible solution for complex coronary anatomy such as 180° coronary ostia in bicuspid aortic stenosis; and (7) bacterial endocarditis with destruction of aortic-ventricular continuity.

Although connective tissue disorders such as Marfan's syndrome have been listed as contraindications for the use of allografts for freehand aortic valve replacement, allografts have been used for aortic root replacement with suture-line reinforcement using Teflon felt or Dacron graft material to prevent later distortion.[33] It remains to be seen whether splinting an allograft in such disorders prevents the later development of aortic insufficiency, as was seen in the early experience of Barratt-Boyes and associates.[3, 31b]

Sizing

Aortic root replacement solves some of the problems inherent in a hypoplastic left ventricular outflow tract. Excision of the aortic root down to the fibrous skeleton and onto the septum allows "expansion" of the ventricular outflow orifice. A myomectomy, as in the Morrow operation for idiopathic hypertrophic subaortic stenosis (IHSS), can be added to further enlarge the left ventricular outflow in the presence of a markedly hypertrophied septum.[34] Once excision of the native aorta has been accomplished, the outflow tract can be sized with Hegar dilators and the same-sized internal diameter allograft chosen. It can be "up-sized" for children in whom it is desirable to place an adult-sized allograft. For example, if the outflow tract measures 20 mm, a 20-mm (ID) allograft is selected. In children over 15 kg it is usually possible to place an 18-mm or larger allograft. If further enlargement is necessary, a Manouguian-type maneuver can be performed onto the anterior leaflet of the

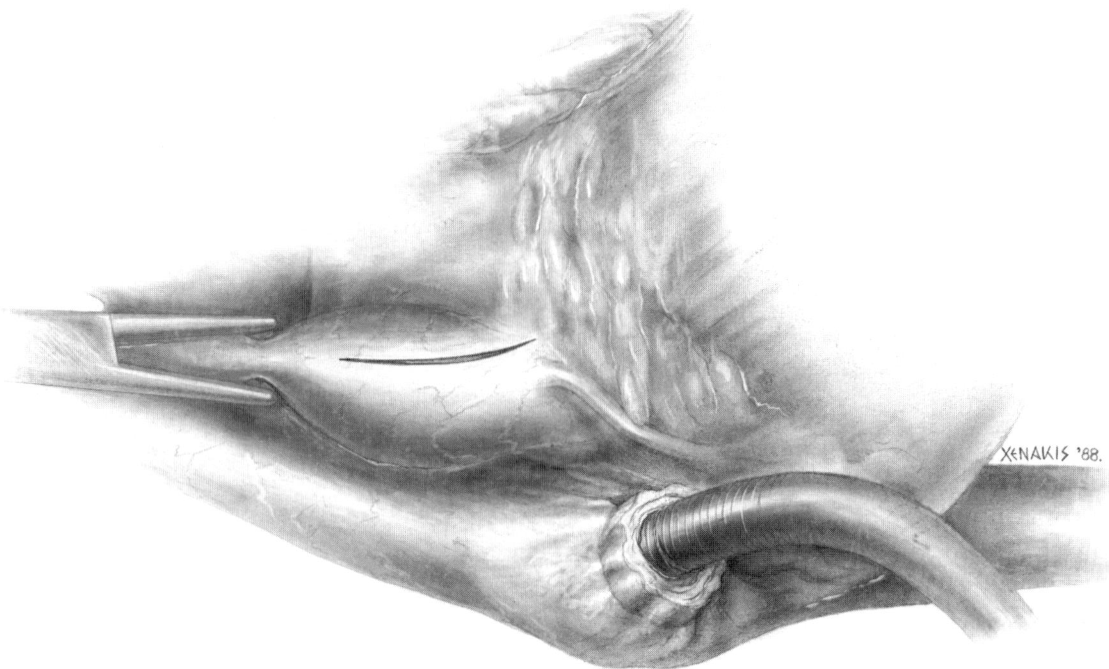

Figure 6.65. The initial incision for aortic root replacement is vertical and deviated to the left of the right coronary ostia.

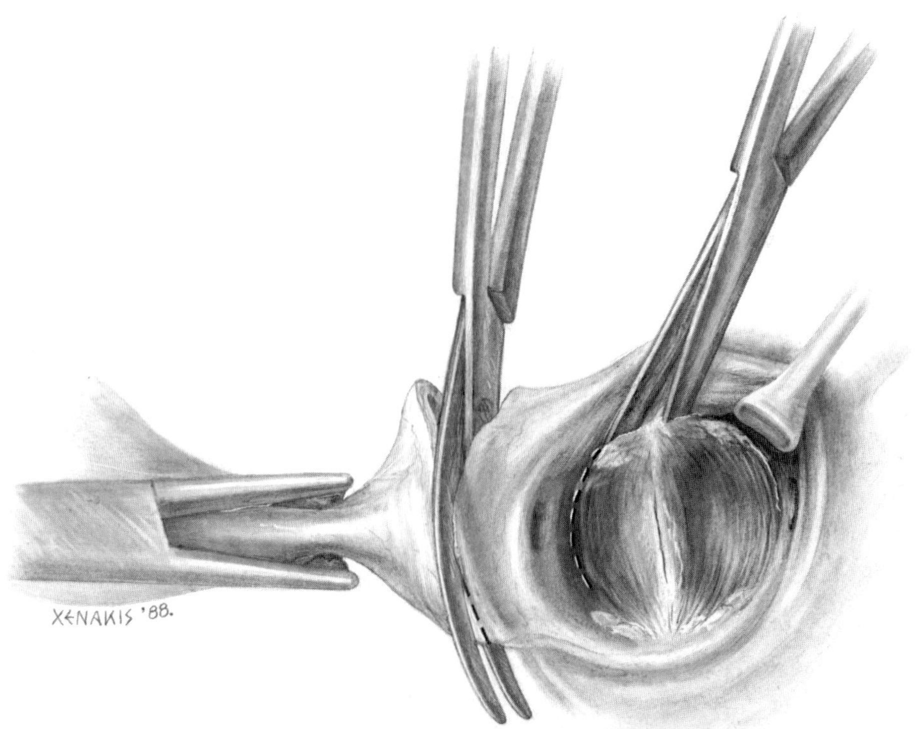

Figure 6.66. The aorta is divided, leaving as long an aortic remnant as possible.

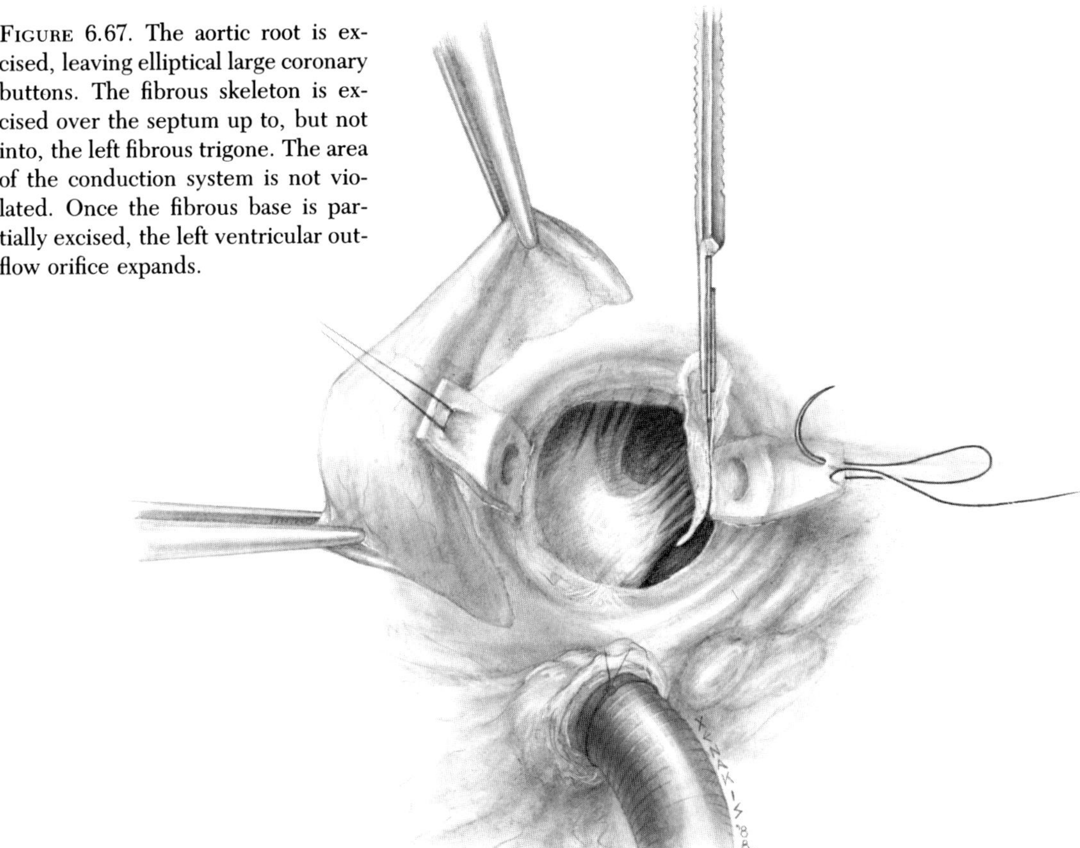

FIGURE 6.67. The aortic root is excised, leaving elliptical large coronary buttons. The fibrous skeleton is excised over the septum up to, but not into, the left fibrous trigone. The area of the conduction system is not violated. Once the fibrous base is partially excised, the left ventricular outflow orifice expands.

patient's mitral valve, which allows further enlargement of 2–4 mm. If additional enlargement of the subvalvular outflow tract is necessary, an aortoventriculoplasty must be performed (see next section).

Preparation and Choice of Allograft

We perform aortic root replacement with an aortic allograft, although a pulmonary allograft would not offer technical problems. (However, a series of such have not been reported to assess the capability of an allograft pulmonary valve performing in the aortic position over the long term.) The valve is thawed in the usual way, and the aortic conduit is left long, to the point of the allograft innominate artery takeoff, where it is transected. The muscle is trimmed and the anterior leaflet of the mitral valve excised 3 mm below the annulus, unless a portion of it is necessary for a Manouguian maneuver.

Surgical Technique for Standard Aortic Root Replacement

As Ross originally devised, we use an interrupted proximal suture line technique.[31b,32] The aortic root is excised and the native coronary ostia left on large buttons of aortic tissue (Figs. 6.65–6.67). An additional septal myomectomy is performed if necessary (Fig. 6.68). The allograft is then oriented in the orthotopic position, with the left coronary ostia comfortably positioned toward the button of the native left coronary ostia. The proximal suture line is constructed of a series of interrupted 4-0 Tycron sutures on a half-circle taperpoint needle, placed 1.0–1.5 mm apart as simple sutures (Fig. 6.69). The allograft is sutured to the fibrous skeleton of the heart at the hinge point of the anterior leaflet of the native mitral valve, and the suture line is brought medially over the top of the membranous septum. A remnant of recipient aortic root is usually left counterclockwise from this region so as to avoid

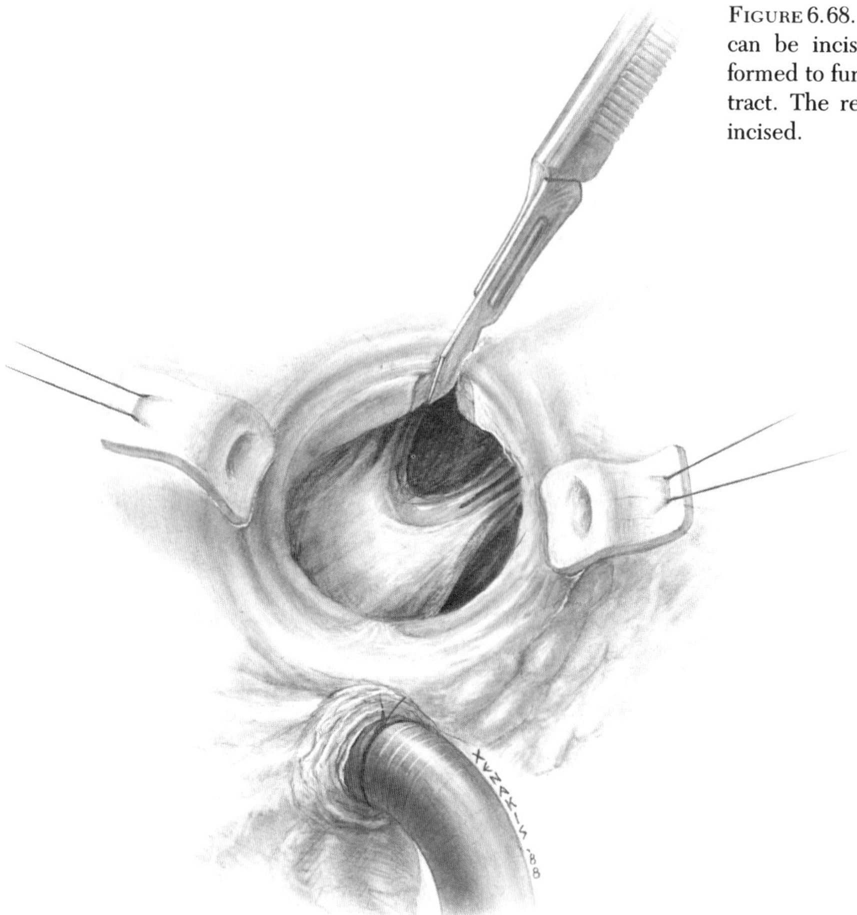

Figure 6.68. A hypertrophied septum can be incised or a myotomy performed to further enlarge the outflow tract. The rest of the septum is not incised.

any encroachment in the region of the AV node, but then the dissection is brought down to the septum. The simple sutures are continued throughout the circumference and placed in individual rubber-shod clamps. A narrow strip of Teflon felt is then inserted through the middle of the simple sutures so that as they are tied down the Teflon felt is positioned as a caulking gusset outside the allograft cardiac anastomosis (Fig. 6.70). The sutures are sequentially tied. Fibrin glue can be used for additional hemostasis.

Now it is easy to see where the coronary buttons need to be positioned on the allograft. They are brought to the region of the allograft coronary ostia, which are excised (Fig. 6.71). These excision buttonholes should be enlarged superiorly so that the tendency is to slightly "stretch" the native coronary ostia up to the orifices to avoid kinking. The patient's buttons are made large to protect the ostia. The stretching to a higher position within the sinus is particularly important when shifting the position of the native coronary ostia in a rotational direction (i.e., moving a bicuspid 180° right coronary ostia slightly to the left into the allograft right coronary sinus). This trick was learned during arterial switch operations for transposition and is also applicable in this setting to avoid coronary kinking. The coronary buttons are sewn to their respective orifices in the allograft utilizing the running 5-0 polypropylene suture technique.

The distal aortic suture line is constructed after checking the length of the allograft. It should usually be cut longer than you might think with a slight anterior posterior bevel (Fig. 6.72). The suture line is accomplished with a running 4-0 polypropylene suture technique uti-

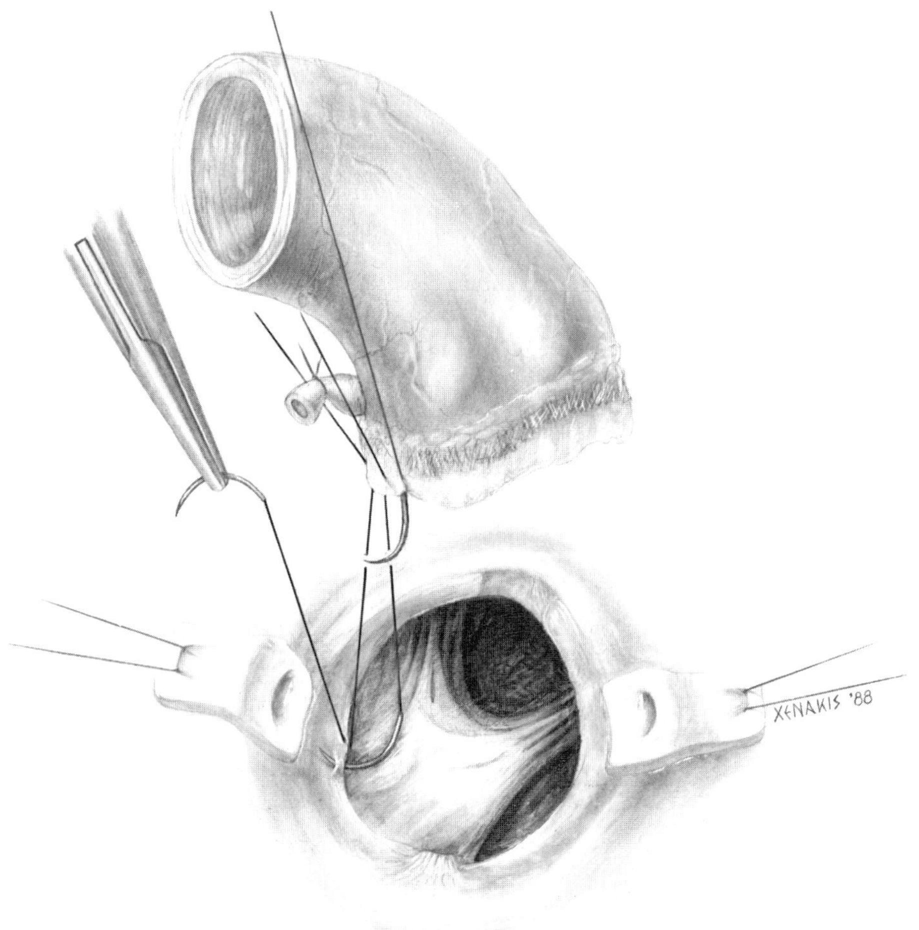

FIGURE 6.69. Proximal suture line constructed of many simple interrupted braided sutures. Each is placed in an individual rubber-shod clamp.

lizing a Teflon felt strip buttress. De-airing maneuvers are performed, and the aortic cross clamp is removed.

Hints

Helpful hints include very high cannulation of the aorta or the use of femoral artery cannulation in adults. In addition, the native aorta should be fully mobilized. Left ventricular venting is always used.

Continuous suture lines have been advocated by some, but we find that the interrupted technique provides better visibility and allows placement of a larger aortic root on top of a smaller heart by spreading the dissimilarity over the entire circumference of the root. Similar reasoning has been advocated by Ross.

We recommend a soft-braided suture rather than monofilament for the interrupted proximal suture line to reduce the risk of cutting through the allograft tissues. Horizontal pledgetted mattress sutures utilized for standard prosthetic valve replacements are discouraged in this setting because the tendency is to narrow the circumference of the native left ventricular outflow orifice. Such narrowing is not a problem in the presence of aortic insufficiency in a large outflow tract for which aortic root replacement has been chosen; but in the usual situation, in which the surgery is done because of a hypoplastic left ventricular outflow tract, this technique is less desirable.

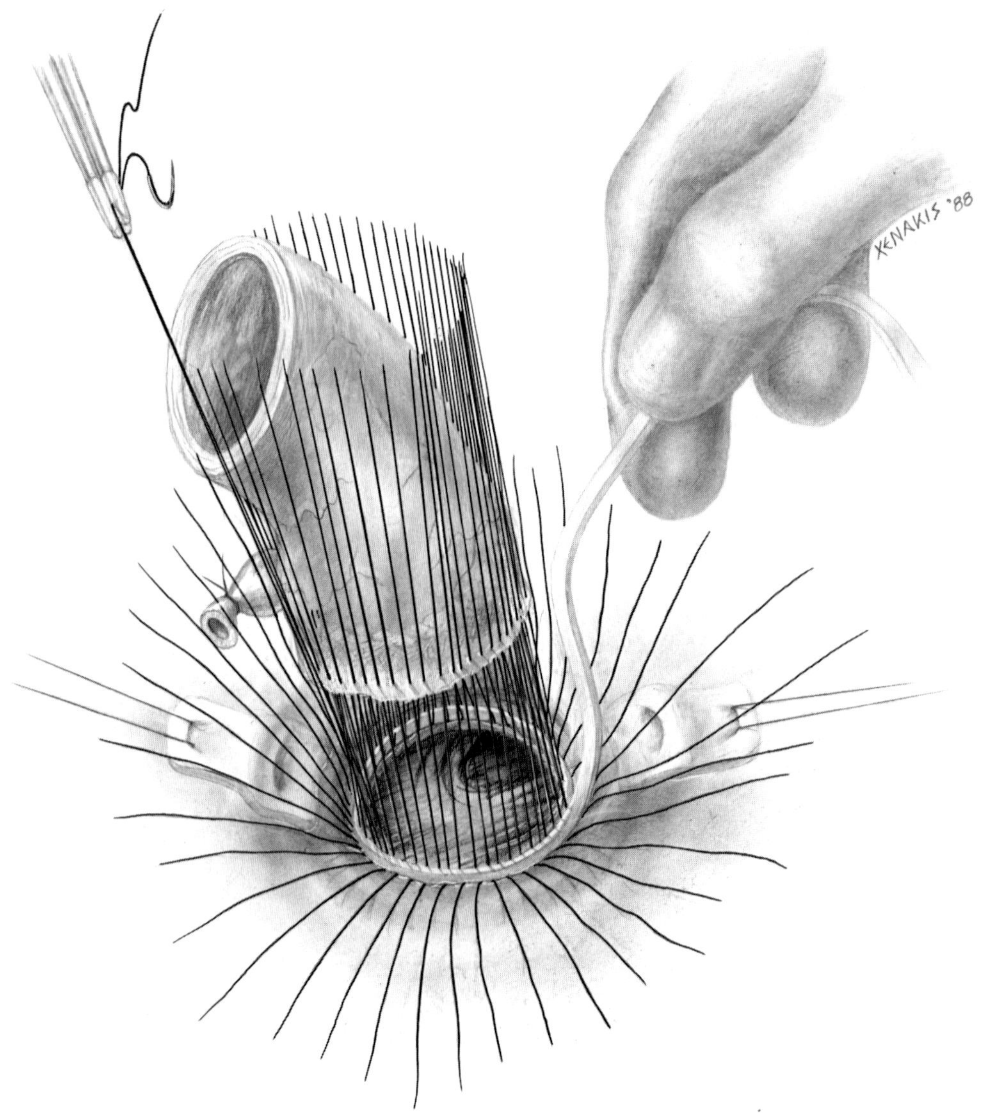

Figure 6.70. Usually around 40 interrupted sutures are placed and then tied over a strip of Teflon felt, which is placed within the circle of sutures *after* seating the allograft, so that it lies external to the tissue closure.

If a pledgetted horizontal mattress suture technique is utilized, pledgets should be placed on both sides of the suture line to prevent narrowing when tying each knot. A variation of this technique has been recommended by the Polish group utilizing Teflon felt strips to stabilize the aortic root in patients with Marfan's syndrome in order to avoid later dilatation of the base of the aorta.[33]

Aortoventriculoplasty with Aortic Allograft (Aortic Root Replacement with Konno)

Indications

In some hearts the entire left ventricular outflow tract is hypoplastic, involving subvalvular, valvu-

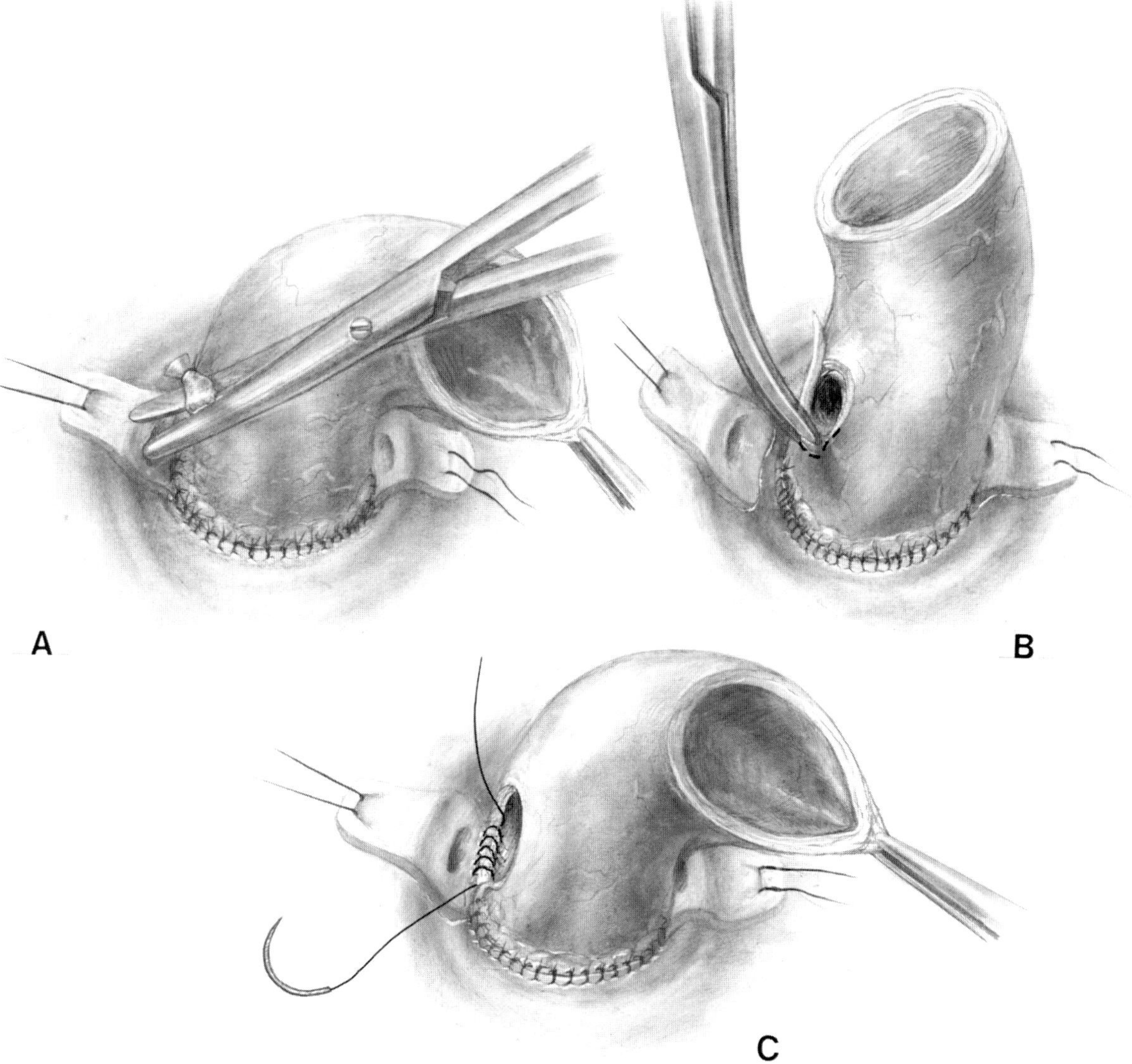

FIGURE 6.71. Preparation and suturing of the coronary buttons. Stay sutures on the buttons improve exposure for the preceding steps as well as the manipulations at this stage.

lar, and even supravalvular stenosis. These patients have various degrees of tunnel aortic stenosis and are typically managed with multiple operations. The final operation usually involves a Konno-type annulus enlargement. Clarke and colleagues have described the extended aortic root replacement for such situations, and we have found it most satisfactory. It combines the concept of the aortoventriculoplasty as described by Konno, Rastan, and their associates with the aortic root replacement of Ross.[15,16,35–39] This procedure is indicated for tunnel aortic stenosis where the annulus is hypoplastic and extensive fibromuscular obstruction involves the subvalvular region. Coexisting supravalvular stenosis may also be excised and replaced with allograft aorta using this technique. Isolated subvalvular aortic stenosis is managed by traditional resection. If complex and extensive subvalvular stenosis is present yet the aortic annulus and valve leaflets

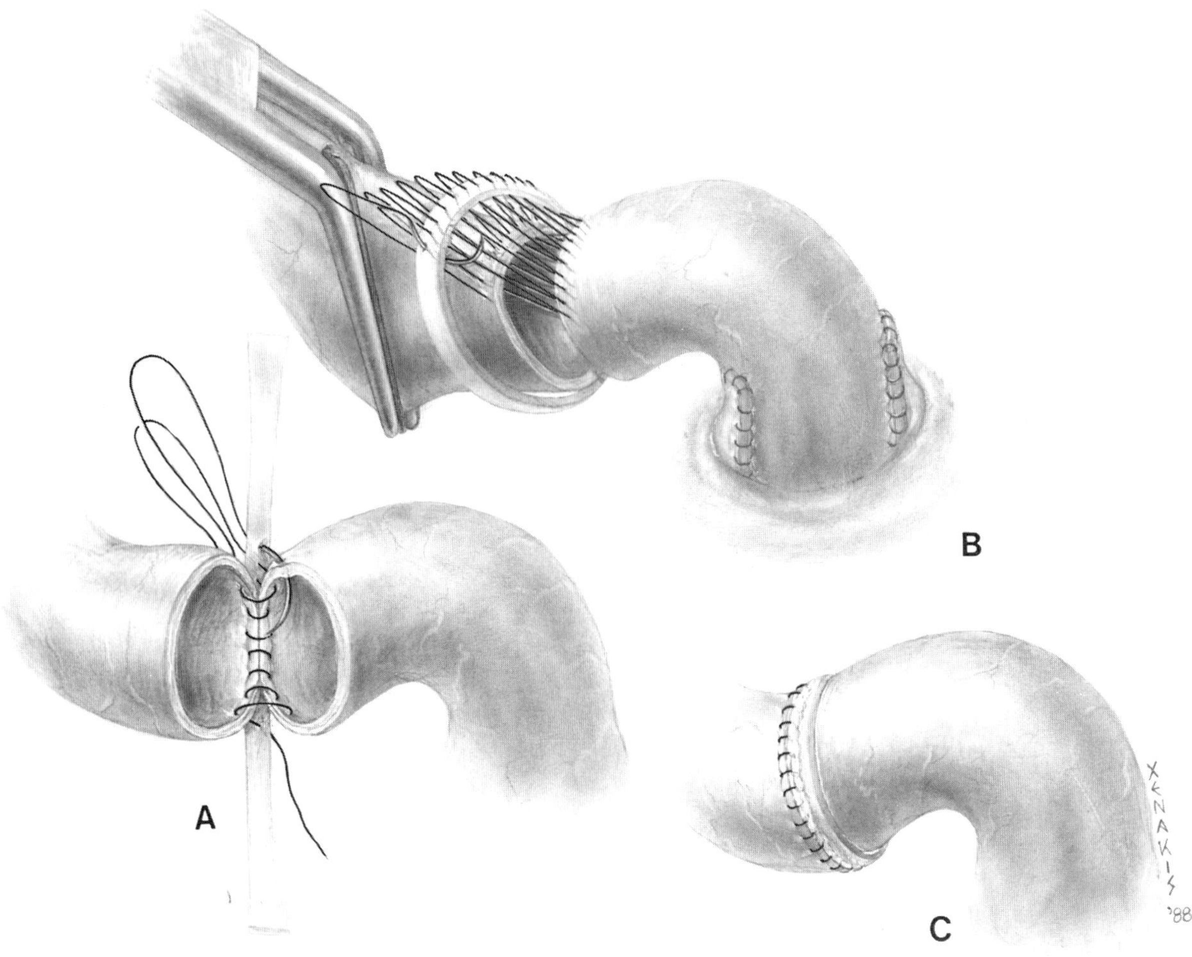

Figure 6.72. Distal suture line of an allograft aortic root replacement. Note the Teflon felt strip positioned on the allograft side.

are normal, the modified subvalvular operation, as described by Kirklin and Barratt-Boyes, is applicable.[40] If the obstruction involves only a hypoplastic annulus with or without sinus/leaflet abnormalities, treatment is with either simple aortic root replacement or aortic valve replacement, with annulus enlargement and augmentation aortoplasty as necessary (vida supra).

Indications for surgical correction of tunnel aortic stenosis are traditional and are performed for onset of symptoms or for gradients exceeding 50–75 torr. Small children may undergo temporizing procedures with subvalvular resections, valvuloplasty, and so on to reduce gradients until body size has increased such that an adult-sized outflow tract can be constructed (15–20 kg or more).

Surgical Technique

The heart is cannulated for cardiopulmonary bypass utilizing ascending aortic cannulation relatively high near the innominate artery and dual vena caval cannulas. Prior to aortic cross-clamping, the aorta and pulmonary artery are fully mobilized. There are usually adhesions from previous operations. After induction of cardioplegic arrest, a vertical aortotomy is performed, begun anteriorly and directed slightly to the left of the right coronary ostia (Fig. 6.73).

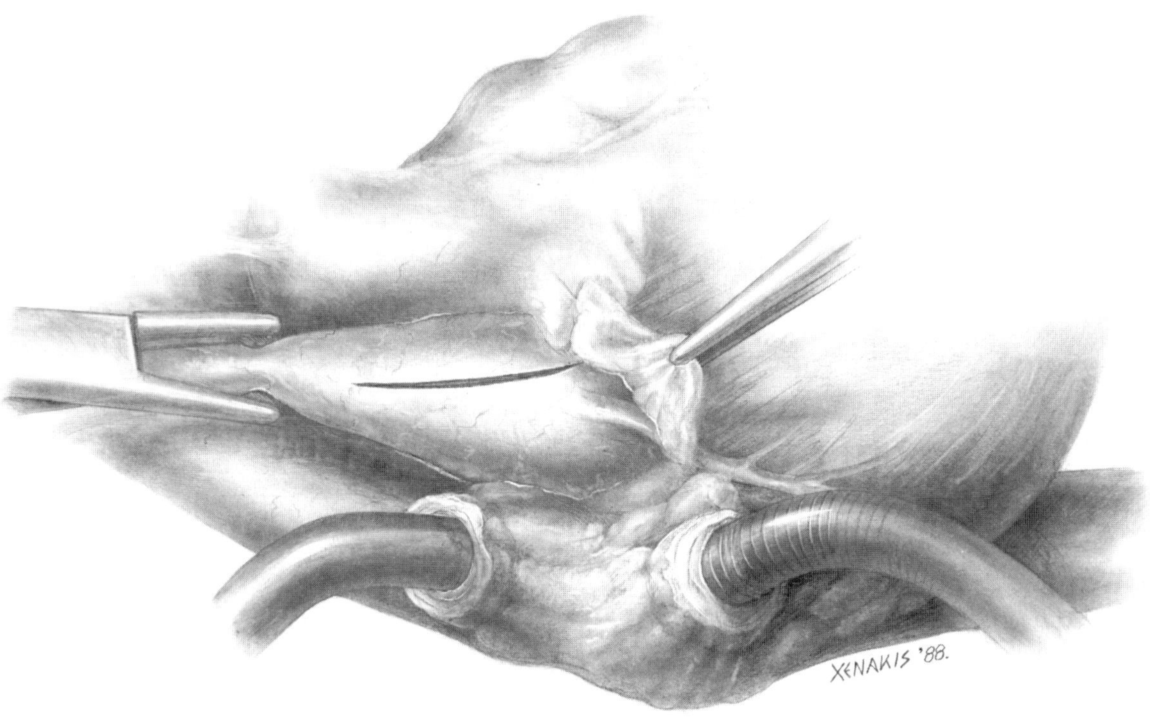

FIGURE 6.73. Aortotomy for aortic root–Konno reconstruction.

The aortotomy is retracted with two stay sutures, and the valve and subvalvular region are examined. If the valve annulus is more than two standard deviations smaller than is normal for that age, it is necessary to enlarge it to an adult size. If the subvalvular obstruction cannot be reasonably handled with a conservative resection, extended aortic root replacement (aortic root–Konno procedure) is performed. The incision in the aorta is extended into the annulus at the point between the left and right coronary ostia, where the commissure is or normally would be. An oblique incision is then made in the right ventricular outflow tract meeting the aortotomy. It is angled toward the apex to avoid the base of the pulmonary valve. These incisions combine to open the top of the septum to view. The septum, which by definition is thick, is incised vertically toward the apex, and the incision is extended until the left ventricular outflow tract is widely open (Fig. 6.74).

The coronary ostia are excised on large buttons and the aorta transected at or above (if narrowed) the level of the sinus ridge. The remainder of the proximal aortic root is excised, however, leaving the fibrous aortic tissue intact just above the membranous septum and not violating the aortic mitral continuity (Fig. 6.75). The incision into the septum allows enlargement to the desired size, which is accomplished with Hegar dilators. The goal is to place, at the minimum, a 19-mm human aortic allograft, which means that a size 21 Hegar should fit generously into the opened left ventricular outflow tract.

The prepared allograft has been trimmed at its base, but coronary windows are not excised at this point. Pledgetted 4-0 monofilament sutures are placed with the pledgets on the ventricular side of the septal incision and passed as horizontal mattress sutures through the anterior leaflet of the mitral valve, the entirety of which is used to fill the septal defect. These sutures are sequentially placed until the level of the "true" annulus is reached (Fig. 6.76).

At this point the suture technique is changed to 3-0 Tycron interrupted sutures in the manner of the aortic root replacement, as described by Ross. They are placed 1–2 mm apart, circumfer-

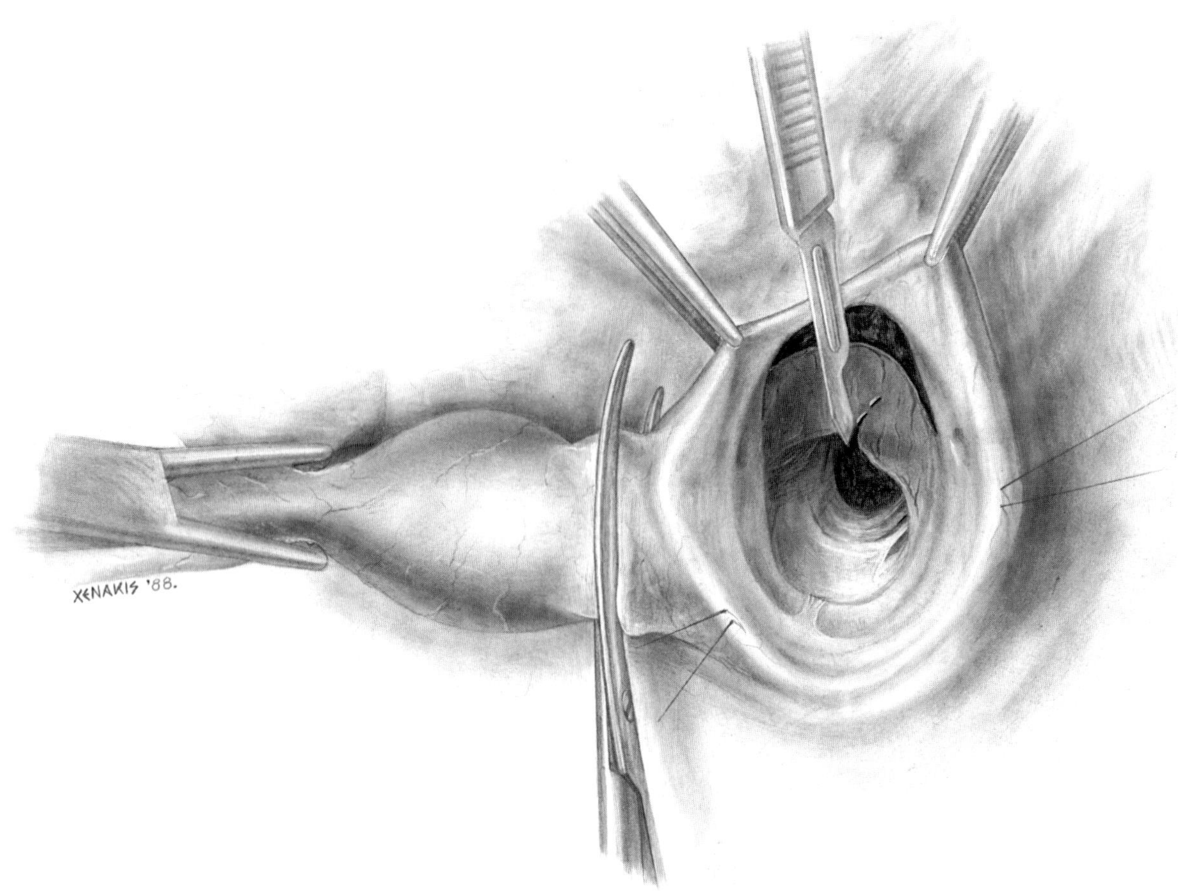

FIGURE 6.74. The incision in the aorta is extended across the annulus to the left of the right coronary ostia and then aimed apically down the free right ventricular wall away from the pulmonary valve. The septum is then incised and excised to open the left ventricular outflow tract.

entially through the annulus of the allograft and recipient. They are not placed as horizontal mattress sutures but, rather, as simple sutures (Fig. 6.77). Particular care is taken at the transition from the septal horizontal mattress sutures to the interrupted simple sutures at the left side of the septal incision so as to ensure excellent hemostasis (Fig. 6.78). Two additional horizontal mattress sutures are placed with the pledget on the right side of the ventricular septotomy and then through the allograft; they are later passed through the pericardial patch closure of the right ventriculotomy and tied, which secures the triangulation points of the closure (Fig. 6.79). All sutures are then sequentially tied, thereby positioning the allograft over the left ventricular outflow. The septal sutures are tied first (Fig. 6.80).

Clarke recommended a running polypropylene suture technique and a double suture technique on the septal portion of the repair.[15] We have not found that necessary and prefer the interrupted technique with multiple pledgetted sutures on the ventricular septum. The allograft mitral leaflet is sutured to the right side of the septum so that the "depth" of the septum contributes to enlargement of the left ventricular outflow tract.

The coronary sinuses are then excised from the allograft to accept the large buttons of the native coronary ostia. The allograft right coronary stump is suture-ligated, as it has been rotated 120° into the noncoronary sinus region. The coronary buttons are made large and usually slightly higher than would be anatomic in order to maintain length and stretch to avoid kinking. The buttons are sutured to the oval defects with running 5-0 monofilament sutures (Figs. 6.81 and 6.82).

FIGURE 6.75. The aortic root is excised, leaving coronary buttons.

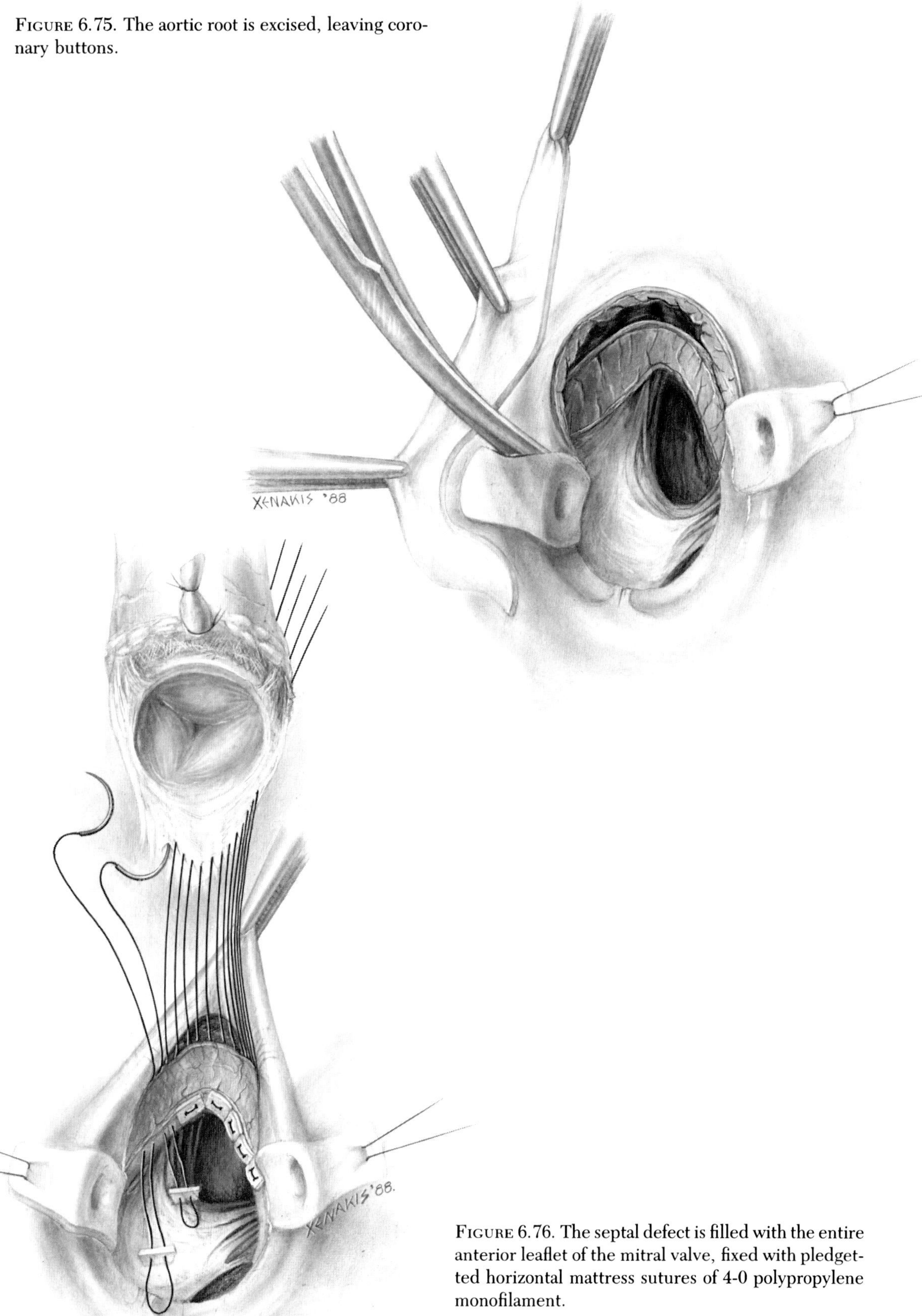

FIGURE 6.76. The septal defect is filled with the entire anterior leaflet of the mitral valve, fixed with pledgetted horizontal mattress sutures of 4-0 polypropylene monofilament.

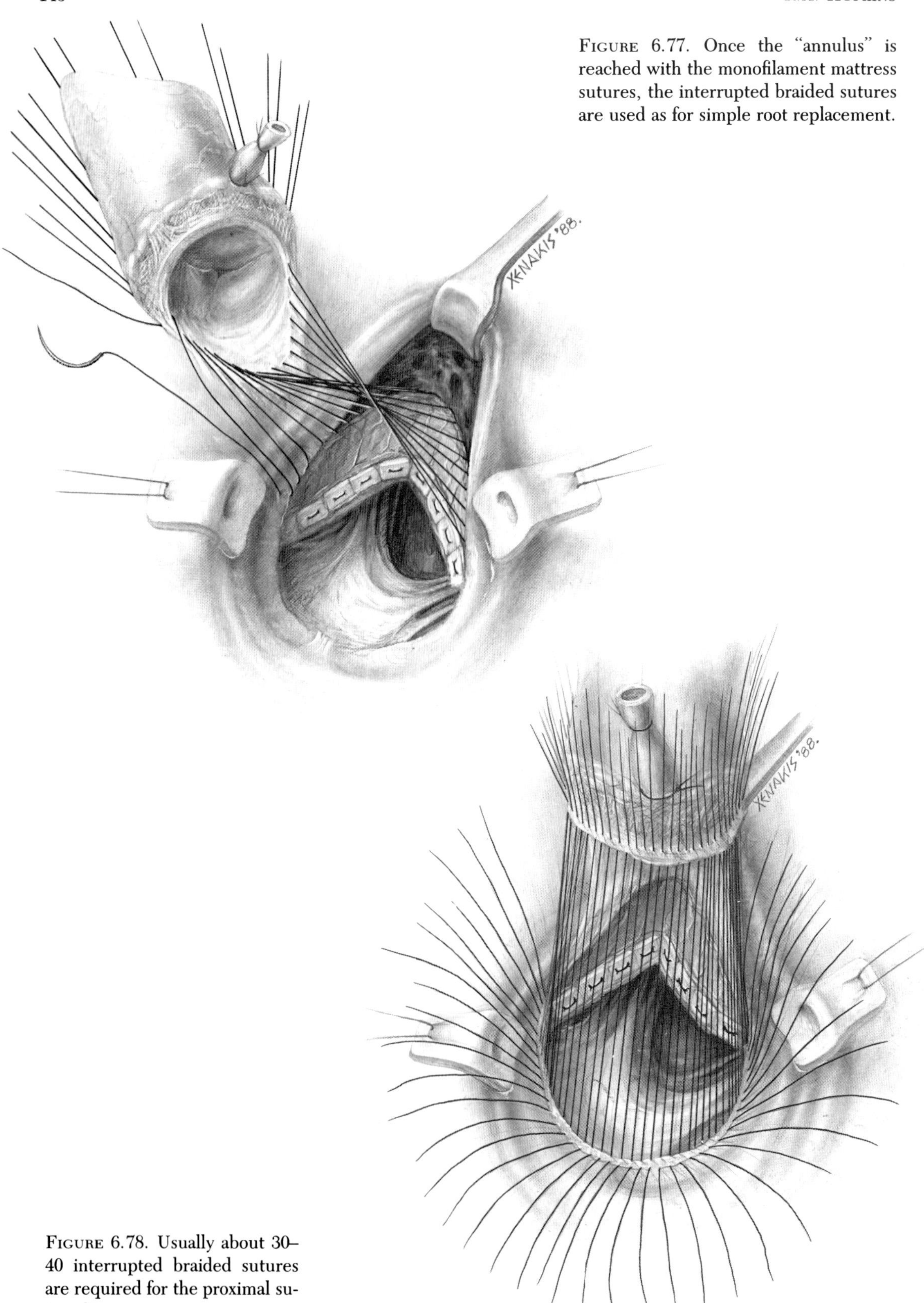

Figure 6.77. Once the "annulus" is reached with the monofilament mattress sutures, the interrupted braided sutures are used as for simple root replacement.

Figure 6.78. Usually about 30–40 interrupted braided sutures are required for the proximal suture line.

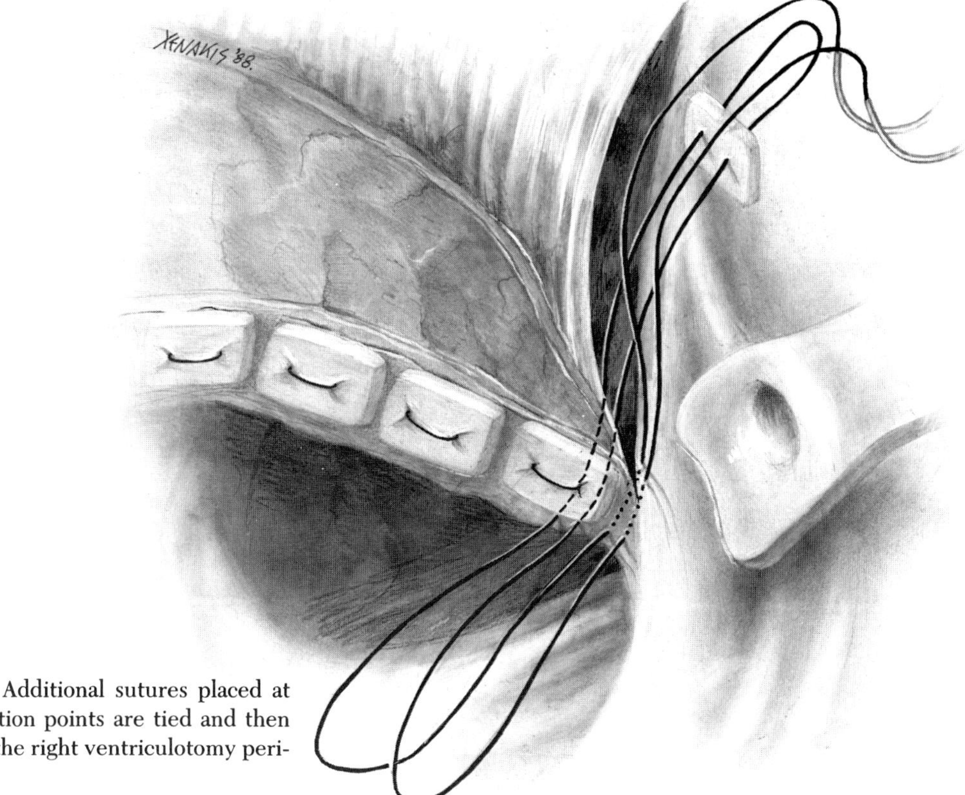

FIGURE 6.79. Additional sutures placed at both triangulation points are tied and then later used for the right ventriculotomy pericardial patch.

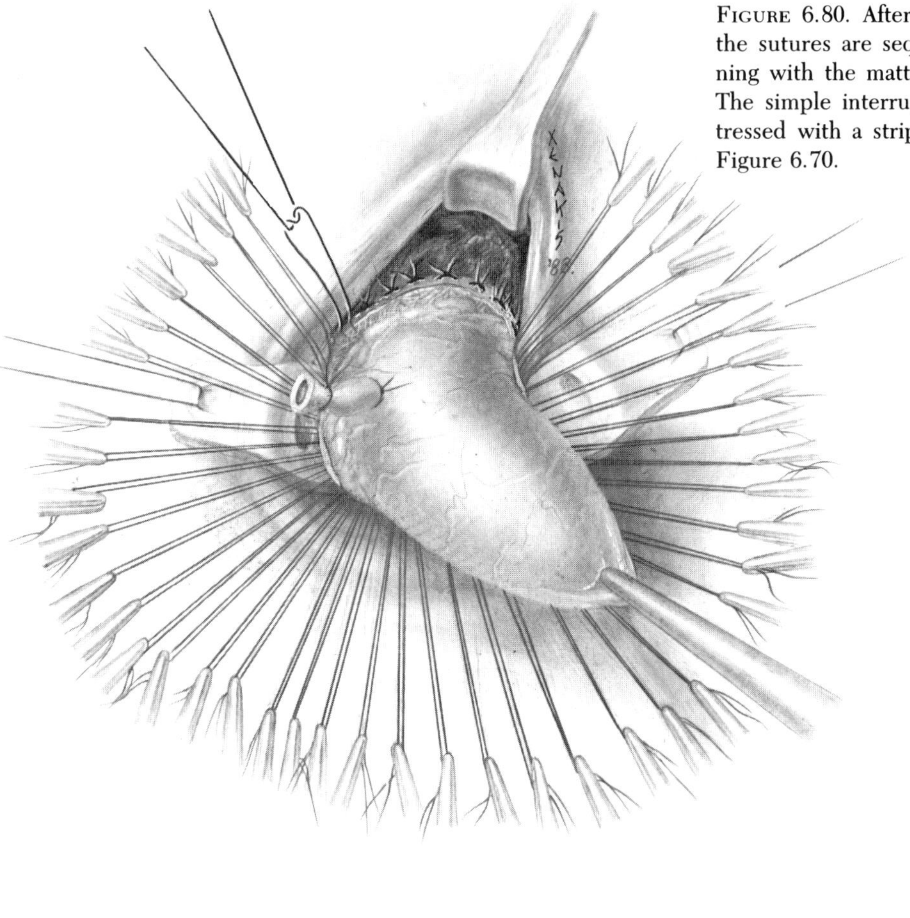

FIGURE 6.80. After seating the allograft, the sutures are sequentially tied, beginning with the mattressed septal sutures. The simple interrupted sutures are buttressed with a strip of Teflon felt, as in Figure 6.70.

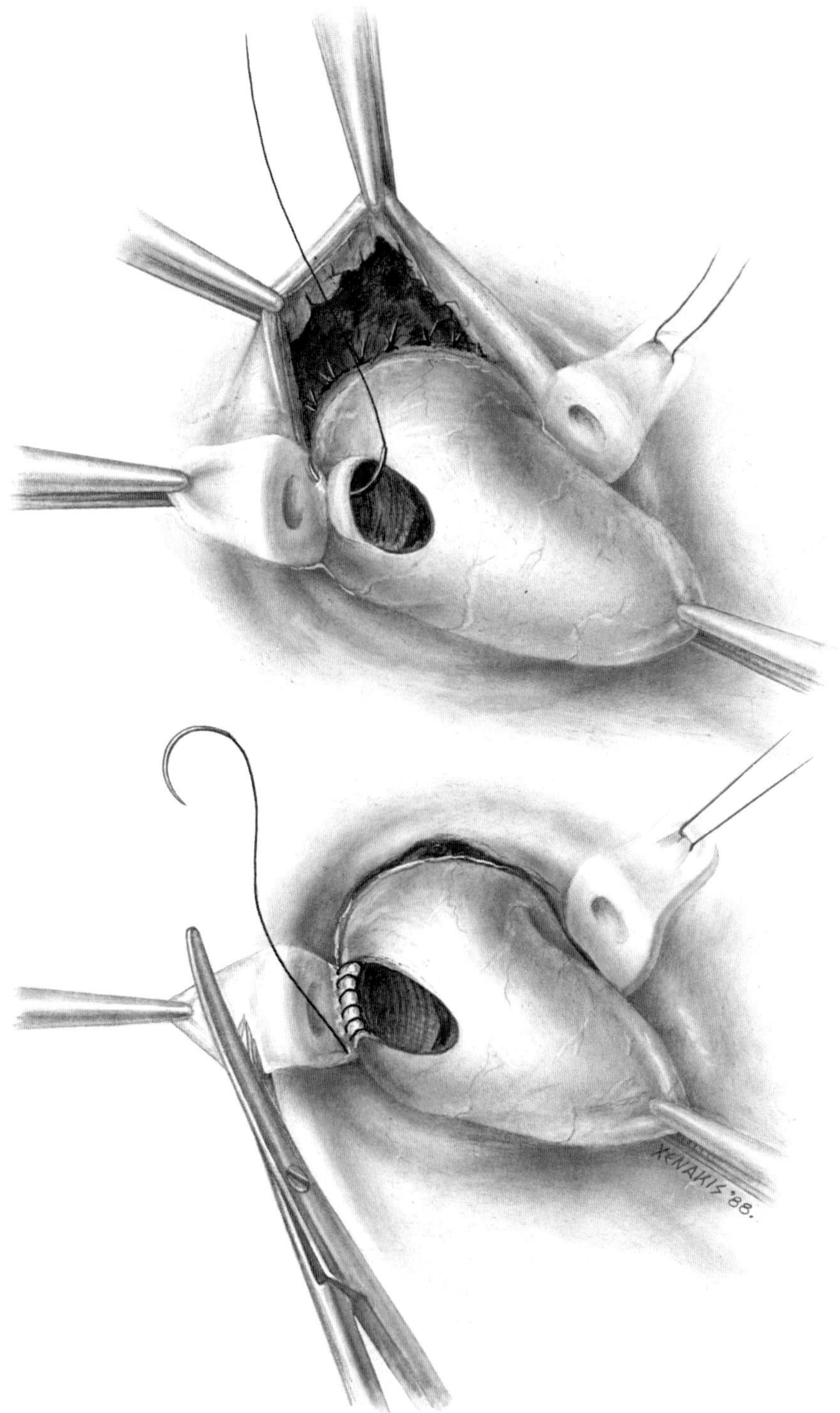

Figure 6.81. Coronary "buttons" sutured with 5-0 polypropylene.

The left ventricular vent is shut off and the left ventricle gradually allowed to fill while the distal aortic suture line is constructed with running 4-0 monofilament suture. This suture line is buttressed with a strip of felt (Fig. 6.83). Because the native curve of the allograft is in a direction reversed from normal, the distal allograft aorta is usually beveled posteriorly. It is also helpful to keep the allograft ascending aortic root relatively short, but of course the incision needs to be above the sinus ridge (Fig. 6.84). Native supravalvular ascending aortic pathology must be excised.

The reconstruction is completed after de-airing the aortic root and removing the aortic cross clamp. As in the Konno operation, the right ventricular free wall defect is repaired with a patch (Fig. 6.85). Clarke recommended a piece of homograft.[15] We have tended to use pericardium for this patch, suturing it to the defect

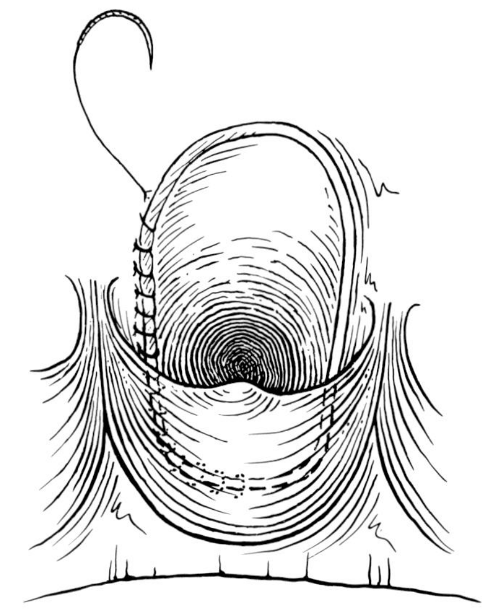

FIGURE 6.82. Large coronary buttons sutured within their new sinuses.

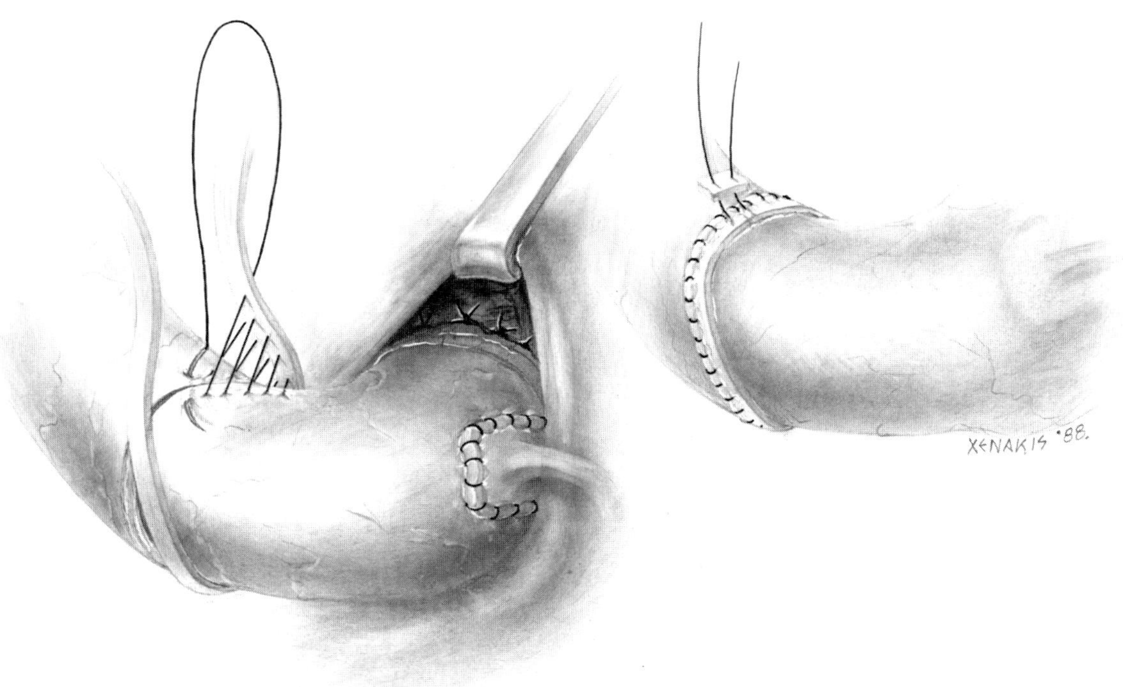

FIGURE 6.83. Distal suture line buttressed with a Teflon felt strip.

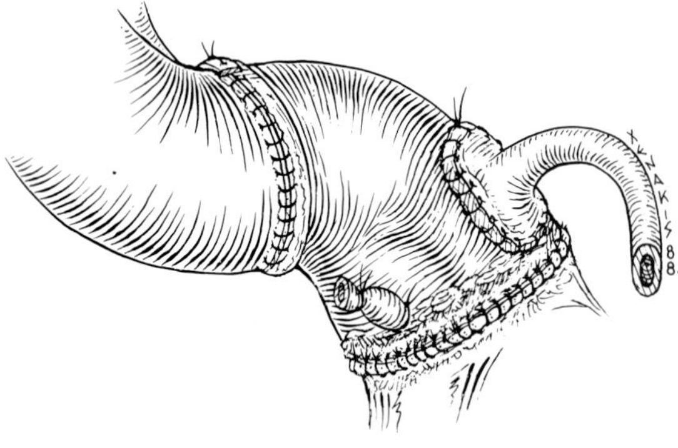

Figure 6.84. A beveled distal suture line is used to increase the anastomosis size and smooth the curvature of the new aortic root.

with a running 4-0 or 5-0 polypropylene suture. The suturing along the annulus of the allograft is, of course, nontransmural, and these sutures need to be carefully placed.

Postoperative Management

Postoperative care is similar to that for any aortic valve replacement. Anticoagulation, if not necessary for other reasons, is limited to daily aspirin (150 mg). The patient is followed, especially looking for murmurs indicating insufficiency. Echocardiography with Doppler is performed prior to discharge for a baseline reading; it is

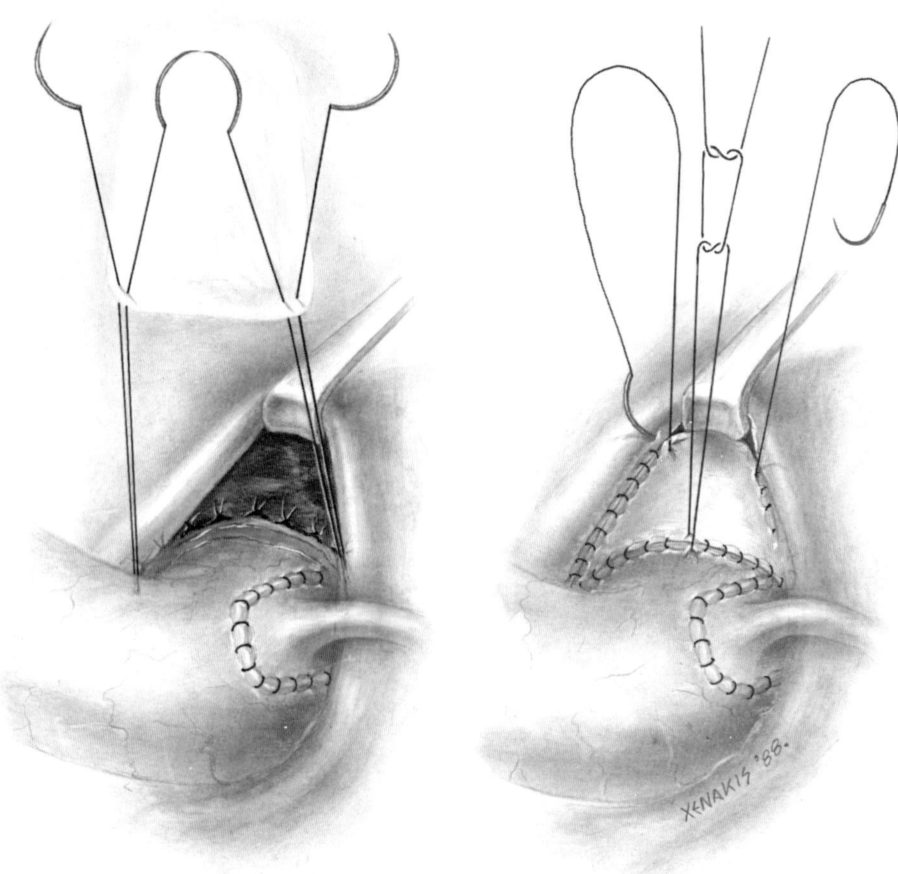

Figure 6.85. Closure of the right ventricular free wall defect completes the reconstruction.

repeated every 6 months for 1 year and then done yearly. Routine prophylaxis for subacute bacterial endocorditis is recommended for all indications, as noted in the prosthetic valve guidelines of the American Heart Association.

References

1. Karp RB: The future of homografts. *J Cardiac Surg* 2(suppl):2–5–308, 1987.
2. Barratt-Boyes BG: The timing of operation in valvular insufficiency. *J Cardiac Surg* 2:435–452, 1987.
3. Barratt-Boyes BG, Roche AHG, Subramanyan R, et al: Long-term follow-up of patients with the antibiotic-sterilized aortic homograft valve inserted free-hand in the aortic position. *Circulation* 75:768–777, 1987.
4. Yankah CA: State of the art. Presented at the First Workshop on Homologous and Autologous Heart Valves. Chicago: Deborah Heart and Lung Center, 5 April 1987.
5. Imamura I, Tomizawa Y, Hashimoto A, et al: A comparative analysis of left ventriculography and root aortography for estimating aortic annulus size. *J Thorac Cardiovasc Surg* 93:592–596, 1987.
6. Bonchek LI, Burlingame MV, Vazales BE: Accuracy of sizers for aortic valve prostheses. *J Thorac Cardiovasc Surg* 94:632–634, 1987.
7. Barratt-Boyes BG, Roche AHG: Review of aortic valve homografts over a six and one-half year period. *Ann Surg* 170:483–487, 1969.
8. Barratt-Boyes BG: Homograft aortic valve replacement in aortic incompetence and stenosis. *Thorax* 19:131–150, 1964.
9. Karp RB: The use of freehand unstented aortic valve allografts for replacement of the aortic valve. *J Cardiac Surg* 1:23–32, 1986.
10. Barratt-Boyes BG: A method for preparing and inserting homograft aortic valve. *Br J Surg* 52:847–856, 1965.
11. Barratt-Boyes BG: A method for preparing and inserting homograft aortic valve. *Br J Surg* 52:847–856, 1965.
12. Ross DN: Application of homografts in clinical surgery. *J Cardiac Surg* 1:175–183, 1987.
13. Doty DB: Replacement of the aortic valve with cyropreserved aortic valve allograft: considerations and techniques in children. *J Cardiac Surg* 1(suppl):129–136, 1981.
14. Doty DB: Aortic homograft technique. In: *Cardiac Surgery*. Chicago: Yearbook, 1986, pp. 12–15.
15. Clarke DR: Extended aortic root replacement for treatment of left ventricular outflow tract obstruction. *J Cardiac Surg* 1(suppl):121–128, 1987.
16. McKowen RL, Campbell DN, Woelfel GF, et al: Extended aortic root replacement with aortic allografts. *J Thorac Cardiovasc Surg* 93:366–374, 1987.
17. Ross DN, Yacoub MH: Homograft replacement of the aortic valve—a critical review. *Prog Cardiovasc Dis* 11:275–293, 1969.
18. Moreno-Cabrol CE, Miller C, Shumway NE: A simple technique for aortic valve replacement using freehand allografts. *J Cardiac Surg* 3:69–76, 1988.
19. Frater RWM: Aortic valve insufficiency due to aortic dilatation: correction by sinus rim adjustment. *Circulation* 74(suppl I):I136–I142, 1986.
20. Bailey WW: A modified freehand technique for homograft aortic valve replacement. *J Cardiac Surg* 2:193–197, 1987.
21. Teoh KH, Fulop JC, Weisel RD, et al: Aortic valve replacement with a small prosthesis. *Circulation* 76(suppl III):III123–III131, 1987.
22. Kirklin JW, Barratt-Boyes BG: *Cardiac Surgery*. New York: Wiley, 1986, pp. 416–418.
23. Manouguian S, Seybold-Epting W: Patch enlargement of the aortic valve ring by extending the aortic incision into the anterior mitral leaflet. *J Thorac Cardiovasc Surg* 78:402–412, 1979.
24. Nicks R, Cartmill T, Bernstein L: Hypoplasia of the aortic root—the problem of aortic valve replacement. *Thorax* 25:339–345, 1970.
25. McAlpine WA: *Heart and Coronary Arteries*. New York: Springer-Verlag, 1975, p. 22.
26. Virdi IS, Monro JL, Ross JK: Eleven year experience of aortic valve replacement with antibiotic sterilized homograft valves in Southampton. *Thorac Cardiovasc Surg* 34:277–282, 1986.
27. Nunez L, Aguado MG, Pinto AG, Larren JL: Enlargement of the aortic annulus by resecting the commissure between the left and non-coronary cusps. *Texas Heart Inst J* 10:301–307, 1983.
28. McAlpine WA: *Heart and Coronary Arteries*. New York: Springer-Verlag, 1975, p. 24.
29. Summerville J, Ross D: Homograft replacement of aortic root with reimplantation of coronary arteries—results after one–five years. *Br Heart J* 47:473–482, 1982.
30. Gula G, Ahmed M, Thompson R, et al: Combined homograft replacement of the aortic valve and aortic root with reimplantation of the coronary arteries. *Circulation* 53/54(suppl II):II150, 1976.

31a. Thompson R, Yacoub M, Ahmed M, et al: The use of "fresh" unstented homograft valves for replacement of the aortic valve. *J Thorac Cardiovasc Surg* 79:896–903, 1980.

31b. Okita Y, Franciosi G, Matsuki O, Robles A, Ross DN. Early and late results of aortic root replacement with antibiotic-sterilized aortic homograft. *J. Thorac Cardiovasc Surg* 95:696–704, 1988.
32. Ross D: Application of homografts in clinical surgery. *J Cardiac Surg* 1(suppl):175–181, 1987.
33. Dziatkowiak A, Pfitzner R, Andres J, et al: Modified techniques for subcoronary insertion of allografts in Yonkah AC, Hertzer R, Miller DC, et al (eds) Cardiac Valve Allografts 1962–1987. New York: Springer Verlag, 1988. pp 141–147.
34. Morrow AG: Hypertrophic subaortic stenosis: operative methods utilized to relieve left ventricular outflow obstruction. *J Thorac Cardiovasc Surg* 76:423–430, 1978.
35. Konno S, Imai Y, Lida Y, et al: A new method for prosthetic valve replacement in congenital aortic stenosis associated with hypoplasia of the aortic valve ring. *J Thorac Cardiovasc Surg* 70:909–917, 1975.
36. Rastan H, Koncz J: Aortoventriculoplasty: a new technique for the treatment of left ventricular outflow tract obstruction. *J Thorac Cardiovasc Surg* 71:920–927, 1976.
37. Rastan H, Abu Aishah N, Rastan D, et al: Results of aortoventriculoplasty in twenty-one consecutive patients with left ventricular outflow tract obstruction. *J Thorac Cardiovasc Surg* 75:659–669, 1978.
38. Somerville J, Ross D: Homograft replacement of aortic root with reimplantation of coronary arteries. *Br Heart J* 47:473–482, 1982.
39. Misbach GA, Turley K, Ullyot DJ, Ebert PA: Left ventricular outflow enlargement by the Konno procedure. *J Thorac Cardiovasc Surg* 94:696–703, 1982.
40. Kirklin JW, Barratt-Boyes BG: Modified Konno operation. In: *Cardiac Surgery*. New York: Wiley, 1986, pp. 996–998.

7—Right Ventricular Outflow Tract Reconstructions

RICHARD A. HOPKINS

The development of the extracardiac conduit for reconstruction of "blue" ventricle to pulmonary artery continuity has revolutionized the surgery of many complex congenital cardiac defects.[1–5] In infants with anomalies such as tetralogy of Fallot, nonvalved reconstruction of the right ventricular outflow has been well tolerated with a low early reoperation rate (e.g., 100% reoperation-free at 4 years in the Boston Children's Hospital series).[6] However, patients developing progressive right ventricular dilatation have required later replacement with a valved prosthesis. Other anatomic situations, particularly that of pulmonary atresia or pulmonary atresia accompanying other defects (e.g., corrected transposition) that have usually been repaired during childhood rather than infancy, have done best with right ventricular outflow tract reconstructions utilizing valved conduits (Rastelli concept). There are neonatal and infant reconstructions that are optimally accomplished with valved conduits (e.g., truncus arteriosus, absent pulmonary valve syndrome). The allograft has become the conduit of choice for all right ventricular outflow tract reconstructions.[7]

Symptoms of progressive right ventricular failure due to pulmonary insufficiency include fluid retention, fatigue, and exercise intolerance. Once right ventricular dilatation progresses to the point that tricuspid regurgitation occurs, symptomatology advances rapidly. Right ventricular function has been demonstrated to improve following placement of a pulmonary valve.[8] Tricuspid insufficiency is important as a marker for deteriorating right ventricular function and as a potent hemodynamic burden in the presence of outflow tract abnormalities. As the San Francisco experience has demonstrated, once tricuspid incompetence develops rapid and persistent right ventricular failure follows that is difficult to mitigate medically.[9] There is marked improvement with restoration of pulmonary sufficiency even if a murmur or mild tricuspid regurgitation persists.[10] If pulmonary valve replacement is postponed and tricuspid regurgitation progresses, the reconstructive surgery must include restoration of tricuspid competence.

Performance of most models of mechanical valves in the right side of the heart has been relatively poor, and in general either bioprostheses or allografts have been recommended. In the series from Chicago, more than one-third of the patients developed prosthetic pulmonary valvular dysfunction less than 1 year following insertion of a St. Jude prosthesis.[11] Thus despite the issue of accelerated failure, if an allograft is not available a porcine prosthesis is probably the optimal choice for the right ventricular outflow tract position.

Ideally, anticoagulation in children is avoided. Unfortunately, porcine prostheses have not fared well in the right-sided circulation, although they have done somewhat better in older children and young adults.[12] Mechanical prostheses are associated with a significant rate of dysfunction in the right-sided position.[13] Synthetic right heart *conduits* have been noted to require replacement 100% of the time by 10 years following insertion, although initial early results are good.[6] Thus the allograft is the ventricular outflow valve of choice in the pediatric and young adult population and is clearly the conduit of choice for right ventricular outflow tract reconstructions in all age groups.

Fontan and colleagues have reported on more than 100 allograft aortic valve conduits with only one replacement for allograft valve dysfunction and no thromboembolism or hemolysis; in the same series, a pressure gradient (13–85 mm Hg, mean 39 mm Hg) was present in only 14 ventricle-dependent conduits.[14] In this series from France, gradients across the allograft conduits occurred at three sites in the prevalvular region, five sites in the valvular or undetermined region, and five sites in the postvalvular (presumably distal anastomosis) region.[15] In the United States Kirklin and associates have demonstrated a 94% actuarial freedom from reoperation for obstruction in cryopreserved allograft conduits at 3.5 years.[15]

Indications

A functioning right ventricular outflow valve is recommended for either primary or secondary reconstructions when there is (1) symptomatic right ventricular dysfunction, (2) fixed pulmonary hypertension, (3) hypoplastic pulmonary arteries, (4) pulmonary insufficiency with right ventricular dilatation, (5) tricuspid regurgitation, (6) echocardiographic evidence of small right ventricular volume or poor performance, (7) absent pulmonary valve syndrome, (8) peripheral pulmonary stenoses, (9) highly reactive pulmonary circulation (e.g., neonatal truncus).[16]

If there were a perfect valve substitute that could grow or be of adult size when placed in the pulmonary position, it could be argued that a valved reconstruction of the right ventricular outflow tract could be applicable in all cases to (1) protect against the long-term effects of pulmonary insufficiency including right ventricular dysfunction and dilatation, (2) accomplish right ventricular outflow tract reconstruction without relative obstruction, and (3) prevent or mitigate tricuspid dysfunction. At present, we do *not* recommend universal application, e.g., for routine primary tetralogy of Fallot repairs.[17] However, a proportion of patients with nonvalved conduits or transannular patches return with progressive right ventricular dysfunction, especially when additional preload or afterload lesions are present, and require reconstruction with an allograft.[18]

Standard Right Ventricle to Pulmonary Artery Aortic Allograft Conduit in Children and Infants

Sizing

Usually an adult-sized right ventricular conduit (19- to 26-mm aortic allograft) is placed, except in small infants (see Appendix: Valve Diameters). It is generally possible in the patient weighing 3.5–5.0 kg to place a 12-mm conduit, whereas in those weighing less than 3 kg an 8- to 10-mm conduit may be required. A 14- to 16-mm conduit is used in patients who weigh 5–10 kg. These weight guidelines are similar to those used by Kirklin and colleagues; they reported the use of 9- to 12-mm allografts for infants with body surface area (BSA) of 0.2–0.3 m^2, 12- to 14-mm allografts for infants with BSA 0.3–0.4 m^2, and 15- to 17-mm allografts for children with BSA 0.4–0.5 m^2.[15] Once a child weighs more than 20 kg it is almost always possible to place a 20-mm or larger conduit in the right ventricular outflow tract position. The distal anastomosis can be enlarged by sewing obliquely (beveled); the size in the neonates is restricted primarily by the maximum ventriculotomy that can be achieved and secondarily by thoracic volume. Conduit compression by the anterior chest is usually easily avoided.

Interestingly, Mercer presented data suggesting that a 12-mm (inside diameter; ID) pulmonary annulus (not conduit) results in only a 50% reduction in cross-sectioned area and might result in acceptably low gradients even as the child approaches 10 years of age.[19] The 12-mm synthetic conduit has been shown to give superb early results in infants but always results in gradients requiring later replacement; it is also a more difficult material with which to avoid kinking, compression, and so on.[20] An 18-mm or larger allograft is usually free of significant obstruction and is a perfectly adequate size into which a child can grow. This implant is achievable in most children exceeding 15 kg in weight. This discussion presupposes a ventricular-sup-

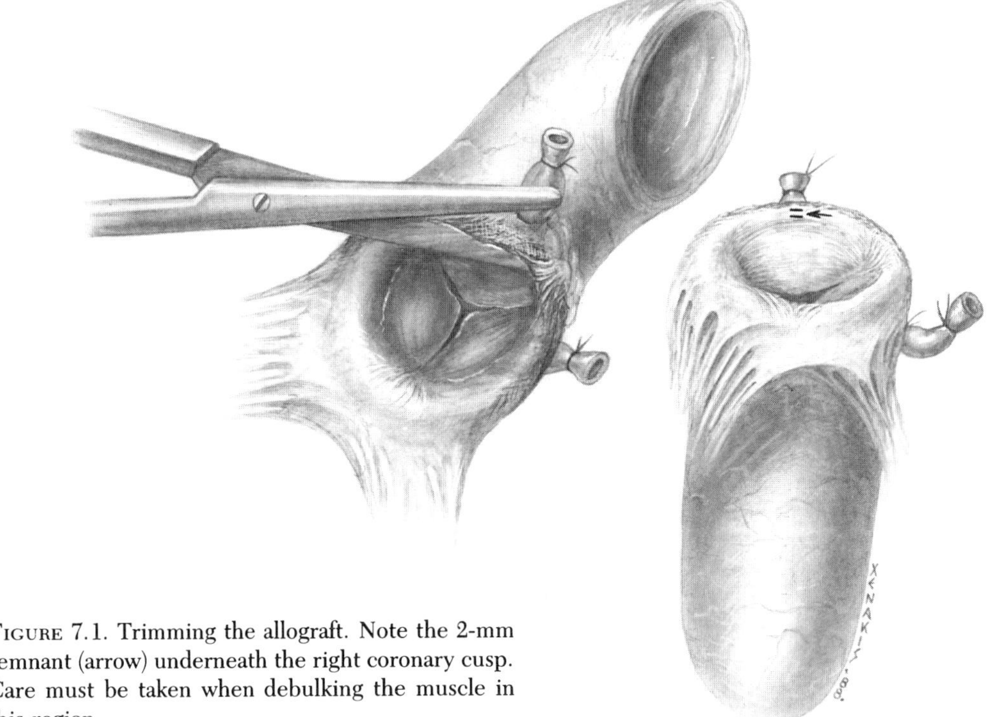

FIGURE 7.1. Trimming the allograft. Note the 2-mm remnant (arrow) underneath the right coronary cusp. Care must be taken when debulking the muscle in this region.

ported pulmonary circulation; atrial-dependent pulmonary circulations require pulmonary inflow geometry to approximate normal tricuspid valve areas in order to avoid obstructive hemodynamics.

Principles

A number of principles are emphasized to optimize the result of allograft insertions for right ventricular outflow tract reconstructions[21]: (1) avoidance of the use of synthetic material on either end of the conduit; (2) placement that avoids compression by the sternum; (3) use of nonrestrictive ventriculotomy; (4) use of the anterior leaflet of the mitral valve to complete the exit from the ventriculotomy into the conduit; (5) oblique suturing of the distal suture line with polypropylene monofilament surgical technique; (6) slight "stretching" of the conduit to enhance semilunar suspension, and (7) avoiding an excessively long ventriculotomy, which tends to flatten the anterior mitral leaflet closure and distort the new outflow valve.

If extensions of the conduit are necessary, they should usually be constructed at the proximal end with pericardium. (We rarely have to use this procedure.) If an allograft pulmonary valve is used rather than an aortic valve, it should be recognized that the postvalvular segment of the allograft is shorter.[22] When so used, the pulmonary allograft requires a patch of pericardium to close the ventriculotomy in order to avoid distortion of the valve (analogous to use of the aortic allograft anterior mitral leaflet).

Technique

Patients are placed on cardiopulmonary bypass utilizing dual caval cannulation. Hypothermia and cardioplegic cardiac arrest allow optimal visualization of the pulmonary arteries for reconstruction during the distal anastomosis. The proximal anastomosis is usually accomplished during rewarming. The conduit is selected and thawed. It is trimmed, debulking the muscle and leaving the anterior leaflet of the mitral valve attached. Care is taken underneath the right coronary ostia where the right leaflet base is usually close to the muscle being trimmed (Fig. 7.1).

A ventriculotomy is performed high in the

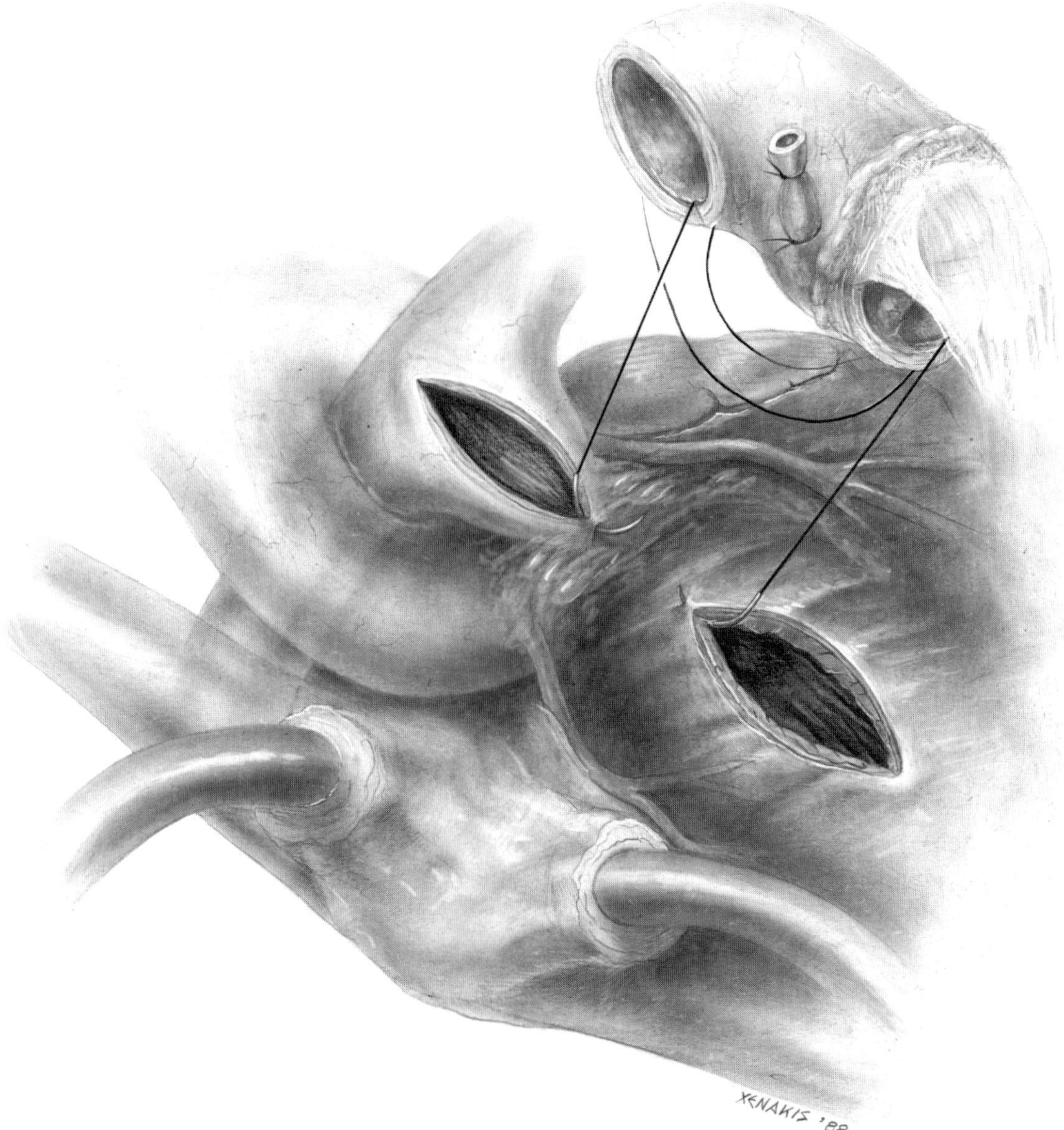

Figure 7.2. Distal anastomosis of aortic allograft (conduit) is performed in an oblique fashion to the pulmonary artery for pulmonary atresia when the main pulmonary artery is reasonably well developed.

infundibulum, placed so as to avoid the coronary arteries and to minimize right ventricular dysfunction. It is extended out the main pulmonary artery when the artery is in continuity with the base of the heart. When there is no main pulmonary artery continuity with the base of the heart, the confluence or whatever element of the main pulmonary artery is present is opened longitudinally and the incision extended toward the confluence or into either, or both, right and left pulmonary arteries if necessary to relieve a stenosis. The length of the conduit is adjusted so that the annulus of the allograft valve seats at the upper edge of the right ventriculotomy. The distal anastomosis is accomplished with a running 5-0 or 6-0 polypropylene suture end-to-

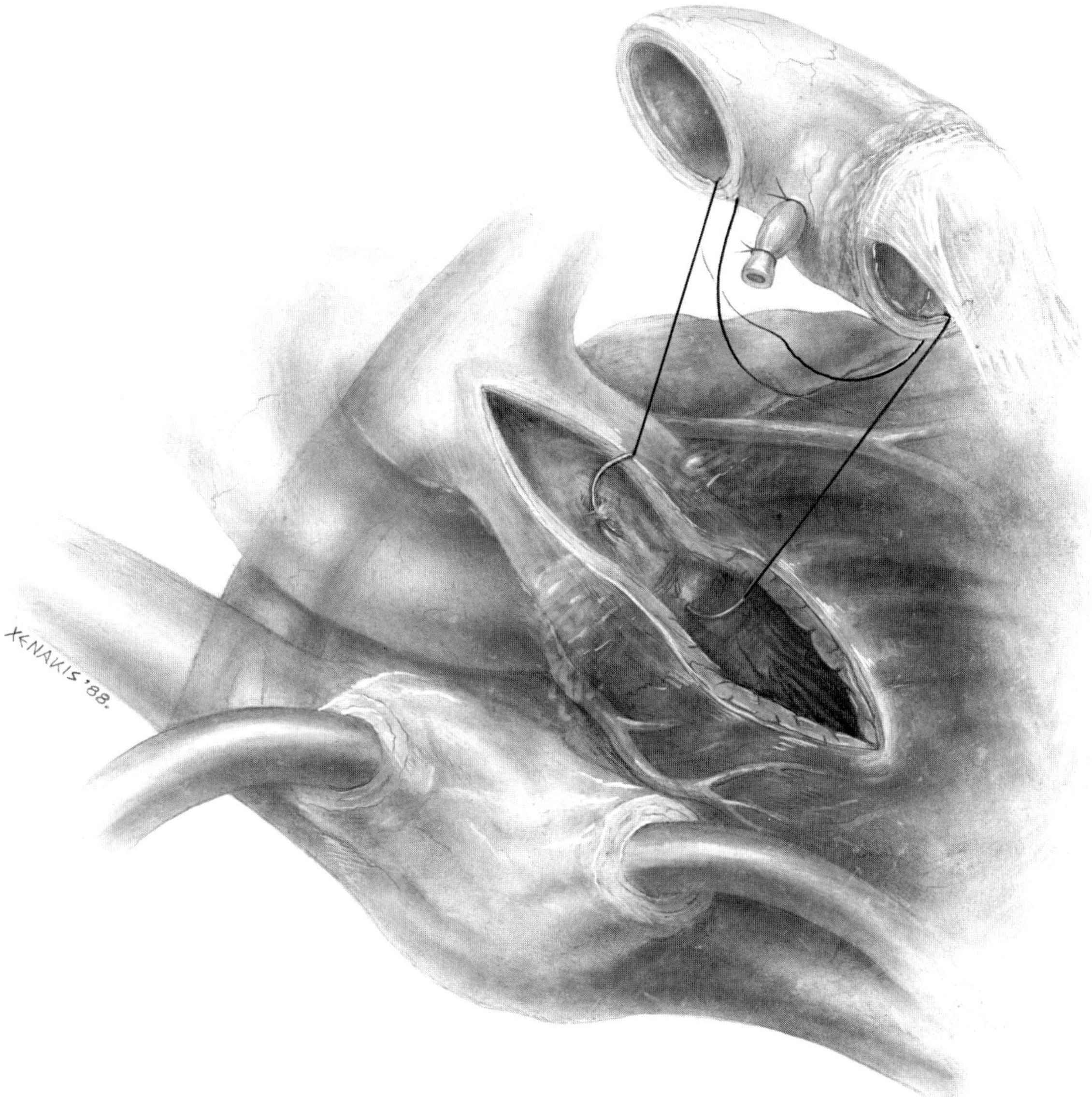

FIGURE 7.3. End-to-end anastomosis in an oblique manner when pulmonary ventricular-arterial continuity is present (e.g., valvular atresia).

end or with an oblique or beveled fashion (Fig. 7.2). An end-to-side technique can be used when the main pulmonary artery is of adequate caliber and there is pulmonary valve atresia or when bypassing a hypoplastic but competent pulmonary valve that exits the pulmonary ventricle (i.e., some continuity exists) (Fig. 7.3). If the native pulmonary valve exits the systemic ventricle, complete division is performed and the stump oversewn.

The proximal anastomosis is accomplished with either a running 4-0 or 5-0 polypropylene suture technique. The allograft should be trimmed of excessive muscle to the point that the fibrous skeleton can be seen. The anterior leaflet of the mitral valve is preserved. The membra-

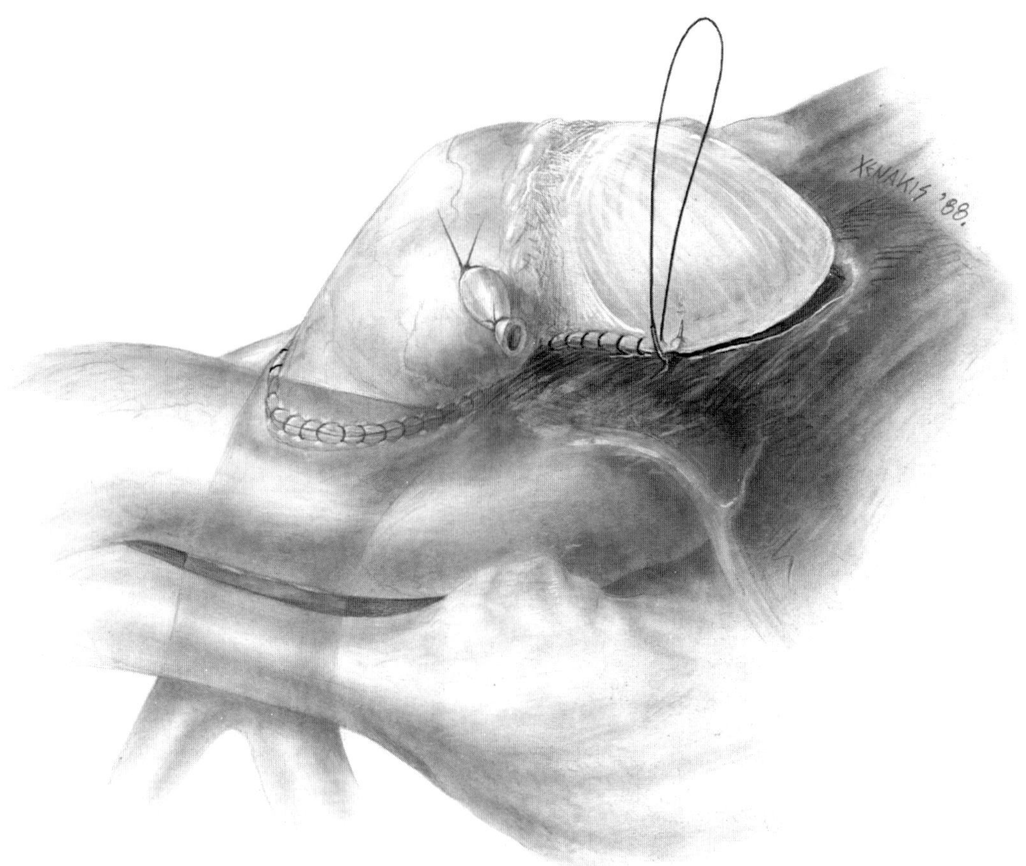

Figure 7.4. Proximal anastomosis completed with a single running polypropylene suture. Note the additional tie on the allograft coronary stumps.

nous septum is usually retained on the allograft. The suture line is begun posteriorly and run to the tip of the anterior leaflet of the mitral valve (Fig. 7.4).

When there is a native pulmonary annulus, even hypoplastic (e.g., normally related great arteries), the posterior allograft annulus is inset and sewn at the level of the recipient "annulus" (Fig. 7.5). Otherwise, the ventriculotomy is made high on the infundibulum, and the proximal anastomosis is accomplished between ventricular muscle and allograft (Fig. 7.6). The ventriculotomy is not made so long that there is flattening of the entrance into the allograft; rather, it is somewhat "short" so that suturing the anterior leaflet of the mitral valve allows the aortic valve to "sit up," leaving a wide-open outflow from the ventricle (Fig. 7.7). Retention of the allograft membranous septum enhances this orientation (Fig. 7.8). If there is marked hypertrophy of the ventricular muscle, undercutting can enlarge the orifice without lengthening the ventriculotomy (Fig. 7.9).

When operating on such lesions as truncus arteriosus, a pledget is often placed in the suture line beginning at the middle posteriorly, as there is often a relative deficiency of myocardial tissue and sutures have been placed nearby for ventricular septal defect closure (Fig. 7.10).

As with the use of Dacron conduits, positioning is arranged to minimize sternal compression. When necessary, the left pericardium can be incised to allow rotation of the heart to the left. In any case, some sternal compression is much better tolerated by the allograft tissue than rigid Dacron conduits, and it rarely seems to present postoperatively as the heart size decreases.

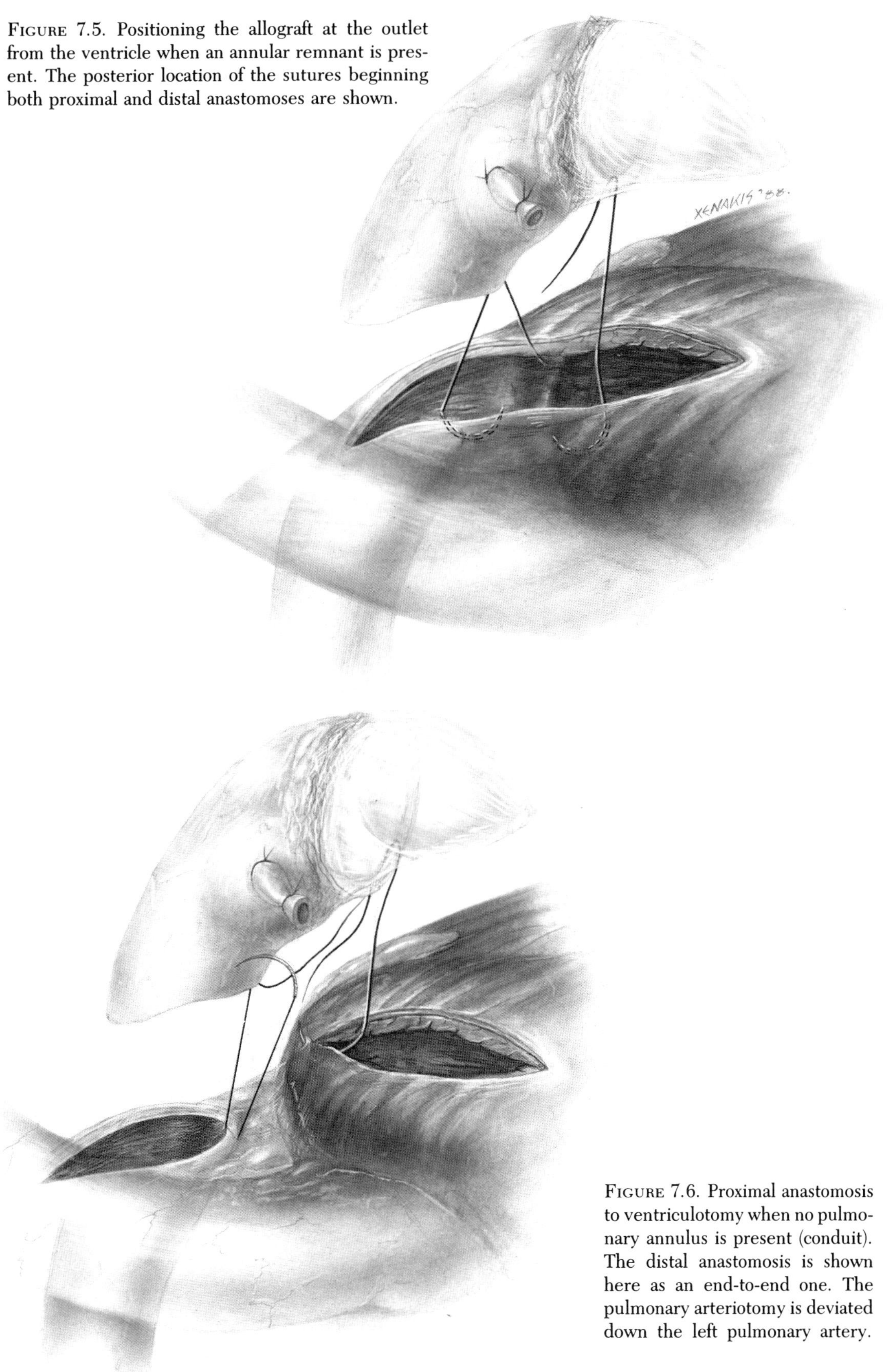

FIGURE 7.5. Positioning the allograft at the outlet from the ventricle when an annular remnant is present. The posterior location of the sutures beginning both proximal and distal anastomoses are shown.

FIGURE 7.6. Proximal anastomosis to ventriculotomy when no pulmonary annulus is present (conduit). The distal anastomosis is shown here as an end-to-end one. The pulmonary arteriotomy is deviated down the left pulmonary artery.

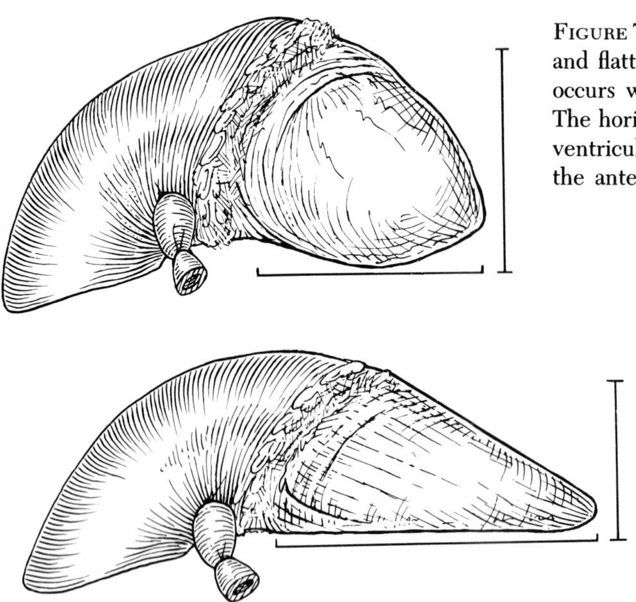

FIGURE 7.7. This drawing demonstrates the narrowing and flattening of the ventricular outflow orifice that occurs when the ventriculotomy is made too long. The horizontal lines represent the dimensions of the ventriculotomy and the vertical lines the height in the anteroposterior diameter of the allograft valve.

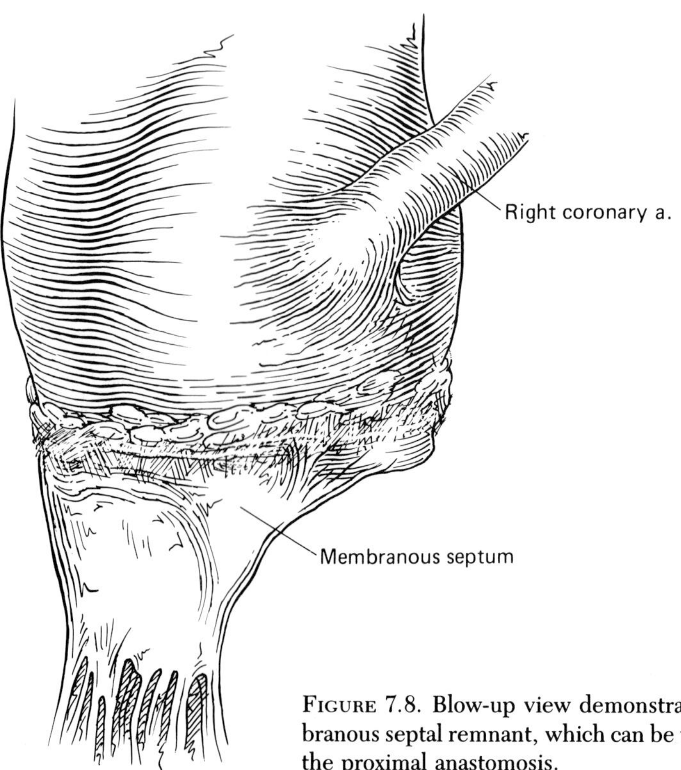

FIGURE 7.8. Blow-up view demonstrating the membranous septal remnant, which can be used to enlarge the proximal anastomosis.

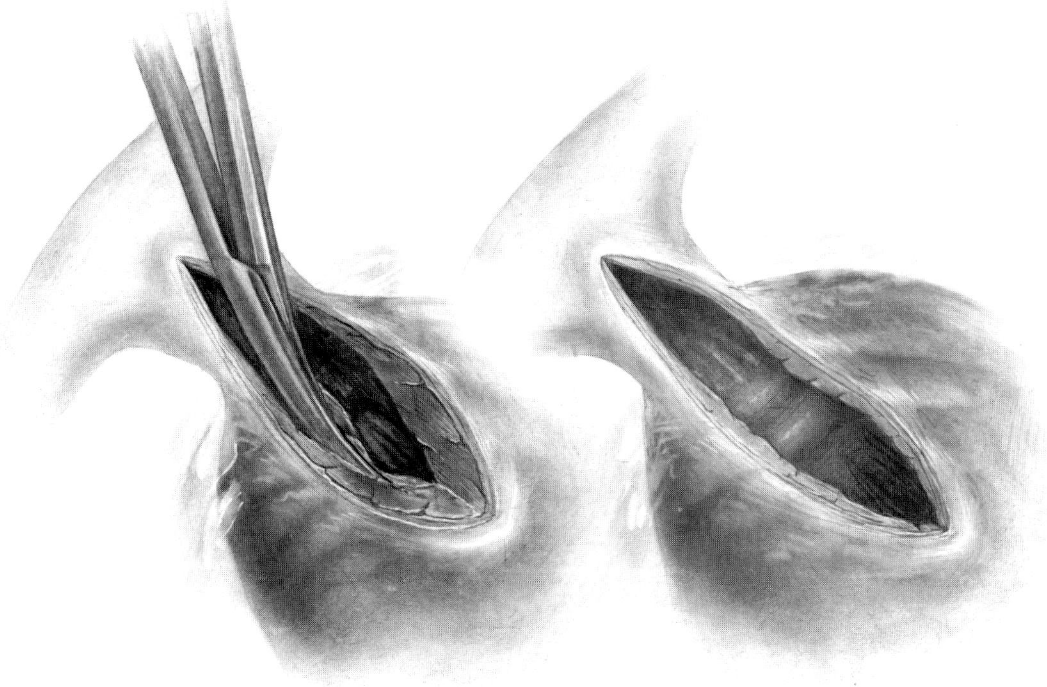

FIGURE 7.9. Enlargement of the ventricular outflow by resecting hypertrophied anterior ventricular myocardium.

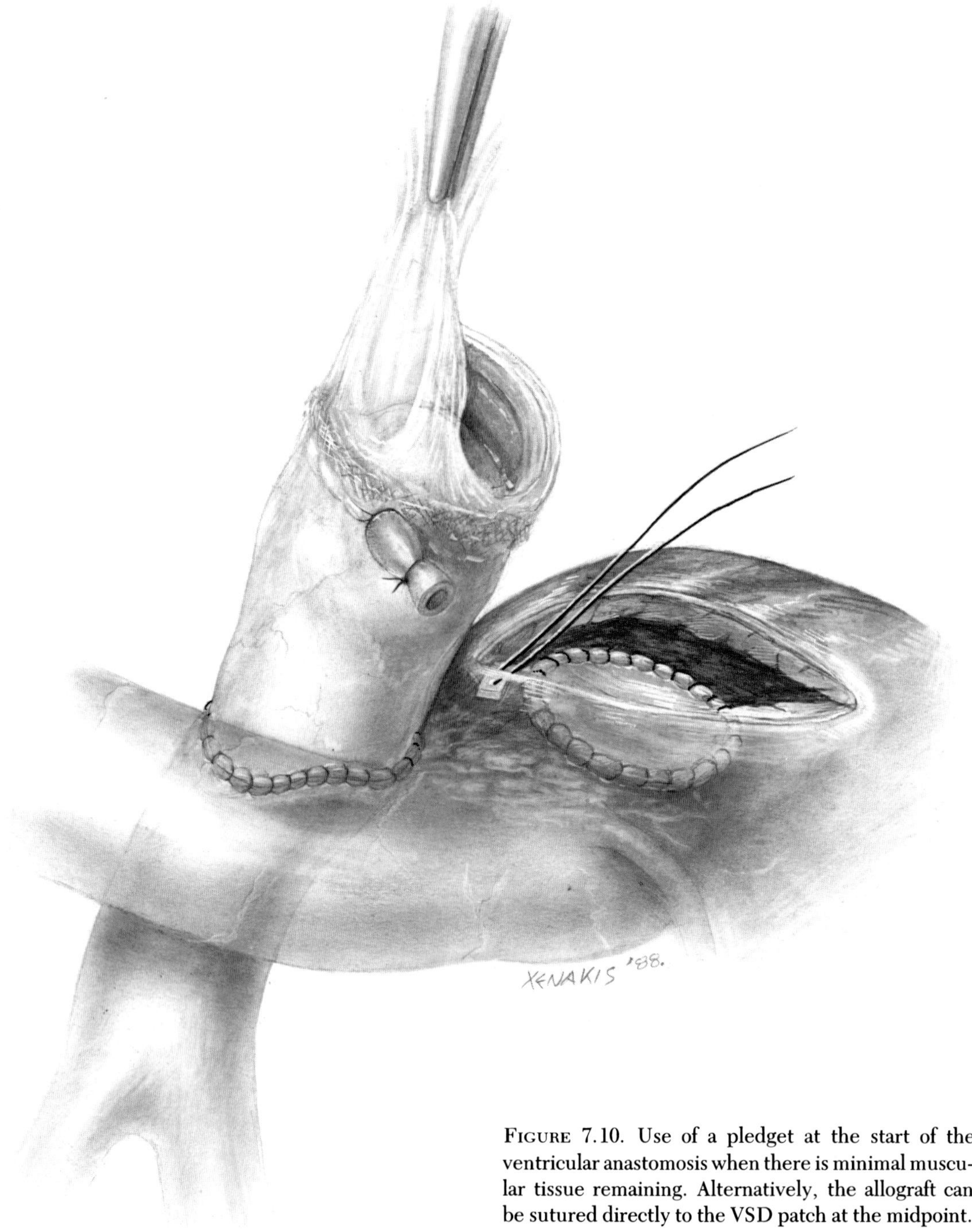

Figure 7.10. Use of a pledget at the start of the ventricular anastomosis when there is minimal muscular tissue remaining. Alternatively, the allograft can be sutured directly to the VSD patch at the midpoint.

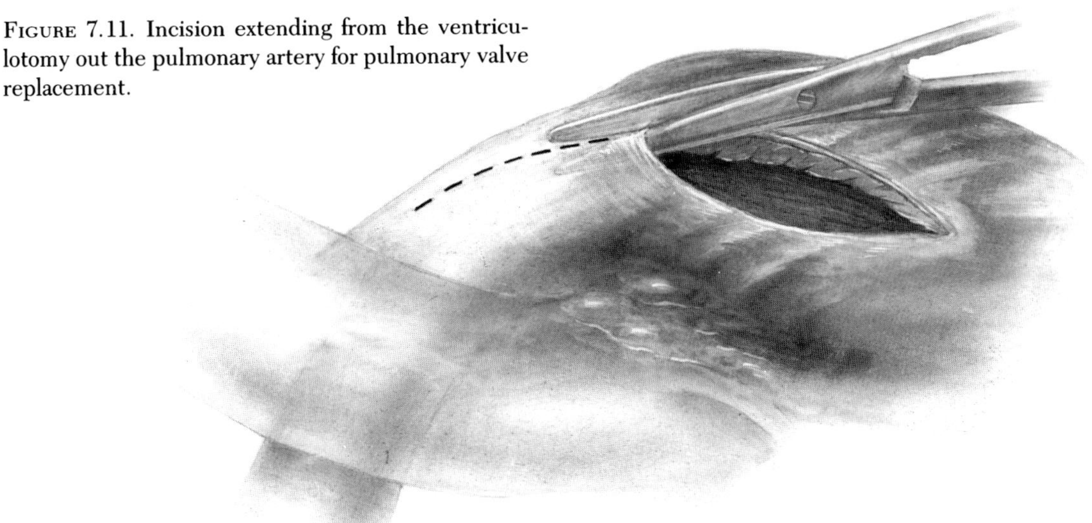

FIGURE 7.11. Incision extending from the ventriculotomy out the pulmonary artery for pulmonary valve replacement.

Pulmonary Valve Replacement in Adults

Indications

Pulmonary valve replacement is usually contemplated in adults in the setting of previous right ventricular outflow tract surgery for pulmonary hypoplasia or atresia. In most cases valve insertion is for symptomatic pulmonary insufficiency that has resulted in right ventricular dysfunction with incipient or manifest tricuspid insufficiency (e.g., tetralogy of Fallot).[8,10,11,23–25a]

Sizing

Sizing is easy in adult pulmonary valve replacements. There is a broad tolerance in the size of aortic allografts that can be placed. An allograft of 22–26 mm is usually selected (see Appendix: Valve Diameters). In general, the tendency is to upsize. The conduit is chosen to allow a large oblique distal anastomosis, and the ventriculotomy is made to accommodate the chosen allograft. If there are any pulmonary arterial stenoses, they are managed at the time of the same operation.

Technique with Aortic Allograft

The patient is placed on cardiopulmonary bypass usually with dual caval cannulas, but a single right atrial cannula can also be used if the only operation to be performed is pulmonary valve replacement. In the absence of septal defects, cardioplegia is not necessary unless pulmonary arterioplasty is contemplated on the branch pulmonary arteries. The right ventricular outflow tract is approached initially with an incision in the proximal pulmonary artery, which is extended across the region of the annulus. The incision is extended into the right ventricular muscle for a short distance (approximately 3–4 cm). Any residual valve leaflet tissue is excised. The incision is then extended for a distance of approximately 5 cm distally on the pulmonary artery (Fig. 7.11).

The prepared aortic allograft is positioned. The distal anastomosis is accomplished in an oblique end-to-end fashion with a running 5-0 or 4-0 polypropylene suture technique (Fig. 7.12). The allograft is positioned so that the allograft annulus is at the level of the native pulmonary annulus. When the recipient annular region is dilated, the positioning is similar to the "inlay technique" of Meisner, Hagl and Sebening.[25b]

The proximal anastomosis is then accomplished with a single running suture begun posteriorly. Each suture is run along the annulus to the surface of the right ventriculotomy, which usually approximates the fibrous trigone on each side of the allograft (Fig. 7.13). If the allograft sits higher than this point, the anterior leaflet

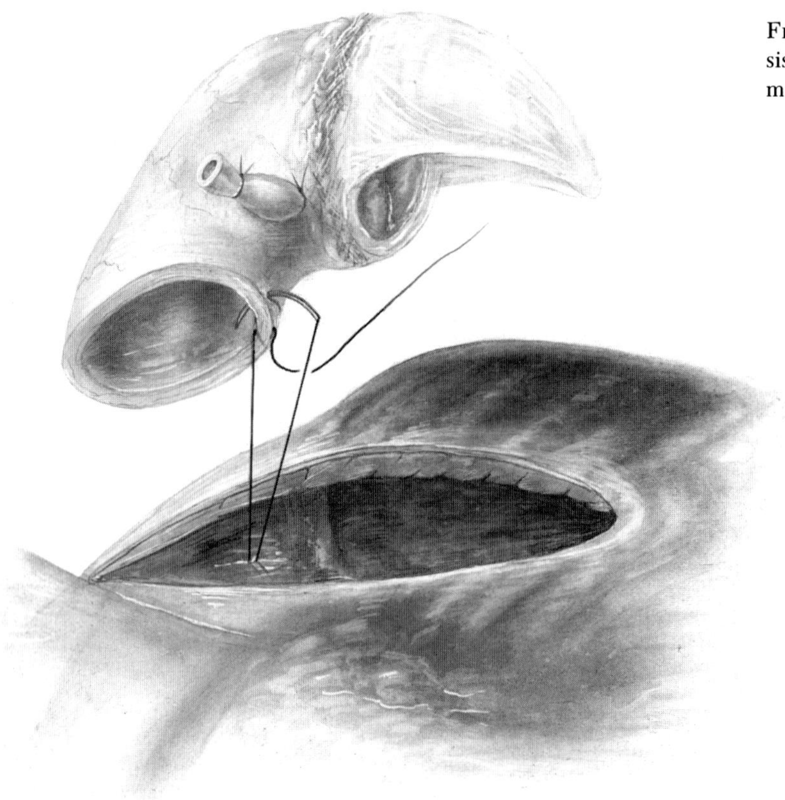

Figure 7.12. Distal anastomosis for pulmonary valve replacement with an aortic allograft.

Figure 7.13. Proximal anastomosis begun at midpoint posteriorly with suturing of annulus to annulus.

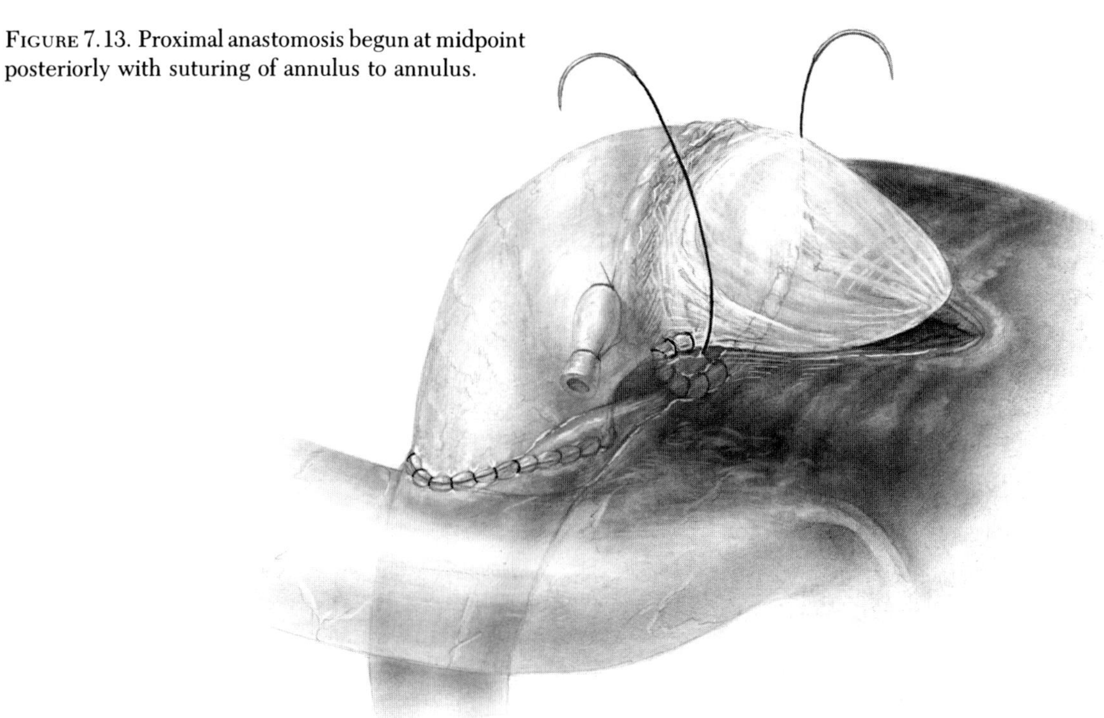

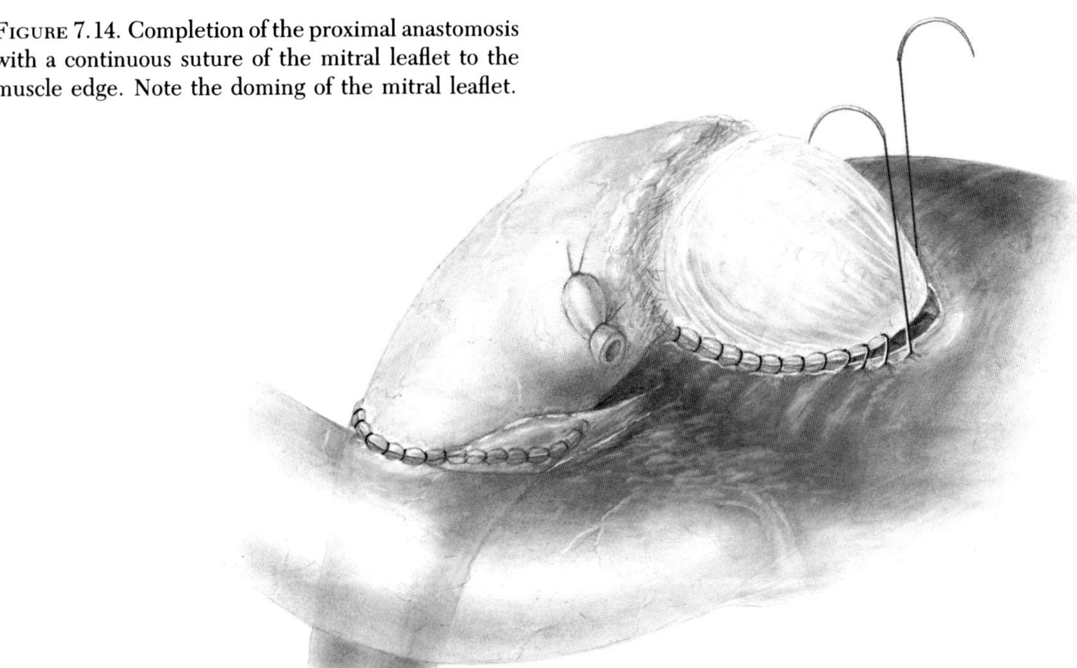

FIGURE 7.14. Completion of the proximal anastomosis with a continuous suture of the mitral leaflet to the muscle edge. Note the doming of the mitral leaflet.

of the mitral valve can be deviated so as to cover this region or an additional piece of pericardium utilized.

The suture line is then continued from the right and left fibrous trigones of the allograft down the short ventriculotomy to the anterior leaflet of the mitral valve. The anterior leaflet of the mitral valve is allowed to bow slightly anteriorly to fully open the pathway to the neopulmonary valve (Fig. 7.14). When the allograft is replacing a previously positioned Dacron conduit, the latter is always completely removed.

Technique with Pulmonary Allograft

Pulmonary allografts can be used as conduits or orthotopic valve replacements.[22] The technique is similar to aortic allograft in the pulmonary position except that the role of the anterior leaflet of the mitral valve is replaced with a trapezoidal patch of pericardium. This patch is kept generous so as to not deform the annulus of the pulmonary valve with tightening during ventricular contractions (Fig. 7.15). The distal anastomosis is usually not as oblique as with an aortic allograft, as the amount of conduit available distal to the sinus ridge (tops of commissures) of the pulmonary valve is not as great and the elasticity and diameter of the pulmonary allograft is usually greater. Thus the arteriotomy in the main pulmonary artery is kept shorter and closer to the heart than when an aortic allograft is utilized.

The pulmonary valve allograft appears to function well in the right ventricular outflow position.[26a] Autotransplants to the aortic position have been reported by Ross and others to function well and with excellent durability. Thus portending even better durability in the low pressure position.[26b,c] Both Ross and McGrath have noted that implantation of the allograft pulmonary valve into both the pulmonary and the aortic positions is, if anything, technically easier than with an aortic allograft: There is less bulk at the proximal suture line, and the wall is thinner.[26a] An extensive series has yet to be reported that supports the use of the allograft pulmonary valve in the aortic position. Pieces of cryopreserved allograft pulmonary artery tissue have been used to augment recipient pulmonary arteries during reconstructions of the pulmonary artery bifurcation and, as reported by Ziemer and colleagues, can be combined with

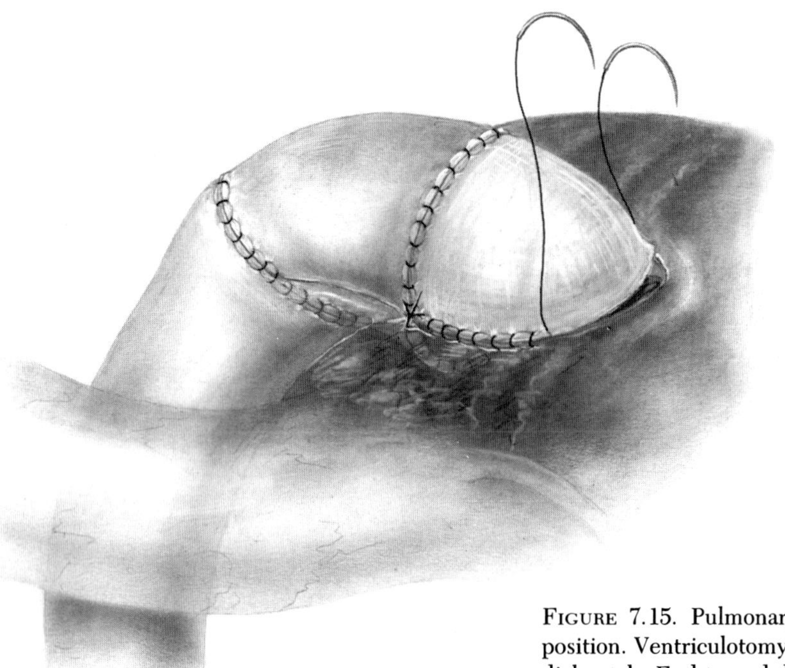

FIGURE 7.15. Pulmonary allograft in an orthotopic position. Ventriculotomy is completed with a pericardial patch. End-to-end distal anastomosis for pulmonary artery in continuity with ventricle.

an allograft pulmonary valve to accomplish total right ventricular outflow tract reconstructions with allograft pulmonary tissue.[27]

Anterior Ventricle to Pulmonary Artery Allograft Conduit in Corrected Transposition

The relief of associated pulmonary stenosis or atresia in the anomaly of corrected transposition (atrioventricular discordance and ventriculoarterial discordance) requires attention to special anatomic features. The correction is usually but not always associated with closure of a ventricular septal defect.[28] The position of the conduction system mandates a different technique for closure of a ventricular septal defect, as well as for care when performing the ventriculotomy for relief of the pulmonary outflow obstruction from the morphologic left ventricle.[29] In general, we close the ventricular septal defect through the defect with sutures placed on the morphologic right side.[29] It is usually accomplished through the ventriculotomy. The emphasis of this section is on the correct performance of the ventriculotomy and construction of the allograft pathway to the pulmonary arteries.

The conduction bundle courses anterior to the pulmonary artery just below the annulus. Thus a ventriculotomy placed high on the morphologic left ventricle (pulmonary ventricle) places the conduction bundle at risk. In addition, retraction of the superior border of the ventriculotomy can induce conduction blocks. There are usually large coronary arteries coursing across the upper portion of this anterior but morphologically left ventricle from the circumflex coronary artery that must be avoided (Fig. 7.16).

Technique

The patient is placed on cardiopulmonary bypass with bicaval cannulation. Hypothermic cardioplegic arrest is induced. The best way to create the ventriculotomy is to place a finger through the mitral valve so as to palpate the location of the papillary muscles (Fig. 7.17) and perform the ventriculotomy relatively low on the ventricle, cutting to the surgeon's finger (Fig. 7.18). The anterior papillary muscle is usually located just to the right of this ventriculotomy.[30] This technique is designed to protect the mitral valve support, the conduction system, and to allow

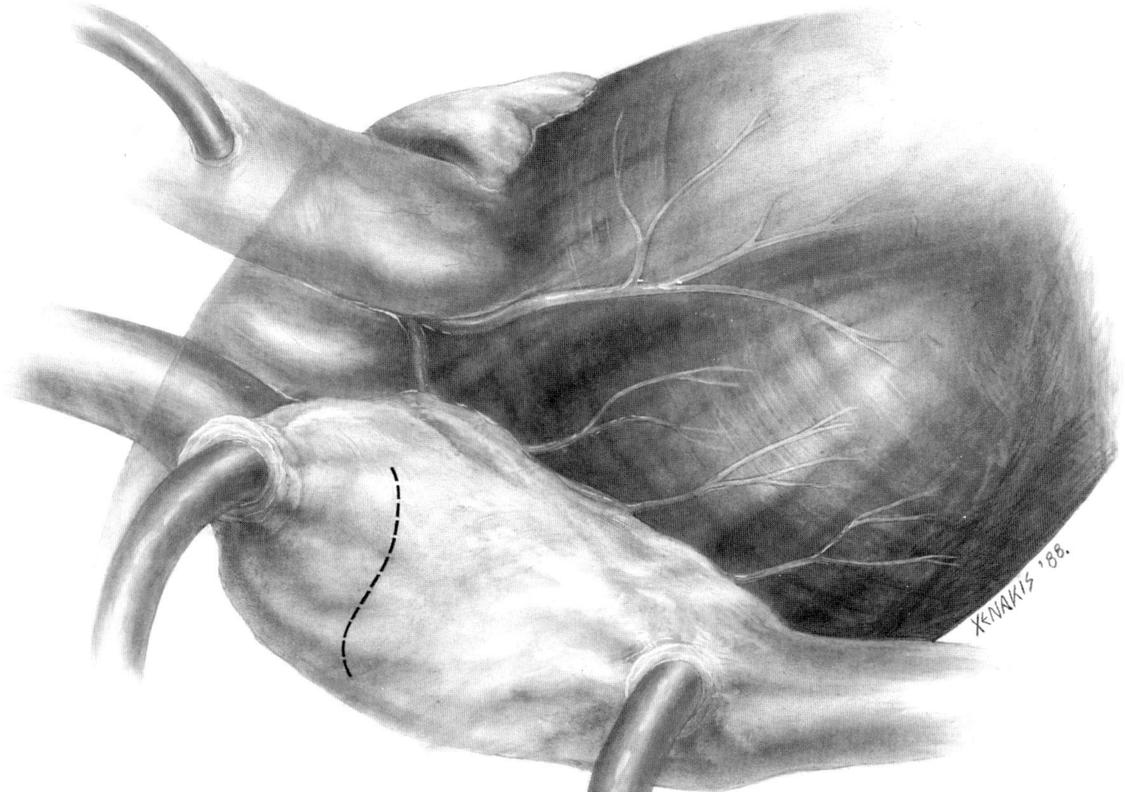

FIGURE 7.16. Cannulation and atriotomy for corrected transposition. Note the location of the coronary arteries.

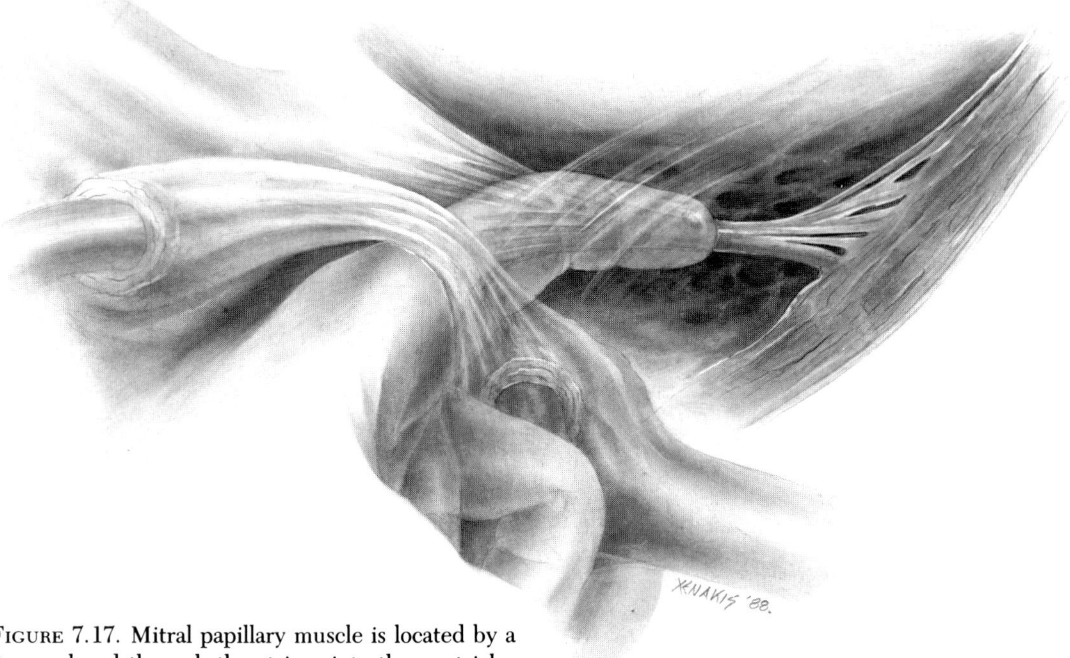

FIGURE 7.17. Mitral papillary muscle is located by a finger placed through the atrium into the ventricle.

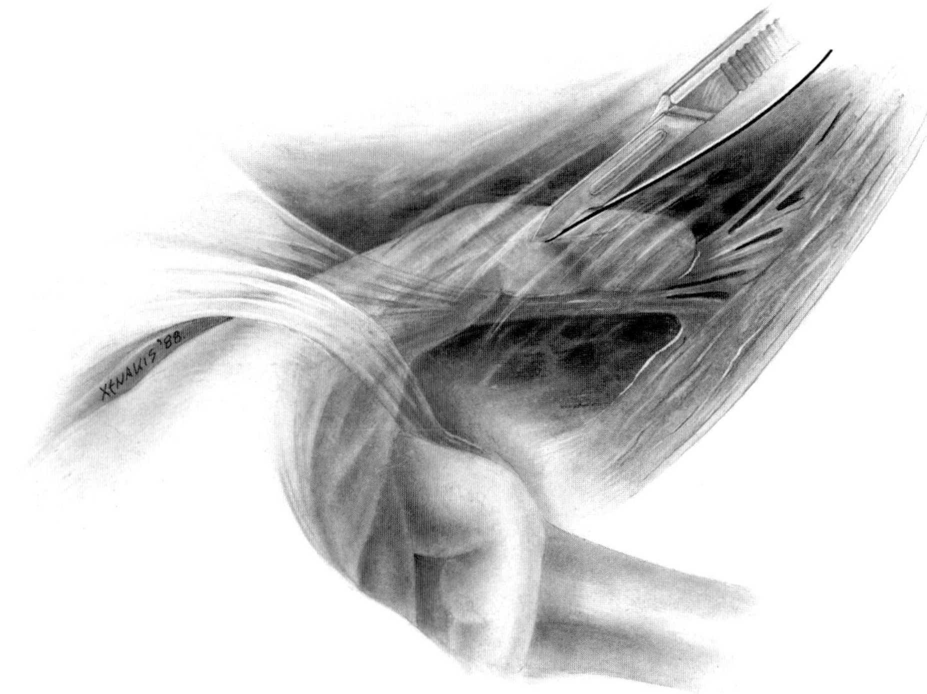

Figure 7.18. Ventriculotomy is made toward the apex, cutting to the surgeon's finger to avoid the atrioventricular subvalvular apparatus.

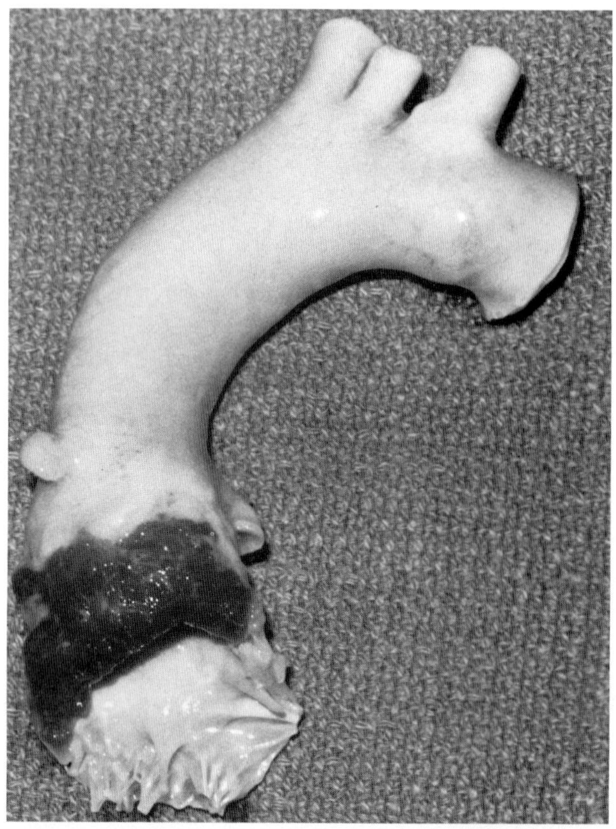

Figure 7.19. Aortic allograft conduit is chosen with a long segment to avoid use of prosthetic extensions. (Courtesy of Virginia Tissue Bank)

FIGURE 7.20. Distal native pulmonary artery to allograft anastomosis is performed first.

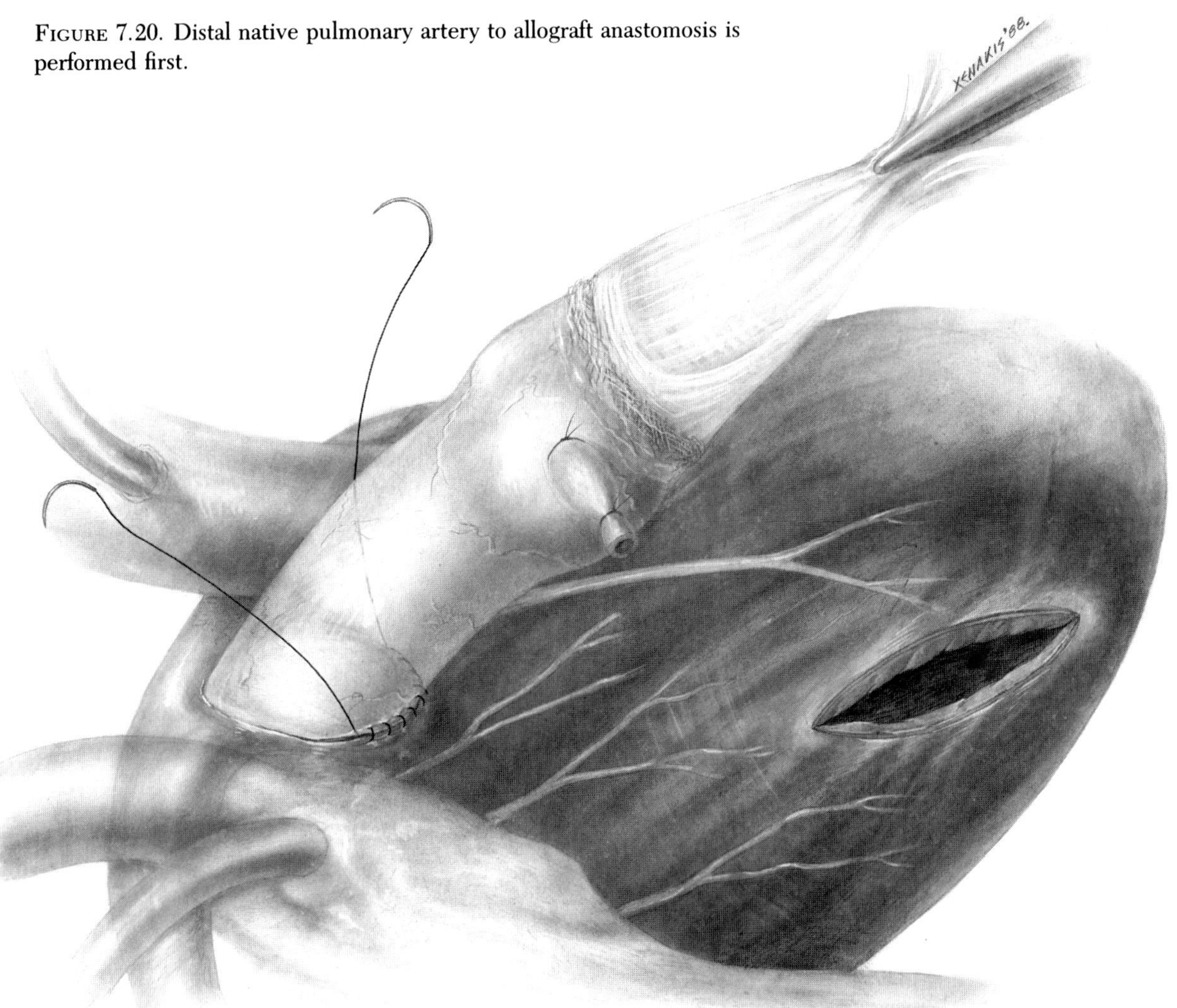

adequate egress from the pulmonary ventricle. An allograft aortic valve conduit must be selected that is of adult size and that has a long conduit (6 cm or more), at least to the level of the innominate artery (Fig. 7.19). An allograft this large can usually be placed without the addition of prosthetic material. The direct suturing of the aortic allograft to the ventriculotomy is thus placed in a relatively low position, where the heart is curving away from the sternum, and there is no difficulty with compression of the prosthesis. The ventriculotomy is positioned adjacent and fairly far apically. Ventriculotomy is begun and then, under direct vision, enlarged to the point that, for a typical-sized patient, a 22- to 24-mm allograft valve can be sewn to the ventriculotomy. The ventricular septal defect is then closed as described by deLeval and associates.[29]

The allograft is prepared, leaving the anterior leaflet of the mitral valve attached with the chordae trimmed. Trimming of the muscular base of the allograft valve is relatively vigorous, but tissue underneath the fibrous skeleton of the valve is usually left to a distance of 2 mm. The membranous septum is left attached to the allograft. This additional material, with the anterior leaflet of the mitral valve, allows suturing of the allograft directly to the ventriculotomy such that it "sits up" on the ventriculotomy.

The length of the allograft required between the ventriculotomy and the pulmonary arteriotomy is assessed. If there is continuity between the pulmonary artery and the pulmonary ventricle, an end-to-side anastomosis is utilized to the main pulmonary artery in an oblique fashion. If there is complete pulmonary atresia, an end-to-end oblique anastomosis is accomplished.

The distal anastomosis is accomplished first with a running 5-0 polypropylene suture line

Figure 7.21. Proximal anastomosis in corrected transposition.

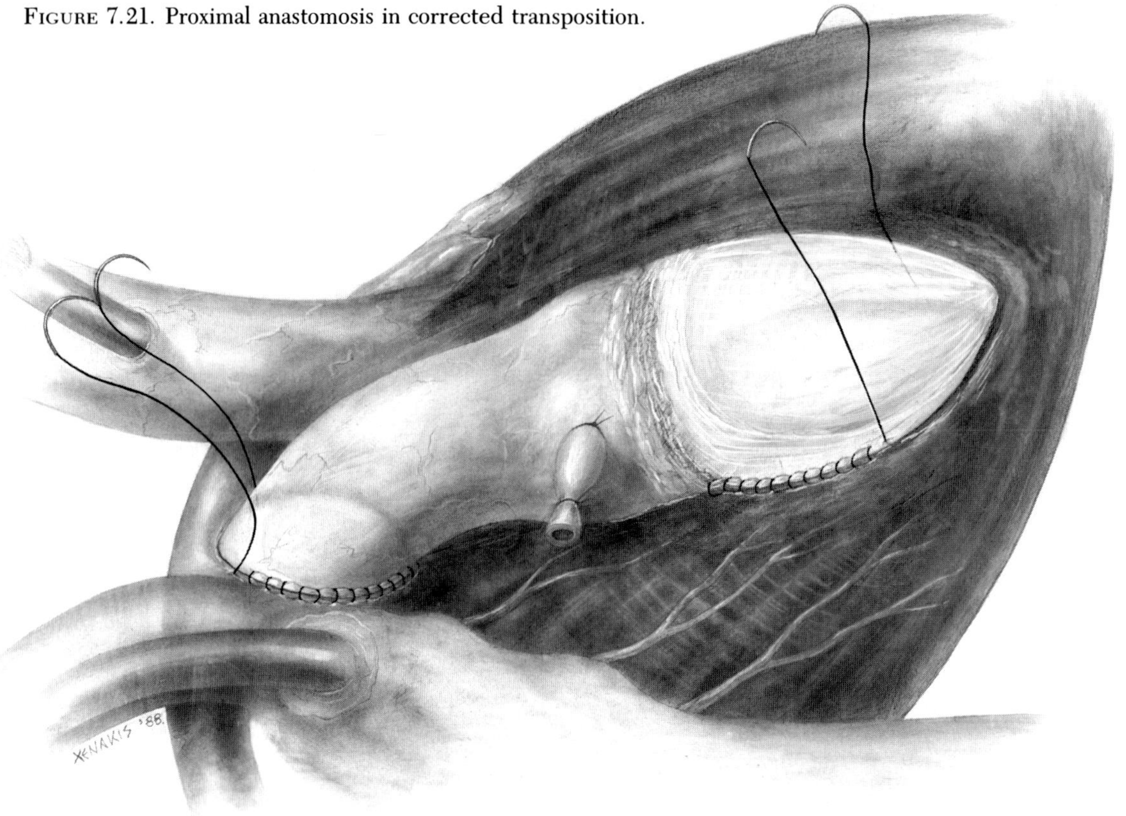

(Fig. 7.20). The conduit is cut at the appropriate length to allow an easy reach to the ventriculotomy. It has not been necessary, in our experience, to extend it into the midarch of the allograft. Such extension is certainly possible, when necessary, to avoid synthetic material extensions. We have never needed to extend conduits proximally or distally, purely for length reasons as our procurement team usually obtains the allograft aortic valve with aorta complete to the distal arch.

After the distal suture line is completed, we normally remove the aortic cross clamp, perform

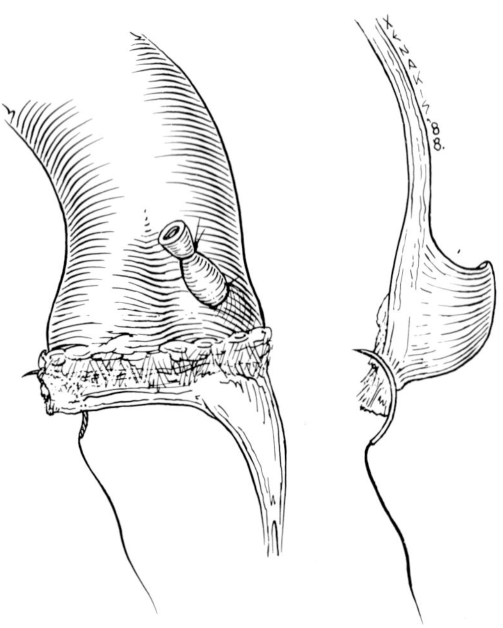

Figure 7.22. Angle of entry for the needle to take advantage of both the inner fibrous base underneath the valve cusps and the fibrous rim externally on the aortic root, which is higher than the base of the leaflet insertions.

FIGURE 7.23. Stenosis extending to the origin of the right pulmonary artery involving the confluence. The incision completely opens the stenotic area. ▷

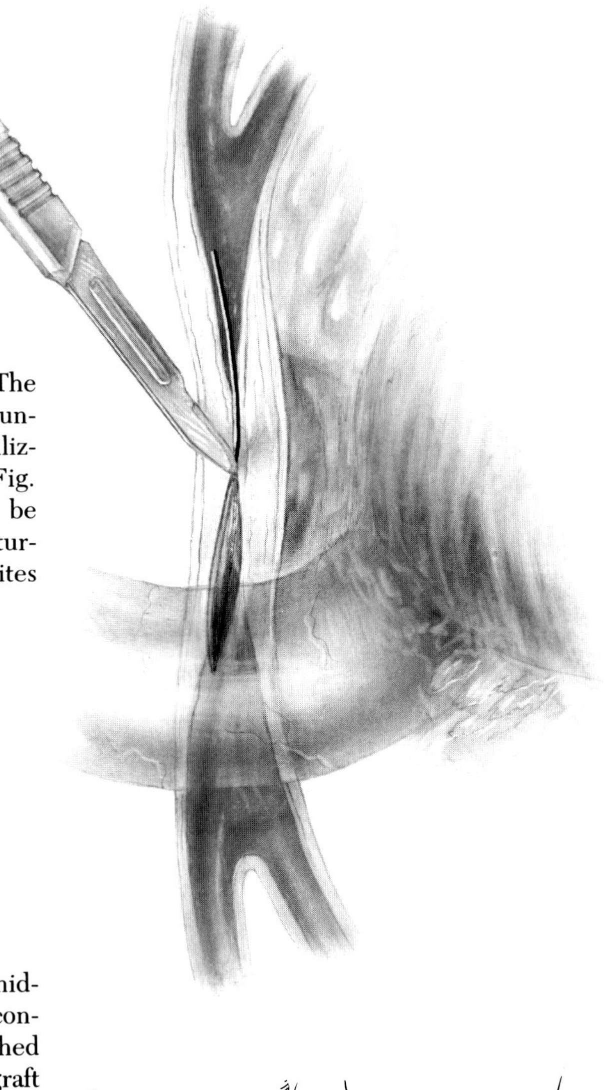

de-airing maneuvers, and begin rewarming. The proximal anastomosis is accomplished with a running 5-0 polypropylene suture technique utilizing the anterior leaflet of the mitral valve (Fig. 7.21). Some subvalvular muscle tissue may be left on the allograft to provide bulk to the suturing. However, care is taken with all suture bites to enter fibrous material (Fig. 7.22).

Reconstruction of Right Ventricular Outflow with Abnormal Pulmonary Arteries

Stenoses in Confluent Pulmonary Arteries

Proximal Stenoses

If a short stenosis is present near or at the midpoint of the pulmonary artery bifurcation, reconstruction of the confluence can be accomplished with primary anastomosis of the distal allograft to the pulmonary artery. The pulmonary artery is split through the level of the stenosis (Fig. 7.23 and 7.24). The distal end of the allograft is slightly rounded (Fig. 7.25). The allograft is sutured to the native pulmonary arterial tissue, with the midpoint of the allograft being shifted to the point of greatest stenosis. This anastomosis is accomplished with running 5-0 monofilament suture technique (Fig. 7.26). Alternatively, the distal anastomosis can be enlarged by cutting the distal allograft somewhat obliquely in the

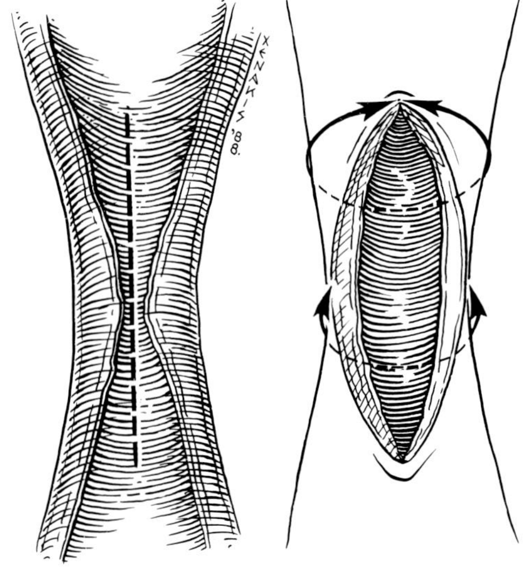

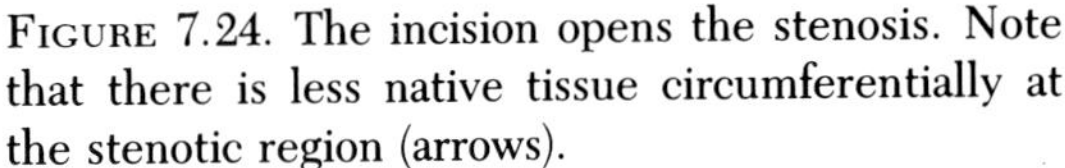

FIGURE 7.24. The incision opens the stenosis. Note that there is less native tissue circumferentially at the stenotic region (arrows).

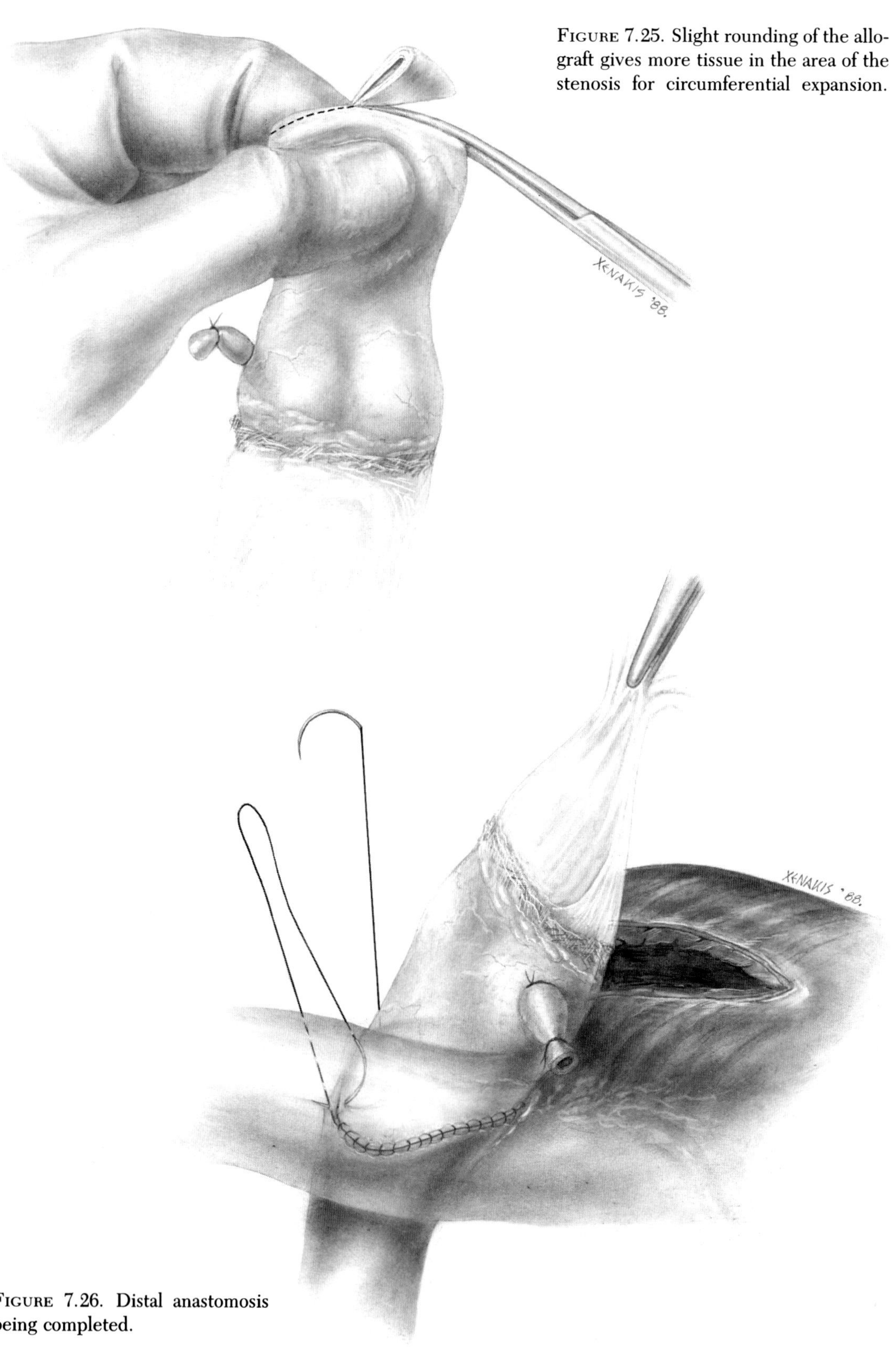

FIGURE 7.25. Slight rounding of the allograft gives more tissue in the area of the stenosis for circumferential expansion.

FIGURE 7.26. Distal anastomosis being completed.

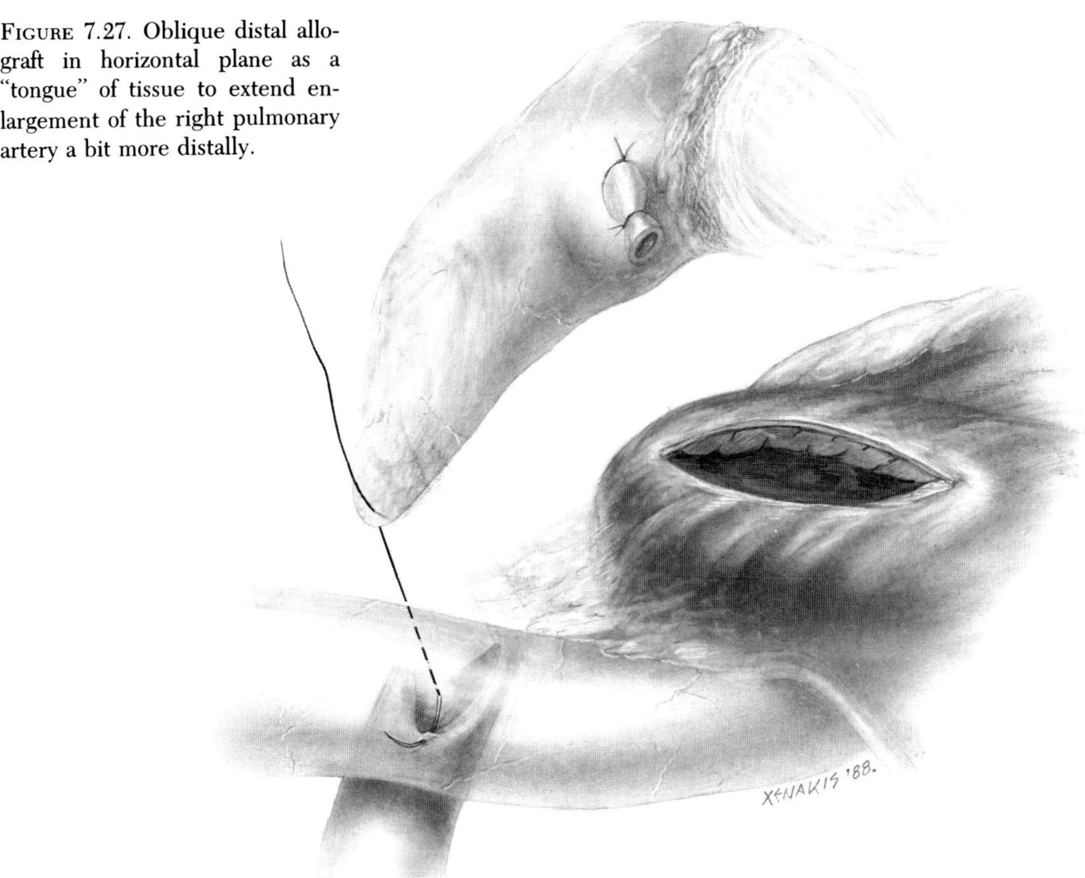

FIGURE 7.27. Oblique distal allograft in horizontal plane as a "tongue" of tissue to extend enlargement of the right pulmonary artery a bit more distally.

transverse plane to provide a "tongue" of tissue to extend the distal anastomosis laterally. During this procedure care must be taken to align the allograft so the mitral leaflet is positioned anteriorly (Fig. 7.27).

The "height" of the reconstructed pulmonary artery bifurcation is also accomplished by utilizing an allograft that is large (in diameter) for the patient (e.g., 23-mm allograft for a 1.5-m^2 BSA individual) and by making the conduit slightly long. This reconstruction of the bifurcation with the distal conduit avoids any interposition of foreign material. A conduit length distal to the aortic valve of around 6 cm is usually required for this kind of reconstruction, and even longer conduit lengths are needed for large individuals. By selecting longer conduits, a proximal anastomosis can be accomplished *without* the need for augmentation with prosthetic material.

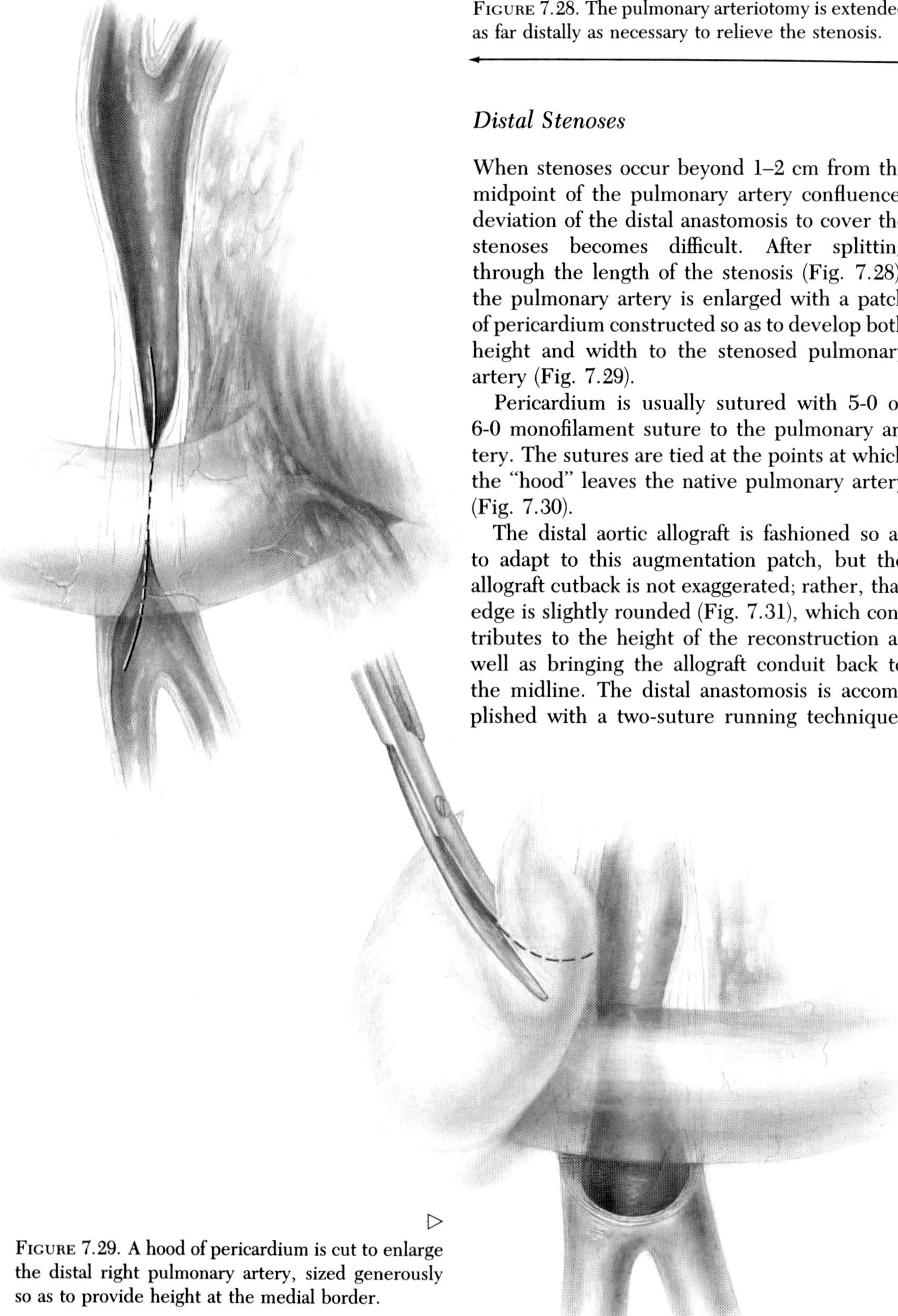

FIGURE 7.28. The pulmonary arteriotomy is extended as far distally as necessary to relieve the stenosis.

Distal Stenoses

When stenoses occur beyond 1–2 cm from the midpoint of the pulmonary artery confluence, deviation of the distal anastomosis to cover the stenoses becomes difficult. After splitting through the length of the stenosis (Fig. 7.28), the pulmonary artery is enlarged with a patch of pericardium constructed so as to develop both height and width to the stenosed pulmonary artery (Fig. 7.29).

Pericardium is usually sutured with 5-0 or 6-0 monofilament suture to the pulmonary artery. The sutures are tied at the points at which the "hood" leaves the native pulmonary artery (Fig. 7.30).

The distal aortic allograft is fashioned so as to adapt to this augmentation patch, but the allograft cutback is not exaggerated; rather, that edge is slightly rounded (Fig. 7.31), which contributes to the height of the reconstruction as well as bringing the allograft conduit back to the midline. The distal anastomosis is accomplished with a two-suture running technique.

FIGURE 7.29. A hood of pericardium is cut to enlarge the distal right pulmonary artery, sized generously so as to provide height at the medial border.

FIGURE 7.30. Pericardial patch sutures are tied.

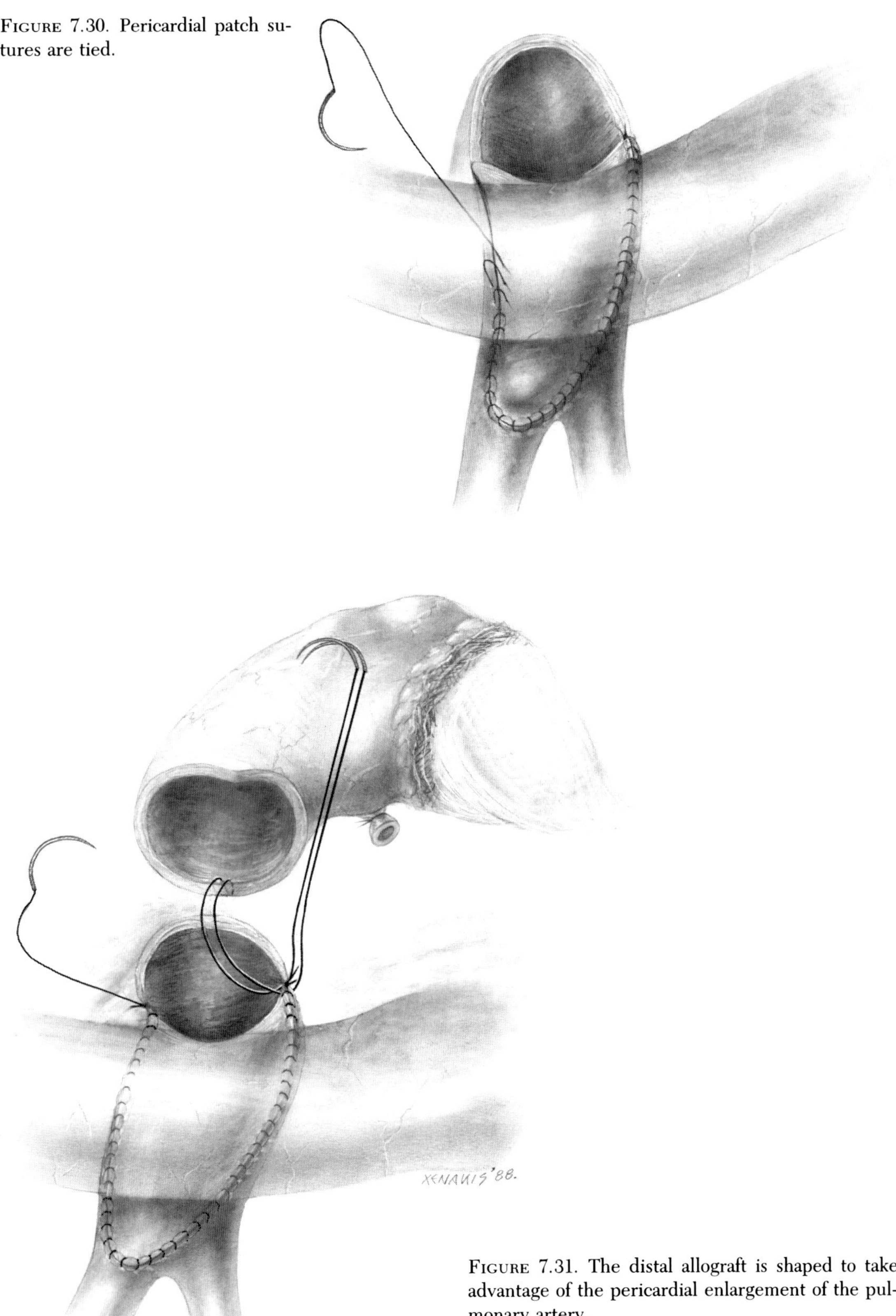

FIGURE 7.31. The distal allograft is shaped to take advantage of the pericardial enlargement of the pulmonary artery.

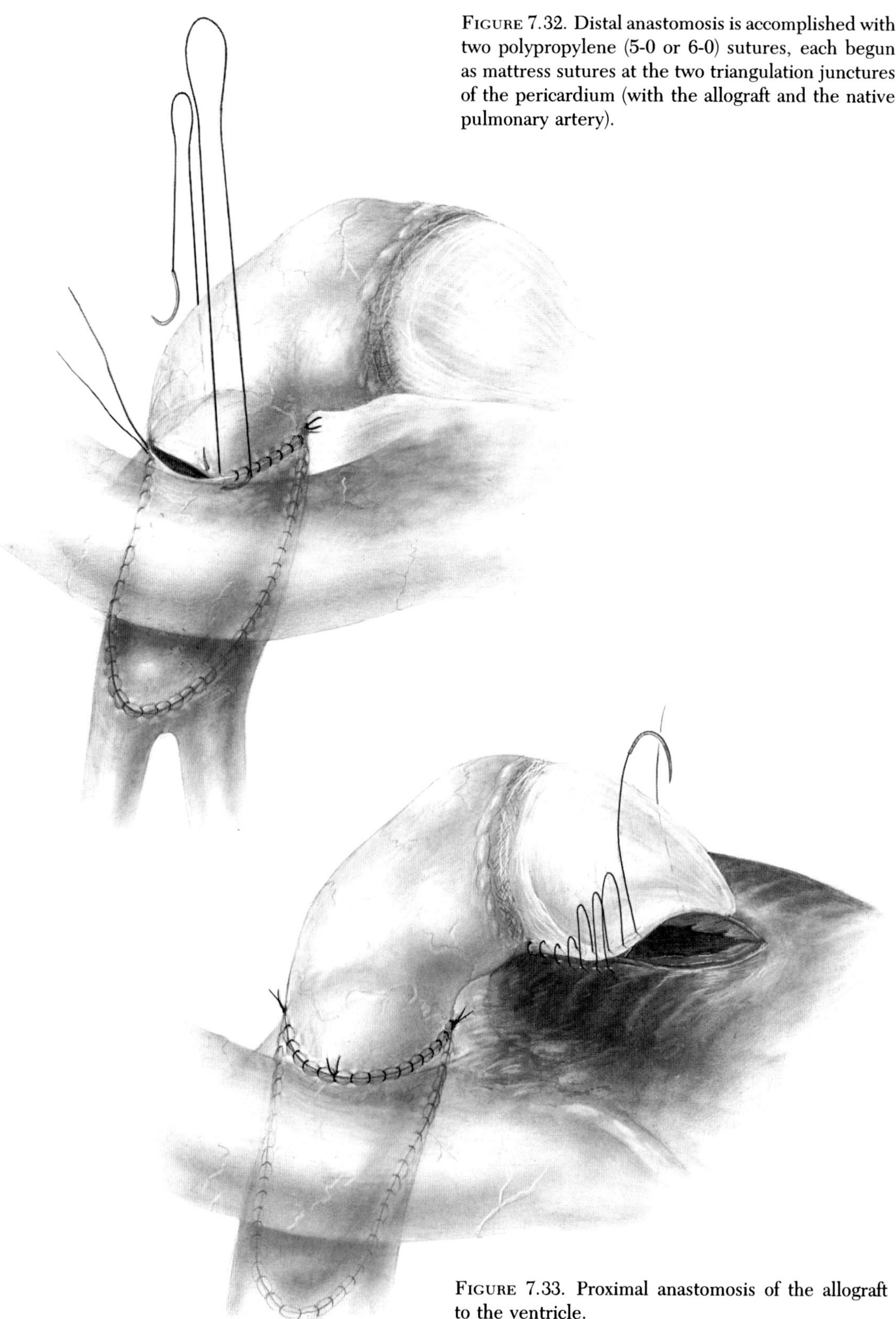

Figure 7.32. Distal anastomosis is accomplished with two polypropylene (5-0 or 6-0) sutures, each begun as mattress sutures at the two triangulation junctures of the pericardium (with the allograft and the native pulmonary artery).

Figure 7.33. Proximal anastomosis of the allograft to the ventricle.

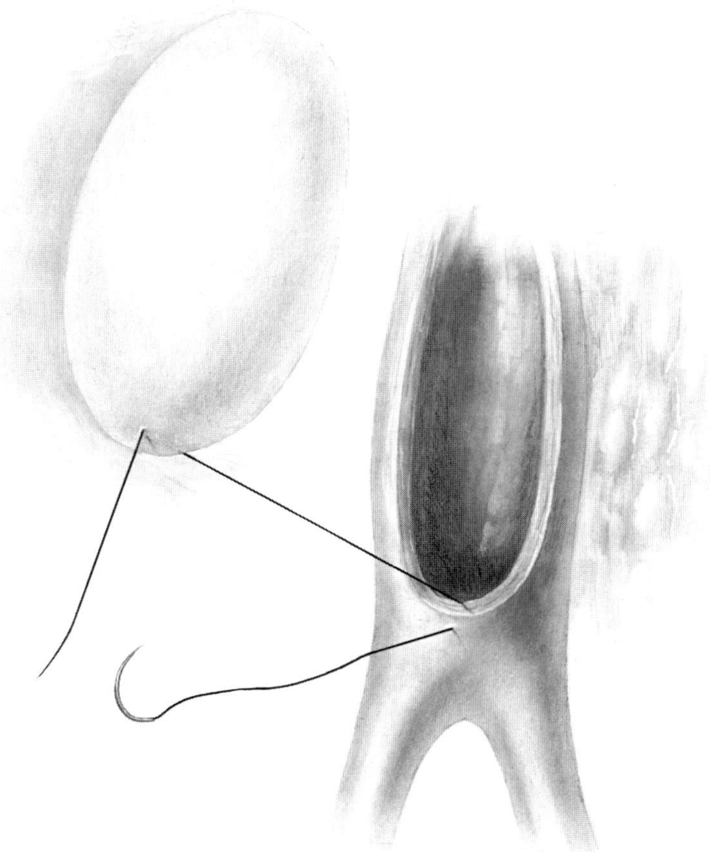

FIGURE 7.34. Incision through the stenotic pulmonary artery confluence and sizing of the oval piece of pericardium for the "skirt" technique.

The initial suturing is begun by placing a horizontal mattress suture at the junction of the allograft, pericardium, and native pulmonary artery and then running the suture continuously along the inferior border of the anastomosis. A second horizontal mattress suture is placed at the analogous point on the upper border of the anastomosis, and the two suture lines are run to each other and tied (Fig. 7.32). Care must be taken with this anastomosis that (as for all other pulmonary artery suture lines) the posterior suture line is particularly well constructed with narrowly placed bites, as it is difficult to suture any leaks later.

The proximal right ventriculotomy to aortic allograft anastomosis is performed in the usual fashion with 4-0 or 5-0 polypropylene continuous sutures (Fig. 7.33).

Hypoplastic But Confluent Pulmonary Arteries

"Skirt" Technique

With the "skirt" technique an oval piece of pericardium (glutaraldehyde-treated, bovine or autologous) that is generously sized is sutured with a continuous suture to a longitudinal pulmonary arteriotomy (Fig. 7.34). This method is utilized in situations where there is no main pulmonary artery, the confluence is hypoplastic, but the left and right main pulmonary arteries enlarge as they approach the hila. The pulmonary arteriotomy is extended to the more-normal-diameter arteries in the hila. The skirt of pericardium is sutured with a continuous suture to the edges

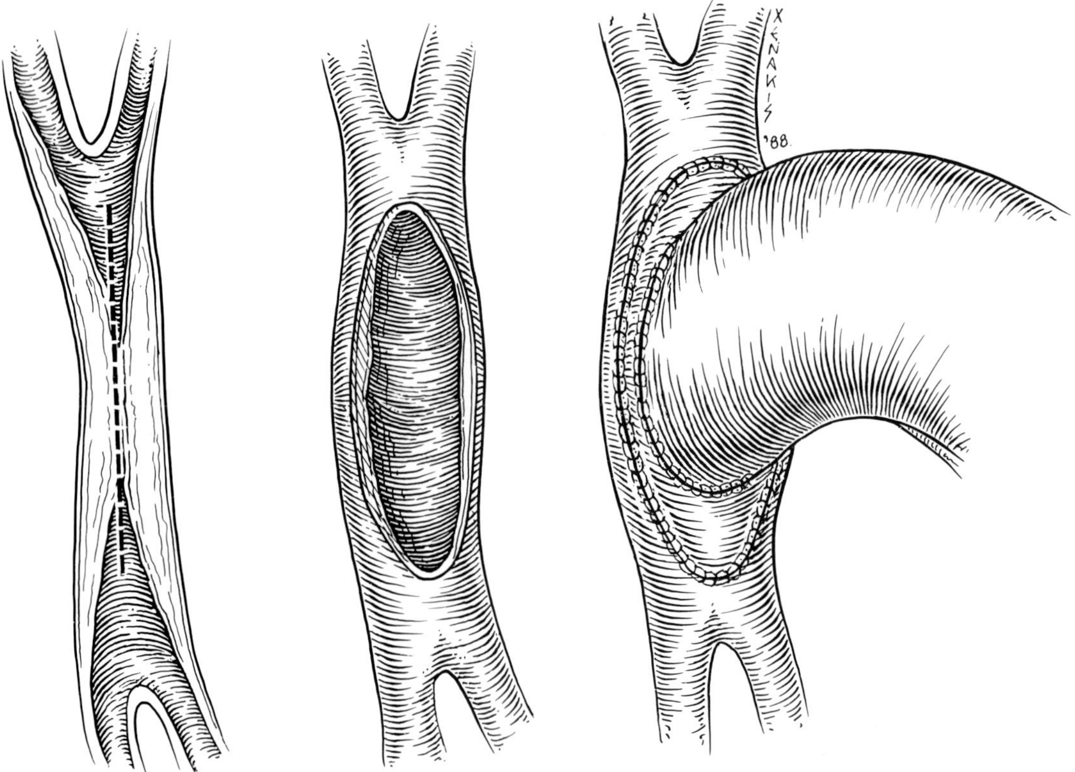

FIGURE 7.35. Enlargement of a stenotic pulmonary artery with a skirt of glutaraldehyde-treated pericardium. Note the circumference added to the pulmonary arterial confluence.

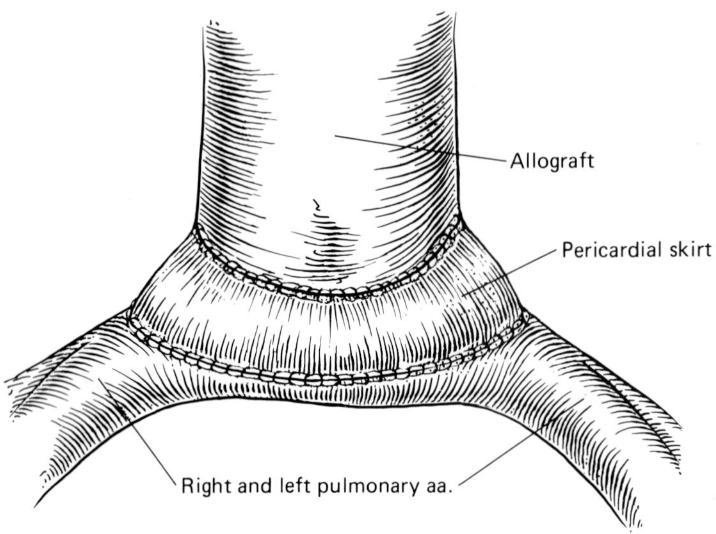

FIGURE 7.36. The pericardial skirt provides height to the bifurcation, enlarging the origins to the right and left pulmonary arteries.

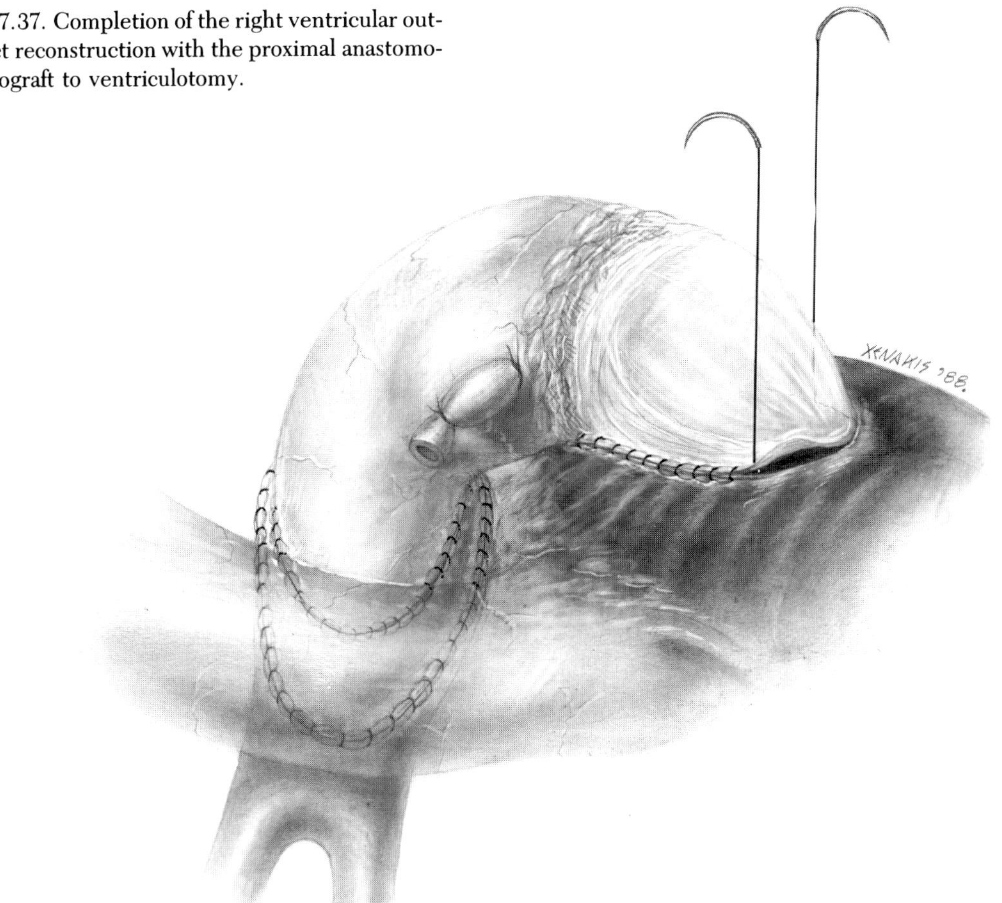

FIGURE 7.37. Completion of the right ventricular outflow tract reconstruction with the proximal anastomosis of allograft to ventriculotomy.

of the arteriotomy (Fig. 7.35). The size of the oval pericardium must be generous and actually almost approaches a circle so as to provide "height" to the final reconstruction. It creates an oblong "cone." The concept of restoration of height (surgeon's view) to the pulmonary artery bifurcation is important, as it avoids the recurrence of stenosis at the pulmonary artery origins. Once the suture line is completed, an incision is made in the midportion of the pericardium. A central piece of the pericardium is excised, and this large aperture is then sutured end-to-end to the distal aortic allograft conduit to complete the reconstruction of the pulmonary artery bifurcation (Fig. 7.36). The proximal suture line to the right ventriculotomy is completed in the usual fashion (Fig. 7.37).

This technique has the advantage of being rapid and geometrically simple. It has the disadvantage that the aortic allograft is not sutured directly to native human tissue, and an intervening piece of nonviable tissue exists. This situation creates the possibility of calcification and peel formation, which might lead to late obstruction. It often occurs when Dacron is used in this position but may not be as great a problem with pericardium. Nevertheless, direct suturing of allograft to native tissue is preferred whenever feasible.

Pulmonary Artery Bifurcation Allograft

Another, and to us more satisfying, technique for reconstructing the hypoplastic but confluent pulmonary arteries is to utilize a pulmonary artery allograft with its bifurcation and combine it with a right ventricular outflow reconstruction using an aortic allograft. An adult-sized pulmo-

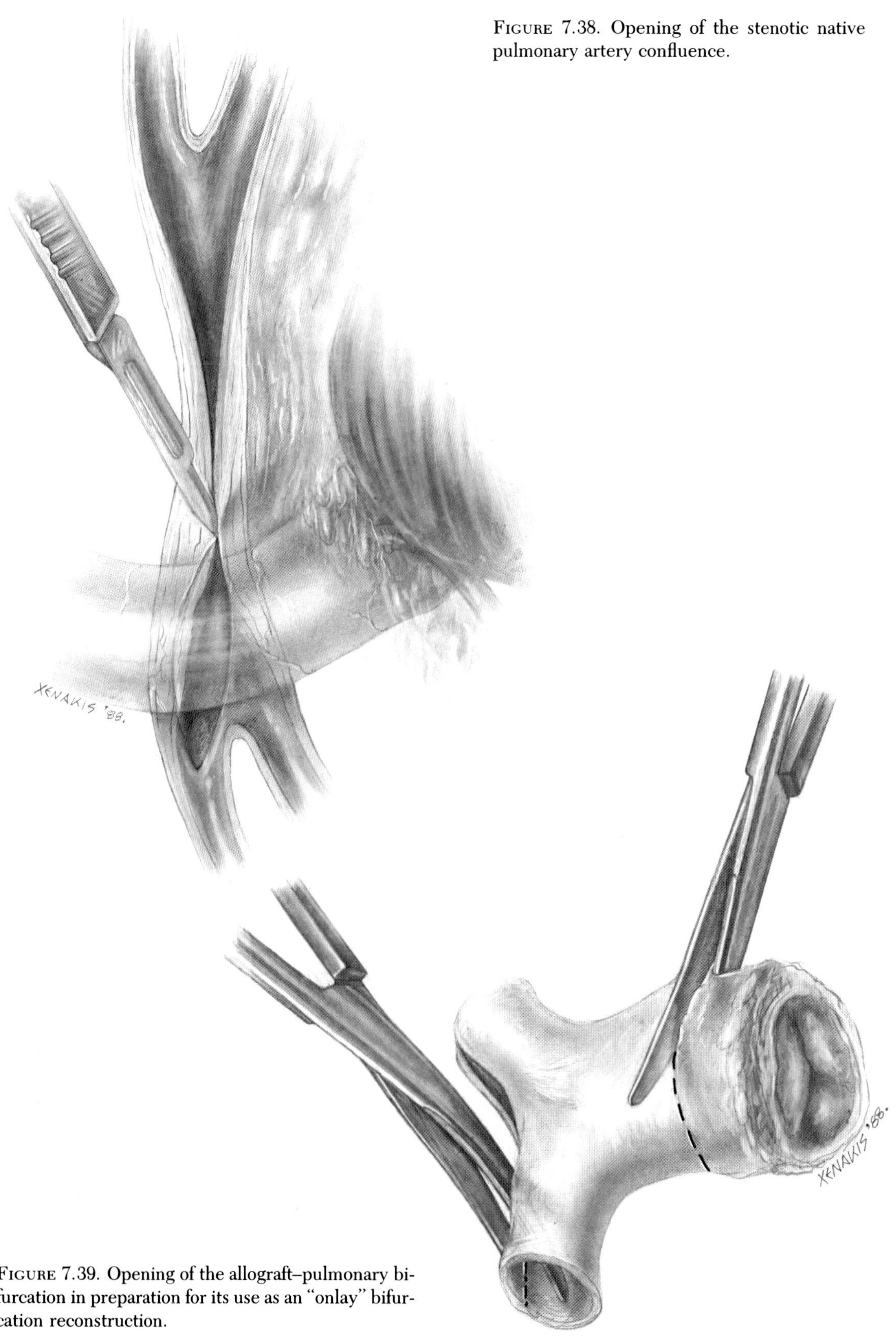

Figure 7.38. Opening of the stenotic native pulmonary artery confluence.

Figure 7.39. Opening of the allograft–pulmonary bifurcation in preparation for its use as an "onlay" bifurcation reconstruction.

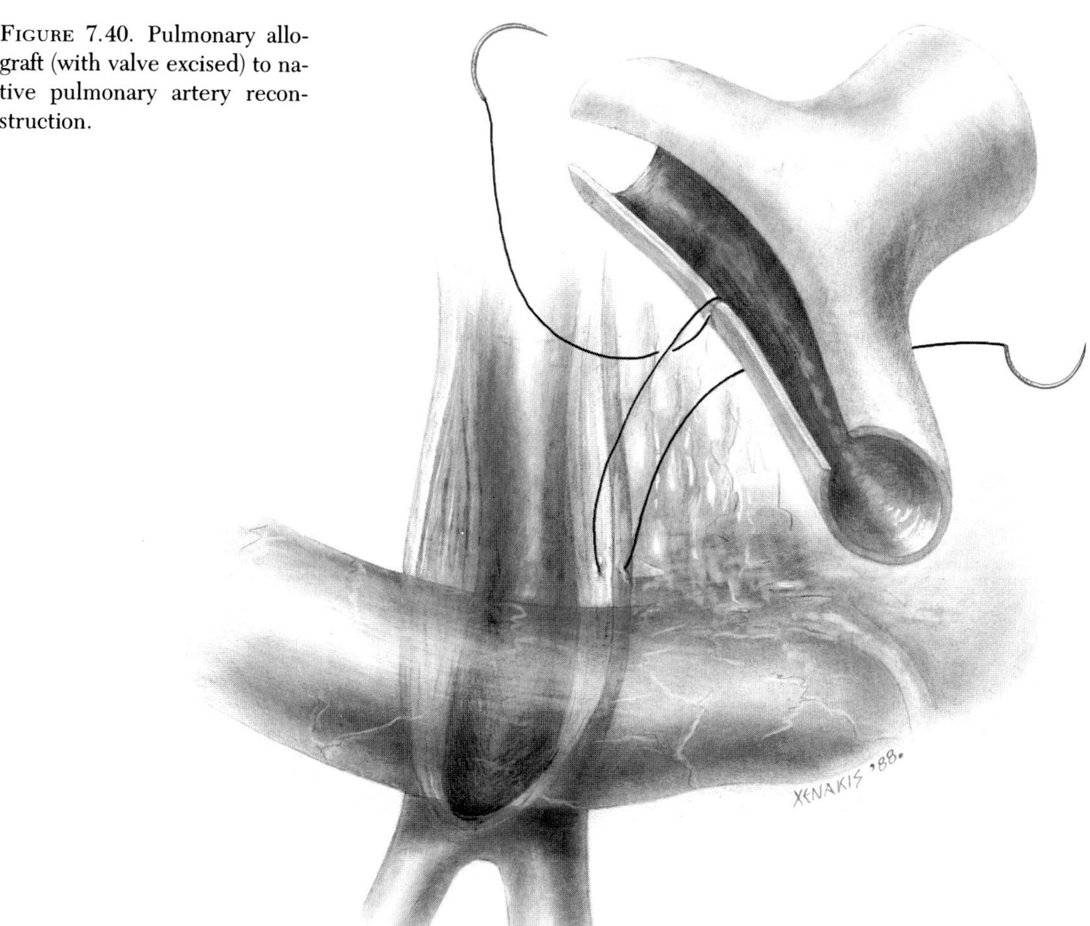

FIGURE 7.40. Pulmonary allograft (with valve excised) to native pulmonary artery reconstruction.

nary artery allograft, as usually harvested, has a right arterial length of 1.0–2.0 cm, a left arterial length of 1.5–3.0 cm, and a segment of main pulmonary artery between the sinus ridge (top of the pulmonary valve pillars) attachments and takeoff of the left and right pulmonary arteries of 3–5 cm. Although this pulmonary arterial segment is often not long enough to reconstruct the entire conduit from right ventriculotomy to distal pulmonary arteries without the addition of prosthetic material, it can be used to greatly enlarge and reconstruct the patient's pulmonary artery bifurcation. This method has the advantage of joining allograft material directly to human tissue. It also greatly enlarges the pulmonary artery bifurcation and utilizes the "height principle." As we apply the technique, it allows use of an aortic valve allograft as the outlet valve from the ventriculotomy and thus primary closure of allograft material to right ventricular native tissue.

The repair is begun just as for the pericardial "skirt" technique, with dissection of the pulmonary artery confluence to the distal pulmonary arteries where adequate diameters are encountered. An arteriotomy is made anteriorly through the pulmonary artery confluence, leaving the posterior wall intact (Fig. 7.38).

The pulmonary bifurcation allograft has been thawed and prepared. The distal right and left main pulmonary arteries are slit with a horizontal incision (Fig. 7.39). The filleted allograft is then sutured to the native pulmonary arteriotomy with a running 5-0 polypropylene suture technique (Fig. 7.40). This method uses the full circumference of the allograft pulmonary arteries

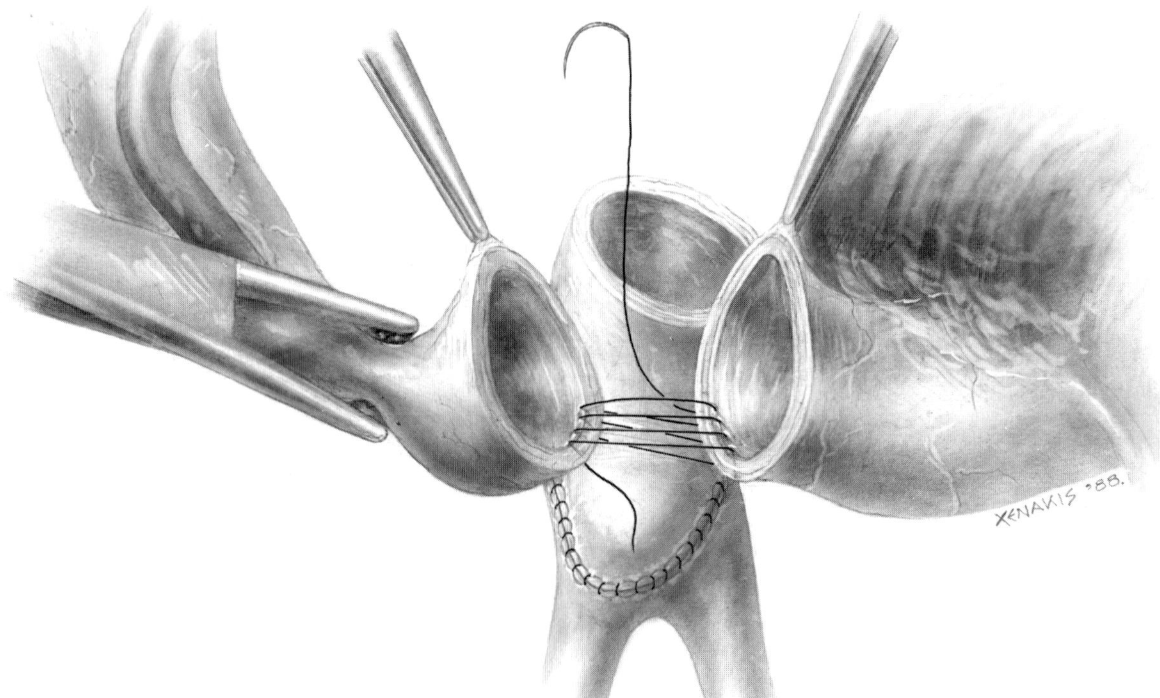

Figure 7.41. The aorta is divided to enhance exposure of the distal right pulmonary artery when dense adhesions prevent safe exposure.

to augment the anterior recipient confluence, thereby enlarging the pulmonary artery bifurcation significantly. If necessary, exposure of the right main pulmonary artery is enhanced by dividing the aorta, which can then be rejoined (Fig. 7.41). (This maneuver is particularly helpful when previous scarring, due to Dacron patch enlargement of the right pulmonary artery, makes dissection behind the aorta risky.)

On completion of the distal anastomosis, the aortic cross clamp can be removed (if cardioplegic arrest was utilized to enhance visibility and decrease blood return in the pulmonary arterial system). Matching the size of the aortic allograft to the pulmonary allograft is not critical, as the anastomosis is oblique, but in general a 1- to 2-mm larger aortic allograft is selected to match the more elastic pulmonary artery bifurcation. The aortic allograft can be chosen to match the ventriculotomy and length requirements from the right ventricle to the pulmonary artery bifurcation so long as it is an adult size for the BSA of the patient. The pulmonary artery bifurcation can then be matched to the native pulmonary arteries and the allograft-to-allograft anastomosis constructed. The thawed aortic allograft (see Chapter 4) is then sutured end-to-end to the pulmonary allograft with a running 5-0 polypropylene suture technique buttressed with a thin felt strip (Fig. 7.42).

The patient is fully rewarmed and the proximal aortic allograft to right ventriculotomy is accomplished in the usual fashion with a running 4-0 polypropylene suture technique (Fig. 7.43). The pulmonary valve tissue has been totally excised, and only the pulmonary artery distal to that tissue is utilized for the bifurcation reconstruction.

→

Figure 7.42. An aortic allograft containing the valve is used to complete the reconstruction from ventriculotomy to pulmonary arterial allograft bifurcation.

Figure 7.43. The proximal suture line to the ventriculotomy is completed while rewarming the patient.

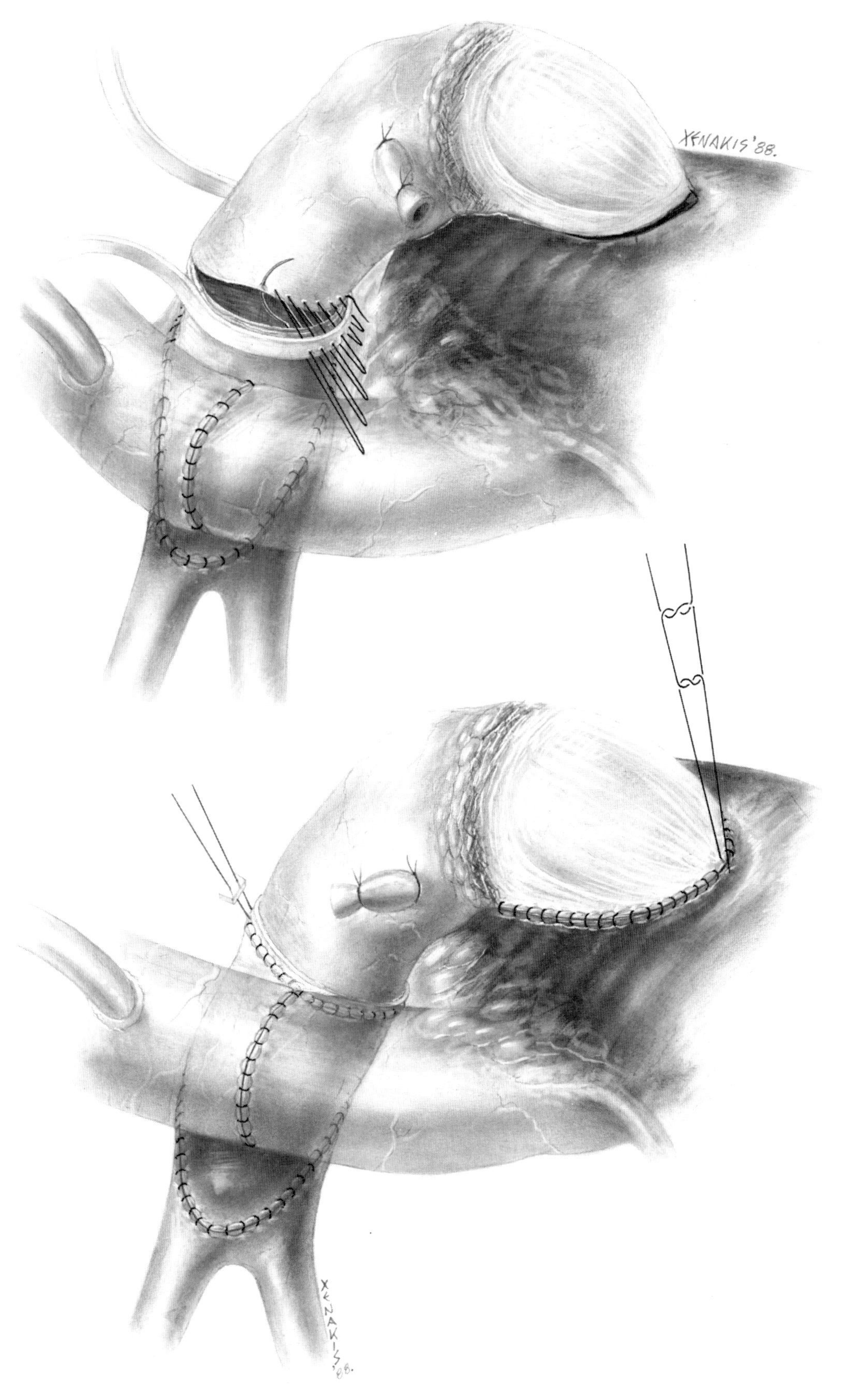
XENAKIS'88.
XENAKIS'88.

Nonconfluent Pulmonary Arteries

Pulmonary Artery Bifurcation Allograft

When the pulmonary arteries are nonconfluent, choices exist for reconstruction. First, the pulmonary artery bifurcation can be reconstructed entirely with a pulmonary bifurcation allograft with separate end-to-end anastomoses right and left, as reported by McGrath and colleagues (we have not personally used this technique), or sewn to an aortic allograft in a manner analogous to the technique just described when the distance is great.[26] Second, the absent posterior wall of native pulmonary arterial confluence can be reconstructed primarily or with pieces of allograft pulmonary artery and then end-to-end anastomoses to an allograft pulmonary or aortic valve.[27] Finally, when right and left pulmonary artery discontinuity extends from hilum to hilum, that lengthy distance can be spanned with a PTFE graft, which is then sutured end-to-side to an allograft. Although this method violates the principle of maximizing allograft to recipient tissue anastomoses, it occasionally is the most feasible reconstruction.

The difficulty with the first method is that the length of allograft spanning the left and right main pulmonary arteries usually available rarely exceeds 5 cm. That method appears to be most applicable in cases of acquired "nonconfluent" pulmonary arteries, resulting from previous shunting procedures, and where at least one of the arteries is relatively centrally located so that the bifurcation can be "cheated" to one side or the other to bridge the gap.

References

1. Rastelli GC, Ongley TA, Davis GD, Kirklin JW: Surgical repair for pulmonary valve atresia with coronary–pulmonary artery fistula: report of a case. *Mayo Clin Proc* 40:521–527, 1965.
2. Ciaravella JM Jr, McGoon DC, Danielson GK, et al: Experience with the extracardiac conduit. *J Thorac Cardiovasc Surg* 78:920–930, 1979.
3. McGoon DC, Danielson GK, Puga FJ, et al: Late results after extracardiac conduit repair for congenital heart defects. *Am J Cardiol* 49:1741–1749, 1982.
4. Moore CH, Martelli V, Ross DN: Reconstruction of right ventricular outflow tracts with a valve conduit in seventy-five cases of congenital heart disease. *J Thorac Cardiovasc Surg* 71:11–19, 1976.
5. Weldon CS, Rowe RD, Gott VL: Clinical experience with the use of aortic valve homografts for reconstruction of the pulmonary artery, pulmonary valve and outflow portion of the right ventricle. *Circulation* 37/38(suppl II):II51–II60, 1968.
6. Jonas RA, Freed MD, Mayer JE Jr, Castaneda AR: Long-term follow-up of patients with synthetic right heart conduits. *Circulation* 72(suppl II):II77–II83, 1985.
7. Kay PH, Ross DN: Fifteen years' experience with the aortic homograft: the conduit of choice for right ventricular outflow tract reconstruction. *Ann Thorac Surg* 40:360–364, 1985.
8. Bove EL, Kavey REW, Byrum CJ, et al: Improved right ventricular function following late pulmonary valve replacement for residual pulmonary insufficiency or stenosis. *J Thorac Cardiovasc Surg* 90:50–55, 1985.
9. Ebert PA: Second operations for pulmonary stenosis or insufficiency after repair of tetralogy of Fallot. In Engle MA, Perloff JK (eds): *Congenital Heart Disease After Surgery: Benefits, Residua, Sequelae*. New York: Yorke, 1983, pp. 202–209.
10. Ebert PA: Second operations for pulmonary stenosis or insufficiency after repair of tetralogy of Fallot. *Am J Cardiol* 50:637–640, 1982.
11. Ilbawi MN, Idriss FS, DeLeon SY, et al: Factors that exaggerate the deleterious effects of pulmonary insufficiency on the right ventricle after tetralogy repair. *J Thorac Cardiovasc Surg* 93:36–44, 1987.
12. Ilbawi MN, Idriss FS, DeLeon SY, et al: Long-term results of porcine valve insertion for pulmonary regurgitation following repair of tetralogy of Fallot. *Ann Thorac Surg* 41:478–482, 1986.
13. Ilbawi MN, Idriss FS, DeLeon SY, et al: Valve replacement in children: guidelines for selection of prosthesis and timing of surgical intervention. *Ann Thorac Surg* 44:398–403, 1987.
14. Fontan F, Choussat A, Deville C, et al: Aortic valve homografts and the surgical treatment of complex cardiac malformations. *J Thorac Cardiovasc Surg* 87:649–657, 1984.
15. Kirklin JW, Blackstone EH, Maehara T, et al: Intermediate-term fate of cryopreserved allograft and xenograft valved conduits. *Ann Thorac Surg* 44:598–606, 1987.
16. Ebert PA: The role of valves in pulmonary conduits. In Dunn JM (ed): *Cardiac Valve Disease in Children*. New York: Elsevier, 1988, pp. 147–152.
17. Hopkins RA: Right ventricular outflow tract re-

constructions—the role of valves in the viable allograft era. *Ann Thorac Surg* 45:593–594, 1988.
18. Finck SJ, Puga FJ, Danielson GK: Pulmonary valve insertion during reoperation for tetralogy of Fallot. *Ann Thorac Surg* 45:610–613, 1988.
19. Mercer JL: Acceptable size of the pulmonary valve ring in congenital cardiac defects. *Ann Thorac Surg* 20:567–570, 1975.
20. Boyce SW, Turley K, Yee ES, et al: The fate of the 12 mm porcine valved conduit from the right ventricle to the pulmonary artery. *J Thorac Cardiovasc Surg* 95:201–207, 1988.
21. Bull C, MacArtney FJ, Horvath P, et al: Evaluation of long-term results of homograft and heterograft valves and extracardiac conduits. *J Thorac Cardiovasc Surg* 94:12–19, 1987.
22. Bailey WW: Cryopreserved pulmonary homograft valved external conduits: early results. *J Cardiac Surg* 1(suppl):199–204, 1987.
23. Misbach GA, Turley K, Ebert PA: Pulmonary valve replacement for regurgitation after repair of tetralogy of Fallot. *Ann Thorac Surg* 36:684–691, 1983.
24. Bove EL, Byrum CJ, Thomas FD, et al: The influence of pulmonary insufficiency on ventricular function following repair of tetralogy of Fallot. *J Thorac Cardiovasc Surg* 85:691–696, 1983.
25a. Ilbawi MN, Lockhart G, Idriss FS, et al: Experience with St. Jude medical valve prosthesis in children. *J Thorac Cardiovasc Surg* 93:73–79, 1987.
25b. Meisner H, Hagl S, Sebening F: Technique of inlay allografts into the RVOT to prevent pulmonary insufficiency in Yonkah AC, Hetzer R, Miller DC, et al (eds): Cardiac Valve Allografts 1962–1987. New York: Springer-Verlag, 1987, pp. 205–213.
26a. McGrath LB, Gonzalez-Lavin L, Graf D: Pulmonary homograft implantation for ventricular outflow tract reconstruction: early phase results. *Ann Thorac Surg* 3:273–277, 1988.
26b. Wain WH, Greco R, Ignegeri A, Bodnar E, Ross DN. 15 years experience with 615 homograft and autograft aortic valve replacements. *Int J. Artif Organs* 3:169–172, 1980.
26c. Gonzales-Lavin L, Robles A, Graf D: The Ross Operation: The Autologous Pulmonary Valve in the Aortic Position. *J. Card. Surg* 3:29–43, 1988.
27. Ziemer G, Luhmer I, Siclari F, Kallfelz HC: Truncus arteriosus type A3: complex repair with cryopreserved pulmonary homograft. *Eur J Cardiothorac Surg* 1:110–115, 1987.
28. Danielson GJ, McGoon DC, Wallace KB, et al: Surgery of corrected transposition. In Anderson RH, Shinebourne EA (eds): *Pediatric Cardiology 1977*. Edinburgh: Churchill Livingstone, 1978, pp. 224–230.
29. DeLeval M, Bastos P, Stark J, et al: Surgical technique to reduce the risks of heart block following closure of ventricular septal defect in atrioventricular discordance. *J Thorac Cardiovasc Surg* 78:515–526, 1979.
30. Danielson GK: Atrioventricular discordance. In Stark J, deLeval M (eds): *Surgery for Congenital Heart Defects*. London: Grune & Stratton, 1983, pp. 387–395.

Appendix—Valve Diameters

BSA	Mean value diameters (mm)							
	Mitral valve		Tricuspid valve		Aortic valve		Pulmonary valve	
	RRL[a]	GOS[a]	RRL	GOS	RRL	GOS	RRL	GOS
0.25	11.2	16.0	13.4	19.2	7.2	10.3	8.4	12.0
0.30	12.6	18.0	14.9	21.3	8.1	11.6	9.3	13.3
0.35	13.6	19.4	16.2	23.2	8.9	12.7	10.1	14.4
0.40	14.4	20.6	17.3	24.7	9.5	13.6	10.7	15.3
0.45	15.2	21.7	18.2	26.0	10.1	14.4	11.3	16.2
0.50	15.8	22.6	19.2	27.5	10.7	15.3	11.9	17.0
0.60	16.9	24.2	20.7	29.6	11.5	16.4	12.8	18.3
0.70	17.9	25.6	21.9	31.3	12.3	17.6	13.5	19.3
0.80	18.8	26.9	23.0	32.9	13.0	18.6	14.2	20.3
0.90	19.7	28.2	24.0	34.3	13.4	19.2	14.8	21.2
1.0	20.2	28.9	24.9	35.6	14.0	20.0	15.3	21.9
1.2	21.4	30.6	26.2	37.5	14.8	21.2	16.2	23.2
1.4	22.3	31.9	27.7	39.6	15.5	22.2	17.0	24.3
1.5	23.1	33.0	28.9	41.3	16.1	23.0	17.6	25.2
1.8	23.8	34.0	29.1	41.6	16.6	23.6	18.0	25.7
2.0	24.2	34.6	30.0	42.9	17.2	24.6	18.2	26.0

Standard deviations

Mitral valve	BSA 0.3 = ±1.9
	BSA 0.3 = ±1.6
Tricuspid valve	BSA 1.0 = ±1.7
	BSA 1.0 = ±1.5
Aortic valve	All 1.0
Pulmonary valve	All 1.2

[a] RRL: data derived from Rowlatt and associates.[1,2] GOS: = Great Ormond Street "normalized" diameters.[3]
Adapted from de Leval.[2]

The table lists mean "normal" valve diameters. The first column for each valve comes from the data measured by Rowlatt and associates.[1,2] The Great Ormond Street (GOS) group have found that these valve measurements tend to underestimate the true in vivo sizes. The data from Rowlatt and co-workers (RRL data) were derived from a large series of normal hearts examined at autopsy. The Great Ormond Street group noted that there was a shrinkage factor due to formalin. Their angiographic estimates correlated to fresh autopsy material and suggested that the atrioventricular valves were certainly underestimated by the earlier techniques. The London (GOS) workers suggested that the RRL measurements should be multiplied by a factor of 1.43 to equal their fresh measurements (C. Bull, personal communication). Thus this table includes both the original data of Rowlatt and co-workers and the larger estimates of "normal."[3,4]

The way we use this table relative to ventricular outflow valves is to consider the RRL valve diameters as the minimum acceptable diameter for a given body surface area and the GOS diameters as the mean to upper limits of achievable valve transplants. From a practical standpoint, it means that we would try to place, for an "adult"-sized freehand aortic valve implant, an allograft of 20 mm (internal diameter) for an individual with a body surface area (BSA) of 1 m^2 and a valve as large as a 24.6 mm for a 2-m^2 individual. Once a patient reaches approximately 20 kg in weight, an aortic valve of 17 mm or larger is usually implantable in the aortic position with the techniques described in the foregoing chapters, which is within the acceptable range.

The pulmonary outflow tract is optimally reconstructed with a 22-mm pulmonary valve for a 1-m^2 individual and could be as large as 26 mm for a 2-m^2 individual adult. In most patients a valve between the upper and lower sizes is almost always achievable. On the right ventricular outflow tract side, a 14-mm (internal diameter) aortic valve can usually be placed in a 5-kg child; once a child weighs more than 10 kg, a right ventricular allograft conduit of 16 mm or larger is implantable; and in children above 20 kg it is almost always possible to place a 20-mm or larger conduit in the right ventricular outflow tract position. Mercer has argued that a more than 50% reduction in pulmonary valve orifice size is required before significant gradients occur.[5] However, with right-sided *conduits* (which have length as well as diameter), sizes below the RRL values are not recommended.

References

1. Rowlatt UF, Rimoldi HJA, Lev M: The quantitative anatomy of the normal child's heart. *Pediatr Clin North Am* 10:499–588, 1963.
2. De Leval M: Tricuspid valve. In Stark JS, de Leval M (eds): *Surgery for Congenital Heart Disease.* London: Grune & Stratton, 1983, p. 460.
3. Bull C, de Leval M, Mercanti C, et al: Pulmonary atresia and intract ventricular septum: a revised classification. *Circulation* 66:266–271, 1966.
4. De Leval M, Bull C, Hopkins R, et al: Decision making in the definitive repair of the heart with a small ventricle. *Circulation* 72(suppl II):II52–II60, 1985.
5. Mercer JL: Acceptable size of the pulmonary valve ring in congenital cardiac defects. *Ann Thorac Surg* 20:567–570, 1975.

Index